Pediatric Obesity

Prevention, Intervention, and Treatment Strategies for Primary Care

2nd Edition

Sandra G. Hassink, MD, FAAP

Director, Nemours Obesity Initiative
Nemours/Al duPont Hospital for Children
Wilmington, DE

Associate Professor of Pediatrics
Thomas Jefferson University Medical School
Philadelphia, PA

American Academy of Pediatrics
141 Northwest Point Blvd
Elk Grove Village, IL 60007-1098

American Academy of Pediatrics Department of Marketing and Publications Staff

Maureen DeRosa, MPA
Director, Department of Marketing and Publications

Mark Grimes
Director, Division of Product Development

Jeff Mahony
Manager, Digital Strategy and Product Development

Jennifer McDonald
Manager, Online Content

Regina Moi
Manager, Patient Education

Sandi King, MS
Director, Division of Publishing and Production Services

Leesa Levin-Doroba
Manager, Publishing and Production Services

Linda Diamond
Manager, Art Direction and Production

Julia Lee
Director, Division of Marketing and Sales

Linda Smessaert, MSIMC
Brand Manager, Clinical and Professional Publications

Library of Congress Control Number: 2013939938
ISBN: 978-1-58110-656-5
eISBN: 978-1-58110-827-9
MA0621

The recommendations in this publication do not indicate an exclusive course of treatment or serve as a standard of medical care. Variations, taking into account individual circumstances, may be appropriate.

Statements and opinions expressed are those of the author and not necessarily those of the American Academy of Pediatrics.

All original forms, worksheets, and patient handouts included herein may be reproduced for noncommercial, educational use with acknowledgment of source.

Listing of resources does not imply an endorsement by the American Academy of Pediatrics (AAP). The AAP is not responsible for the content of external resources. Information was current at the time of publication.

Current Procedural Terminology (CPT®) 5-digit codes, nomenclature, and other data are copyright 2013 American Medical Association (AMA). All Rights Reserved.

1 2 3 4 5 6 7 8 9 10

To my husband, Bill, and my children,
Matthew, Stephen, and Alexa,
for your unfailing love and support.
Also to all my friends and colleagues along the way
who have dedicated themselves to improving
the lives of children.

Table of Contents

Foreword

Up to one-third of the childhood population has a body mass index (BMI) greater than 85% for age[1] and more than half of these children have a BMI greater than 95%.[2] These children are at risk for and are often already suffering from obesity-related comorbidities such as type 2 diabetes, non-alcoholic steatohepatitis, polycystic ovarian syndrome, sleep apnea, and Blount disease. They are also at risk for a lifetime of obesity with all its attendant medical and psychosocial consequences.

The evolution of obesity in childhood and adolescence is a complex interplay of gene-environment interactions, child temperament, parenting style, family dynamics, and home, school, and community environments. Children are influenced by parental role modeling, television advertising, and commercial food and entertainment offerings. Obesity and obesity-related comorbidities begin in childhood. Children in many ways are at the epicenter of the epidemic.

What does this mean for us as providers of pediatric health care? Not only can we not ignore the effects of obesity on the children we care for, we need to put ourselves in a position to take positive action in developing prevention, intervention, and treatment strategies for obesity.

This manual will help guide these efforts by providing information, strategies, and suggestions for approaches to prevention, intervention, and treatment at the primary care level. Starting with chapters on assessment and evaluation, each subsequent chapter focuses on a specific developmental stage with strategies for prevention of obesity in the normal weight population, intervention for children at risk for obesity, and treatment approaches for those children and adolescents whose BMIs are already greater than 95%. Families play a central role in modeling behavior, buffering the effects of an obesity-promoting environment and changing nutrition and activity habits to achieve a healthy energy balance for their children. Included in each chapter are questions for parents, self-assessment exercises, and points to touch on to enhance parenting information and skill in making family-based change. Additional information on practice-based changes and school interventions for primary care professionals can be used as a springboard for change in their own communities.

Patient handouts, American Academy of Pediatrics policy statements, and coding and reimbursement information are all collected in the appendices to aid the practitioner in implementing practice change aimed at obesity prevention, intervention, and treatment.

In this new second edition, a new chapter titled "Before Birth: Maternal Health" has been added to spotlight the understanding that maternal obesity increases the risk of pregnancy-related complications for both mother and infant. Data from numerous new studies have been incorporated into all chapters, and references have been updated. The nutrition and activity questions and approaches in each of the Health Supervision Visit chapters have been reviewed and enhanced. In the appendices, the growth charts have been updated to include the World Health Organization (WHO) charts, several new AAP policy statements have been added, coding information has been updated, and a brand new section on AAP obesity resources has been added.

References

1. Ogden CL, Carroll MD, Curtin LR, McDowell MA, Tabak CJ, Flegal KM. Prevalence of overweight and obesity in the United States, 1999-2004. *JAMA.* 2006;295:1549–1555
2. Whitaker RC, Wright JA, Pepe MS, Seidel KD, Dietz WH. Predicting obesity in young adulthood from childhood and parental obesity. *N Engl J Med.* 1997;337:869–873

Acknowledgments

*Thanks for the thoughtful reviews of these chapters
by the following experts:*

Christopher F. Bolling, MD, FAAP

Kimberly C. Avila Edwards, MD, FAAP

Marc S. Jacobson, MD, FAAP

Howard L. Taras, MD, FAAP

1

Childhood Obesity: An Overview

1.1 The Rise in Obesity

Childhood obesity has risen to epidemic proportions. Every day pediatricians are faced with children who are overweight or obese and children who are suffering from the comorbidities of obesity. An overview of the problem will help us begin to create a strategy to respond to the needs of these patients and their families.

What happened to the population in the past 3 decades that has given rise to an increase of childhood and adult obesity of epidemic proportions?

There has been an inexorable shift in energy balance over the past 30 years. A combination of decreased activity, increased inactivity, and consumption of excess calories has contributed to the steadily increasing prevalence rates of childhood and adolescent obesity. From 2007 to 2008, 31.7% of children 2 to 19 years of age were above 85% for body mass index (BMI; classified as overweight), 16.9% were above 95% (classified as obese), and 11.9% were above 97%. This increase in obesity is occurring across the board and is alarmingly affecting our youngest patients; 9.5% of infants and toddlers were at or above 95% for weight/length.[1]

Minority populations are being hit even harder. The proportion of Hispanic and African American children aged 2 to 19 years with BMI values greater than 85% were 38.2% and 35.9%, respectively, as compared with 29.3% for non-Hispanic white children (2007–2009). These disparities are magnified by the number of children 2 to 19 years of age with BMI values greater than 95%: Mexican American (20.9%) and African American (20%), compared with non-Hispanic white children (15.3%).[1]

Genetic and Environmental Factors

What genetic and environmental interactions are involved?

There are hundreds of genes or gene markers associated in some way with energy balance. Predisposition to energy imbalance, increased nutrient partitioning to adipose tissue, and susceptibility to intrauterine programming are among many proposed mechanisms involving gene-environment interaction. Families with 1 or 2 obese parents are at

increased risk for having a child or adolescent with obesity.[2] Predisposition for obesity-related comorbidities may also be inherited. For example, it is common to see type 2 diabetes, hypertension, dyslipidemia, and insulin resistance clustered in families. In most cases of obesity, genetic susceptibility to the environment influences outcome.

The interaction between genetics and environment is complex. Nutritional components may influence gene regulation, the intrauterine environment may affect later susceptibility to an energy-abundant environment, and the environment may have a greater effect during periods of rapid growth.

Societal Effects of Obesity

How does this explosion of obesity and associated comorbidities involve the child, family, community, and society at large?

The societal costs of obesity are increasing. There will be a burden of illnesses in the young adult and adult populations never seen before. More young parents will be chronically ill, and this will affect their children. There will be increasing stress on the health care system in terms of economics, time, and personnel. Children with obesity have almost twice the rate of physician visits as children with a BMI less than 95%, as well as increased prescription drug use and hospital admission rates.[3] The length of stay for discharges associated with obesity is longer than that for overall discharges. Costs associated with childhood obesity are estimated at $14 billion annually in direct and indirect health expenses. Annual obesity-related hospital costs for children and adolescents were $238 million in 2005, nearly doubling between the years 2003 and 2005.[3] The overall health effects on the population and the cost to the larger economy are already threatening to become our nation's biggest health expenditure.

1.2 The Medical Effects of Childhood Obesity

What are the medical effects of having an increasing population of children and adolescents with obesity?

Childhood obesity can be thought of as an accelerator of

adult diseases. Children and adolescents are now experiencing comorbidities, including type 2 diabetes, hypertension, dyslipidemia, obstructive sleep apnea, and nonalcoholic steatohepatitis (NASH), which was previously seen predominantly in adults. In addition, childhood obesity gives rise to serious orthopedic problems, such as slipped capital femoral epiphysis (SCFE) and Blount disease, and increases the incidence of less common but serious obesity-related conditions such as pseudotumor cerebri. These are diseases and complications few of us thought we would see in childhood or even adolescence; they give urgency to our need to institute prevention and early intervention, as well as diagnosis and treatment.

Comorbidities

There are a group of obesity-related comorbidities that require immediate attention: pseudotumor cerebri, SCFE, Blount disease, obstructive sleep apnea syndrome, NASH, cholelithiasis, metabolic syndrome, acanthosis nigricans, polycystic ovarian syndrome (PCOS), and type 2 diabetes.

Obesity occurs in 30% to 80% of children with *pseudotumor cerebri.*[4] Pseudotumor cerebri is defined as increased intracranial pressure with papilledema and normal cerebrospinal fluid in the absence of ventricular enlargement. Papilledema is part of the pathology of pseudotumor cerebri but may not occur initially. Presentation may range from an incidental finding on funduscopic examination to headaches, vomiting, blurred vision, or diplopia. Loss of peripheral visual fields and reduction in visual acuity may be present at diagnosis.[5] Neck, shoulder, and back pain have also been reported.[5] Treatment of pseudotumor cerebri includes acetazolamide, lumboperitoneal shunt in severe cases, and weight loss.[6] Pseudotumor cerebri is a diagnosis of exclusion after other causes of increased intracranial pressure are eliminated. It is important to remember that the neurologic deficits are symmetric in pseudotumor. Patients with asymmetric presentations must have other neurologic conditions.

Slipped capital femoral epiphysis is a slipping of the femoral epiphysis through the zone of hypertrophic cartilage cells, which are under the influence of gonadal and growth hormones.[7] From 50% to 70% of patients with SCFE have obesity.[8] Patients can present with limp or complaints of groin, thigh, or knee pain. The characteristic gait is with the leg abducted and externally rotated. Hips should be examined, and radiographs of both hips should be obtained because bilateral slips occur in 20% of cases. Medial and posterior displacement of the femoral epiphysis is seen through the growth plate relative to the femoral neck.[9] Treatment is surgical pinning of the hip.

The diagnosis of *Blount disease* involves identifying bowing of the tibia and femur. This can affect one or both knees. This condition is thought to result from excessive pressure damage to the medial proximal tibial epiphysis. Obesity is reported in two-thirds of patients with Blount disease.[10] Treatment requires surgical correction and weight loss.

Obstructive sleep apnea syndrome is a common diagnosis associated with obesity. This syndrome is defined as a breathing disorder characterized by prolonged partial upper airway obstruction or intermittent complete obstruction that disrupts normal ventilation during sleep and normal sleep patterns.[11] Symptoms can include nighttime awakening, restless sleep, difficulty awakening in the morning, daytime sleepiness, napping, enuresis, decreased concentration and memory, and poor school performance.[12] Nighttime polysomnography is the diagnostic procedure of choice. If left untreated, obstructive sleep apnea can result in pulmonary hypertension, systemic hypertension, and right-sided heart failure.[11] Weight gain, hypertrophy of the tonsils and adenoids, and intercurrent upper respiratory infections can provoke symptoms.

Nonalcoholic steatohepatitis is suspected when elevated liver enzymes are found in the context of fatty liver discovered by ultrasound in the absence of other causes of liver disease. From 20% to 25% of children with obesity have evidence of steatohepatitis.[13] The definitive diagnosis is made on the basis of the liver biopsy, in which evidence of inflammatory infiltrates and fibrosis can be seen. Nonalcoholic steatohepatitis can progress to cirrhosis and end-stage liver disease.[14] Weight loss reduces fatty infiltration and may decrease fibrosis.

Cholelithiasis symptoms in children include right upper quadrant abdominal pain and tenderness; diagnosis is made on the basis of ultrasound and appropriate laboratory studies. Of cases in adolescents, 50% are associated with obesity.[15]

Metabolic syndrome is a cluster of conditions characterized by insulin resistance. The components in childhood are central adiposity, elevated blood pressure, elevated triglyceride levels, decreased high-density lipoprotein (HDL) cholesterol, increased low-density lipoprotein cholesterol, and impaired glucose tolerance or hyperinsulinemia.

Acanthosis nigricans is often associated with metabolic syndrome, insulin resistance, and type 2 diabetes. This condition is characterized by hyperpigmentation and a velvety thickening that occurs in the neck, axillae, and groin.

Polycystic ovarian syndrome can occur in adolescence and is characterized by insulin resistance in the presence of elevated androgens. Clinical signs and symptoms include oligomenorrhea or amenorrhea, hirsutism, acne, polycystic ovaries, and obesity. There is some evidence that girls with premature adrenarche are at risk for PCOS.[16]

Type 2 diabetes occurs when the diagnosis of hyperglycemia is made in the presence of insulin resistance and an elevated insulin level. Type 2 diabetes can present with hyperglycemic hyperosmolar state (HHS), diabetic ketoacidosis, or symptoms of polyuria, polydipsia, and weight loss. Diagnosis can also be made in a patient with obesity on the basis of symptoms of hyperglycemia, such as abdominal pain, vomiting, dizziness, and weakness.

Obesity Emergencies

Complications of obesity can be life-threatening and even life-ending. Some severe obesity-related emergencies include HHS, diabetic ketoacidosis, pulmonary embolism, and cardiomyopathy of obesity. All of these have been seen in children and adolescents with obesity.

Hyperglycemic hyperosmolar state can rarely be the first manifestation of type 2 diabetes. Patients may initially present with symptoms of vomiting, abdominal pain, dizziness, weakness, polyuria and polydipsia, weight loss, and diarrhea.[17] If unrecognized, patients may develop hyperosmolar nonketotic coma and death.[18] Diagnostic criteria for HHS include a plasma glucose level greater than 600 mg/dL, serum carbon dioxide level greater than 15 mmol/L, small ketonuria, absent to low ketonemia, an effective serum osmolality greater than 320 mOsm/kg, and stupor or coma.[17,18]

Diabetic ketoacidosis can be an initial manifestation of type 2 diabetes even though most pediatricians associate it primarily with type 1. Insulin resistance often accompanies obesity and results in low baseline insulin sensitivity and relative insulin deficiency, which leads to increased lipolysis, increased free fatty acids in circulation, ketonemia, and ketonuria. Diabetic ketoacidosis should be treated as such, with the diagnosis of the diabetes type made when the patient is stabilized.

Pulmonary embolism has been reported as a complication of gastric bypass in adolescence.[19] The risk factors for pulmonary embolism include obesity, obesity-hypoventilation syndrome, obstructive sleep apnea syndrome, and coagulation disorder; symptoms include dyspnea, chest pain, decreased oxygen concentration, and hemoptysis.

Congestive heart failure resulting from obesity has been seen in adolescents with morbid obesity. The effect of obesity on the heart is known as *cardiomyopathy of obesity* and is thought to result from high metabolic activity of excessive fat, which increases total blood volume and cardiac output and leads to left ventricular dysfunction. Dilation, increased left ventricular wall stress, and compensatory left ventricular hypertrophy then occur. Pulmonary hypertension caused by upper airway obstruction can also occur. Signs and symptoms of cardiac failure should point to this diagnosis.[20]

Bariatric Surgery

As more adolescents are undergoing bariatric surgery, pediatricians may see either immediate or late-onset surgical complications (Table 1.1).

1.3 The Pediatrician's Role in the Obesity Epidemic

Today's Children at Risk

How does the obesity epidemic involve individual patients and our interaction with them and their families?
As you end this chapter, ask yourself, "What, as pediatricians, do we want for our patients?" Provide a healthy start in life? A chance to participate in the normal activities of childhood? A childhood free of disease? The vignettes that close this chapter show us how close this problem is to our everyday practice. This manual will help you begin to address the prevention and treatment of obesity in your daily encounters with patients and families.

You are seeing newborns in the nursery and examine Marta, a 1-day-old little girl born of Hispanic parents. Her chances of developing type 2 diabetes over her lifetime is 50%.
The lifetime risk of developing diabetes for an average person born in the United States in 2000 until his or her death is

- Male—1 in 3 chance
- Female—2 in 5 chance
- Hispanic female—1 in 2 chance (high risk)

Progression to diabetes among those with prediabetes is not inevitable. Studies suggest that weight loss and increased physical activity among people with prediabetes prevent or delay diabetes and may return blood glucose levels to normal.[21]

You are seeing Tom, a 14-year-old who wants to play football, for a sports physical. His BMI is 35, which is greater than 97%.
Adolescents who are obese have approximately an 80% likelihood of being obese adults.[22]

Table 1.1. Possible Complications of Bariatric Surgery	
Complication Type	**Complications**
Early onset	• Bleeding • Bowel perforation • Deep vein thrombosis • Pulmonary embolism • Dehydration • Dysphagia • Nausea/vomiting • Dumping syndrome • Small bowel obstruction • Anastomotic leak • Peritonitis • Anastomotic stricture • Abdominal adhesions
Late onset	• Cholecystitis • Dysphagia • Gastroesophageal reflux • Incisional hernia • Malnutrition • Pancreatitis • Ulcers • Renal calculi • Internal hernia • Small bowel obstruction

Deficiencies	• Protein deficiency
	  – Hair loss
	  – Edema
	  – Hypoalbuminemia
	  – Anemia
	  – Fatigue
	
	• Vitamin/mineral deficiencies
	  – B_{12}
	  – Folic acid
	  – Iron
	  – Fat-soluble vitamin

Gastric banding	• Intraoperative conversion to open gastronomy • Hemorrhage • Port infection • Stomal obstruction • Perforation • Late mechanical dysfunction • Hiatal hernia • Erosion • Band or port slippage

Sources: Zitsman JL, Fennoy I, Witt MA, et al. Laparoscopic adjustable gastric banding in adolescents: short-term results. *J Pediatr Surg.* 2011;46(1):157–162; Decker GA, Swain JM, Crowell MD, et al. Gastrointestinal and nutritional complications after bariatric surgery. *Am J Gastroenterol.* 2007;102(11):2571–2580

You are asked to speak at a preschool parents' meeting on nutrition and obesity.

The number of children with obesity has tripled in the past 3 decades.[23] One in 3 children is currently overweight or obese (BMI at 85% or higher).[1]

You meet Mr. and Mrs. Brown for a prenatal visit. Both the Browns are significantly obese.

There is a 75% chance that children will be overweight if both parents are obese—there is a 25% to 50% chance if just 1 parent with obesity.[3]

Parents of a high school sophomore with obesity ask you if there is anything they can do to help him lose weight.

More than 90% of high schools have vending machines, stores, or snack bars, but only 21% sell low-fat yogurt, fruits, or vegetables.[23] Only 50% of schools offer intramural activity or clubs for students.[3] Only 6% to 8% of schoolchildren have daily physical education.[23]

You are interviewed by your local newspaper and asked about the cost of the epidemic of childhood obesity.

Costs associated with childhood obesity are estimated at $14 billion annually in direct and indirect health expenses. Annual obesity-related hospital costs for children and adolescents were $238 million in 2005.[3]

Parents of an 8-year-old who is overweight ask you about her health risks during a well examination.

Children with a BMI greater than 85% are more likely to have elevated cholesterol and triglyceride levels and a lower HDL-C level and higher blood pressure than children of normal weight.[24]

A mother of a 4-year-old boy who is overweight and drinking 5 to 6 cups of juice a day believes that she is giving him a healthy drink.

Children increase their chances of becoming obese 1.6 times for each additional can or glass of sugared beverage they consume each day.[25]

Obesity prevention, intervention, and treatment will be integral to the practice of pediatrics in primary care practices, subspecialty pediatrics, and hospital-based care. Pediatricians are in a primary position to help children and families increase their knowledge and skills to combat obesity and obesity-related comorbidities.

References

1. Carroll MD, Curtin LR, Lamb MM, Flegal KM, Ogden CL. Prevalence of high body mass index in US children and adolescents, 2007-2008. *JAMA.* 2010;303(3):242–249

2. Whitaker RC, Wright JA, Pepe MS, Seidel KD, Dietz WH. Predicting obesity in young adulthood from childhood and parental obesity. *N Engl J Med.* 1997;337:869–873

3. Marder WD, Chang S. Childhood obesity: costs, treatment patterns, disparities in care, and prevalent medical conditions. *Thomson Medstat Research Brief.* 2006. http://www.medstat.com/pdfs/childhood_obesity.pdf

4. Scott IU, Siatkowski RM, Eneyni M, Brodsky MC, Lam BL. Idiopathic intracranial hypertension in children and adolescents. *Am J Ophthalmol.* 1997;124:253–255

5. Lessell S. Pediatric pseudotumor cerebri (idiopathic intracranial hypertension). *Surv Ophthalmol.* 1992;37:155–166

6. Distelmaier F, Sengler U, Messing-Juenger M, Assmann B, Mayatepek E, Rosenbaum T. Pseudotumor cerebri as an important differential diagnosis of papilledema in children. *Brain Dev.* 2006;28:190–195

7. Kempers MJ, Noordam C, Rouwe CW, Otten BJ. Can GnRH-agonist treatment cause slipped capital femoral epiphysis? *J Pediatr Endocrinol Metab.* 2001;14:729–734

8. Wilcox PG, Weiner DS, Leighley B. Maturation factors in slipped capital femoral epiphysis. *J Pediatr Orthop.* 1988;8:196–200

9. Busch MT, Morrissy RT. Slipped capital femoral epiphysis. *Orthop Clin North Am.* 1987;18:637–647

10. Dietz WH, Gross WL, Kirkpatrick JA. Blount disease (tibia vara): another skeletal disorder associated with childhood obesity. *J Pediatr.* 1982;101:735–737

11. Schechter MS, Section on Pediatric Pulmonology, Subcommittee on Obstructive Sleep Apnea Syndrome. Technical report: diagnosis and management of childhood obstructive sleep apnea syndrome. *Pediatrics.* 2002;109:e69

12. Gozal D. Sleep-disordered breathing and school performance in children. *Pediatrics.* 1998;102:616–620

13. Tazawa Y, Noguchi H, Nishinomiya F, Takada G. Serum alanine aminotransferases activity in obese children. *Acta Paediatr.* 1997;86:238–241

14. Harrison SA, Diehl AM. Fat and the liver—a molecular overview. *Semin Gastrointest Dis.* 2002;13:3–6

15. Crichlow RW, Seltzer MH, Jannetta PJ. Cholecystitis in adolescents. *Am J Dig Dis.* 1972;17:68–72

16. Ibanez L, Dimartino-Nardi J, Potau N, Saenger P. Premature adrenarche—normal variant or forerunner of adult disease? *Endocr Rev.* 2000;21:671–696

17. Morales AE, Rosenbloom AL. Death caused by hyperglycemic hyperosmolar state at the onset of type 2 diabetes. *J Pediatr.* 2004;144:270–273

18. Rubin HM, Kramer R, Drash A. Hyperosmolality complicating diabetes mellitus in childhood. *J Pediatr.* 1969;74:177–186

19. Sugerman HJ, Sugerman EL, DeMaria EJ, et al. Bariatric surgery for severely obese adolescents. *J Gastrointest Surg.* 2003;7:102–108

20. Alpert MA. Obesity cardiomyopathy: pathophysiology and evolution of the clinical syndrome. *Am J Med Sci.* 2001;321:225–236

21. Diabetes Public Health Resource. Centers for Disease Control and Prevention Web site. www.cdc.gov/diabetes. Accessed May 25, 2006

22. Guo SS, Wu W, Chumlea WC, Roche AF. Predicting overweight and obesity in adulthood from body mass index values in childhood and adolescence. *Am J Clin Nutr.* 2002;76:653–658

23. Centers for Disease Control and Prevention Web site. www.cdc.gov. Accessed May 25, 2006

24. Freedman DS, Dietz WH, Srinivasan SR, Berenson GS. The relation of overweight to cardiovascular risk factors among children and adolescents: the Bogalusa Heart Study. *Pediatrics.* 1999;103:1175–1182

25. Ludwig DS, Peterson KE, Gortmaker SL. Relation between consumption of sugar-sweetened drinks and childhood obesity: a prospective, observational analysis. *Lancet.* 2001;357:505–508

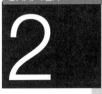

2 Assessment of Obesity

2.1 Introduction

Pediatricians have always focused on helping children maintain normal growth. One of the founding principles of pediatrics is that good nutrition is essential for optimal health and growth. In 1897, L. Emmett Holt, Sr, MD, in *The Diseases of Infancy and Childhood,* wrote, "Nutrition in its broadest sense is the most important branch of pediatrics." In the late 19th and early 20th centuries, cycles of gastroenteritis and resultant malnutrition and recurrent infections caused the death of countless infants. Efforts were made to promote breastfeeding, ensure a safe milk supply, and create formula tailored to infant needs. Vitamin deficiencies were identified and treated, and the government created programs, such as the food stamp program (now known as the SNAP program); the Special Supplemental Nutrition Program for Women, Infants, and Children (commonly referred to as WIC); and school lunch and breakfast programs, to ensure that children's nutritional needs were met.

Pediatricians vigorously identified and treated children with failure to thrive and weight or height deceleration with the knowledge that growth disturbances were often the early signs of significant illness. Growth charts became tools to assess overall health, and there was always a reassurance when children "stayed on the growth chart." Attention to the optimal growth of premature infants, children with chronic disease, and disadvantaged children has all become integral parts of pediatric practice.

With a focus on optimal growth as a cornerstone to preventive care, pediatricians:

- Understand the importance of height, weight, and body mass index (BMI) as measures of overall health.
- Recognize the importance of breastfeeding in supporting healthy growth.
- Give attention to environmental, social, and psychosocial factors as parameters that are crucial to healthy growth.
- Recognize the importance of social supports in maintaining optimal nutrition and growth.
- Recognize the effect of family life events on the growth of children.

- Recognize the link between deviations in growth and disease.

The obesity epidemic challenges us to use these same skills to examine our strategies for prevention, intervention, and treatment to help children stay on the growth curve. We recognize that children with obesity are at risk for and suffer from diseases that were previously seen only in adults. Pediatricians have the opportunity to be involved with children and families from birth throughout adolescence. We have experience in taking a broad approach to growth and can use insights from our experiences to help our patients and families.

2.2 Assessing Obesity

With the onset of the obesity epidemic, assessing the growth status of all children is more important than ever. Preventive efforts that focus on maintaining normal healthy weight gain require that no opportunity be missed to measure height and weight and calculate BMI. Frequent assessment of BMI also makes it possible to identify children who are overweight or obese and allows for early intervention to reinforce and reestablish good nutrition and activity habits. Children who have BMI values greater than 95% require screening for obesity-related comorbidities and intervention to manage obesity.

Identifying excess adiposity in childhood is important for determining risk of obesity-associated comorbidities and future risk of obesity and obesity-related disease in adulthood. Direct measures of adiposity, such as hydrodensitometry, dual-energy x-ray absorptiometry, and magnetic resonance imaging, are used in research. Body mass index (weight/height^2) has been shown to correlate with direct measures of adiposity.[1] Because adipose tissue stores change as children grow and differ between boys and girls, BMI charts are specific for age and gender. Growth charts for 2 to 20 years are included in Appendix A.2; boys on page 123 and girls on page 125.

Body mass index should be calculated at least once a year in all children and adolescents[2] and can be calculated as weight in kilograms divided by height in meters squared or weight in pounds multiplied by 703 and divided by height in inches squared. Once BMI is calculated, BMI classification can be assigned (Table 2.1).

Table 2.1. Current Classification of Weight Status by Body Mass Index (BMI)	
BMI	**Classification**
<5%	Underweight
5%–85%	Normal weight
85%–95%	Overweight
>95%	Obese

Body mass index measurements are an important screening tool, but when applied to an individual patient, they need to be used in the context of that individual. For example, a highly trained, muscular athlete may have an increased BMI but no excess adiposity. History and physical assessment of nutrition and activity and anthropometric measurements, such as skinfold thickness, help put BMI into proper focus for each individual.

For patients younger than 2 years of age, weight-for-length graphs should be used to characterize appropriate growth. Growth charts for birth to 24 months are included in Appendix A.2; boys on page 122 and girls on page 124. If weight is accelerating ahead of height, attention should be paid to identifying any underlying medical or metabolic cause of obesity and ensuring that optimal nutrition and activity habits are being fostered.

Rapid change in BMI can also be used to identify a rate of excessive weight gain relative to linear growth. Sequential BMI measurements should be plotted and compared with BMI charts for age and gender. Often identifying the point at which excessive weight gain begins allows changes in risk factors for obesity to be addressed.

A Case in Point: CS

CS is an 11-year-old girl you are seeing for her yearly checkup. As you plot her height and weight and calculate her BMI, you note that she has gained 20 pounds (9.1 kg) since last year and has a BMI placing her at 90% for her age and gender.

Over the past year she visited your office several times for respiratory illnesses but has no other problems. She is not taking any medications. You ask about school, and she and her mother report that her grades are good but she is experiencing some teasing. When you ask CS about this, she becomes upset and tells you that no one wants to play with her. Mom says she is worried about CS's self-esteem. You acknowledge the difficulty of getting teased and ask CS how she responds. She says she gets upset and usually says something back to the girls who tease her. You briefly discuss some responses to teasing, and CS expresses some interest in trying to ignore their comments and walk away.

You then share the growth and BMI charts with Mom and CS and explain that sometimes eating and activity habits change when someone is being teased and feeling bad. You let them know that staying healthy is important and begin to ask specifically about her eating and activity. Mom notes that CS comes home from school starving and that as soon as she finishes dinner she asks for more food. CS says she is watching television or is on the computer a lot, which Mom translates to about 4 hours a day.

You then begin to explore CS's interest in out-of-school activities to help give her another venue for physical activity and peer interaction. Mom says they have a YMCA membership; you ask CS and Mom to look into 2 or 3 possible activities to join, such as a dance, karate, or swimming, and have CS to choose one of them. You ask Mom if she would prepare an after-school snack for CS instead of having her daughter get her own, to which Mom agrees.

You go over the laboratory studies that you want to order for CS based on her BMI; then you ask CS and Mom to come back in 3 to 4 weeks to review her laboratory studies, to see how the changes in her eating and activity are going, and most important, to see how she is doing with the kids at school.

Second Visit
A month later CS returns to your office. You reviewed the laboratory studies; her triglyceride levels are mildly elevated, but there are no other abnormalities. Her weight decreased by 1 pound (0.5 kg). She joined a karate class at the YMCA and has been going 2 to 3 times a week. Mom prepares an after-school snack, and CS is not asking for extra food. CS seems happier and says she has met some kids at karate that she likes. CS and Mom say they are willing to keep some diet records to address CS's elevated triglyceride levels at the next visit. You schedule the next visit and plan to continue supporting CS and her family with the goal of normalizing her triglyceride levels and returning her to her previous growth trajectory.

Several states now mandate that schools measure or report BMI. This may provide additional opportunities to address risk for obesity and actual obesity in the school-age population if linked with communication with children's pediatricians.

2.3 Identifying Children and Families at Risk for Obesity

Risk factors for obesity can be identified in children and include

- Genetic and medical disorders associated with obesity
- Parental obesity
- Nutrition and activity patterns associated with obesity
- Living in an at-risk environment

Obesity associated with genetic syndromes is a rare but important cause of childhood obesity.[3] Syndromes associated with obesity are frequently characterized by developmental delay, short stature, dysmorphic features, and involvement of specific organ systems.

Prader-Willi syndrome, which most commonly results from a deletion of 15q11q13, is the most common single-gene obesity-associated syndrome, occurring in 1 out of every 10,000 to 15,000 births. Primary features include infantile hypotonia, a poor sucking reflex, developmental delay, mental retardation, short stature, and skin picking. Obesity becomes apparent as early as 2 years of age, along with hyperphagia, hypogonadism, and behavioral difficulties.[4] With early diagnosis and counseling, excessive weight gain can often be controlled. Additional obesity-associated genetic syndromes are listed in Table 2.2.

Medical conditions that may result in obesity include injury to the hypothalamus as a result of trauma or malignancy, surgery, or radiation treatment (Table 2.3). Endocrinologic causes of obesity include Cushing syndrome, hypothyroidism, and growth hormone deficiency. Psychosocial conditions may also be associated with obesity.

Drug therapy can present a risk for weight gain. Table 2.4 shows commonly prescribed drugs that may be associated with obesity.

Children from pregnancies complicated by diabetes and/or cigarette smoking and children born small for gestational age with accelerated catch-up growth have a greater incidence of obesity (see Chapter 3).

Table 2.2. Genetic Syndromes Associated With Obesity

Syndrome	Associated Issues
Prader-Willi syndrome	Infantile hypotonia; poor feeding followed by hyperphagia and weight gain, developmental delay, mental retardation, short stature, skin picking, behavioral and psychosocial problems
Bardet-Biedl syndrome	Polydactyly, cognitive delay, short stature, retinitis pigmentosa, renal disease, hypogonadism
Alström syndrome	Nerve deafness, diabetes, pigmentary retinal degeneration, cataracts
Albright hereditary osteodystrophy	Short stature; may have pseudohypoparathyroidism, ectopic calcifications, hypocalcaemia
Hereditary Cushing syndrome	Carney complex, an autosomal dominant syndrome of multiple neoplasia, spotty skin pigmentation, multiple endocrine neoplasia, testicular neoplasia, ovarian cysts[5]
Isolated growth hormone deficiency	Short stature, central obesity[5]
X-linked syndromic mental retardation	X-linked mental retardation with a high prevalence of obesity from mutations in the *MECP2* gene[5]

Table 2.3. Medical Conditions Associated With Obesity

Condition	Associated Issues
Hypothalamic obesity	• Head injury; central nervous system malignancy, radiation, or surgery
	• Associated neurologic and endocrinologic deficits
Cushing syndrome	• Hypertension, centripetal obesity, striae
	• Elevated cortisol
Hypothyroidism	• Constipation, linear growth delay, myxedema, lethargy
Growth hormone deficiency	• Short stature
Depression or anxiety	• Change in eating and activity behavior or pharmacotherapy
Abuse	• Signs and symptoms consistent with physical, psychological, and/or sexual abuse[3]

Table 2.4. Drugs Associated With Obesity

• Glucocorticoids	• Carbamazepine
• Phenothiazines	• Beta-adrenergic blockers[6]
• Tricyclic antidepressants	• Insulin
• Valproic acid	• Selective serotonin reuptake inhibitors[6]

Parental obesity is a strong predictor of childhood and adolescent obesity. A child of 1 obese parent has a 30% likelihood of becoming and obese adult. A child of 2 obese parents has a 70% chance. The strong predictive value of parental obesity can allow early identification of children at risk for obesity and early intervention in helping families develop good nutrition and activity patterns. This is particularly important because activity and nutritional patterns are formed at a very early age. For example, studies show that preschool-age children from obese or overweight families share food preferences with their parents and prefer sedentary activity.[7]

Nutritional patterns that may increase the risk of obesity include eating meals at restaurants, eating take-out meals, consuming increased portion sizes, snacking, and skipping meals,[8] as well as drinking soda, sugar-sweetened beverages, and juice.[9,10] Other major sources of risk for obesity are increased television watching, decreased physical activity,[2] and decreased sleep.[11] It is important to identify nutritional and activity patterns that increase the risk of obesity because many are directly influenced by parental and family behavior patterns and could be amenable to lifestyle change.

The school environment can increase the risk of obesity if sugar-sweetened beverages and snacks are available. Lack of physical education, longer school days, and a decrease in recess may also contribute to an environment that promotes obesity. Less walking and biking to school have also been implicated in rising obesity trends.[8]

Once obesity is identified, screening for obesity-related comorbidities and intervening to normalize weight need to occur. These topics will be addressed at length in the following chapters.

References

1. Cole TJ, Bellizzi MC, Flegal KM, Dietz WH. Establishing a standard definition for child overweight and obesity worldwide: international survey. *BMJ.* 2000;320:1240–1243

2. Krebs NF, Jacobson MS, American Academy of Pediatrics Committee on Nutrition. Prevention of pediatric overweight and obesity. *Pediatrics.* 2003;112:424–430

3. Hassink S. Problems in childhood obesity. In: Bray GA, ed. *Office Management of Obesity.* Philadelphia, PA: Elsevier; 2004:73–90

4. Cassidy SB. Prader-Willi syndrome. *Curr Probl Pediatr.* 1984;14:1–55

5. Perusse L, Rankinen T, Zuberi A, et al. The human obesity gene map: the 2004 update. *Obes Res.* 2005;13:381–490

6. Malone M, Alger-Mayer SA, Anderson DA. Medication associated with weight gain may influence outcome in a weight management program. *Ann Pharmacother.* 2005;39:1204–1208

7. Wardle J, Guthrie C, Sanderson S, Birch L, Plomin R. Food and activity preferences in children of lean and obese parents. *Int J Obes Relat Metab Disord.* 2001;25:971–977

8. Nicklas TA, Baranowski T, Cullen KW, Berenson G. Eating patterns, dietary quality and obesity. *J Am Coll Nutr.* 2001;20:599–608

9. American Academy of Pediatrics Committee on School Health. Soft drinks in schools. *Pediatrics.* 2004;113:152–154

10. American Academy of Pediatrics Committee on Nutrition. The use and misuse of fruit juice in pediatrics. *Pediatrics.* 2001;107:1210–1213

11. Sekine M, Yamagami T, Hamanishi S, et al. Parental obesity, lifestyle factors and obesity in preschool children: results of the Toyama Birth Cohort study. *J Epidemiol.* 2002;12(1):33–39

Health Supervision Visits:

Prevention, Early Intervention, and Treatment for the At-Risk Child

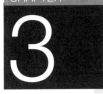

CHAPTER
3

Before Birth: Maternal Health

3.1 What Do We Know?

Improving maternal health before and during pregnancy is a focal point for improving pregnancy outcomes, and it is important to understand that maternal obesity increases the risk of pregnancy-related complications for both mother and infant (Table 3.1).[1,2]

Maternal morbidity increases with increasing body mass index (BMI); therefore, attention to obesity in women in their childbearing years has important implications for maternal health. More than one-third of women between 20 and 39 years of age have a BMI greater than 30. More than 18% have a BMI greater than 35 and 4.2%, greater than 40. In this age group, obesity rates with a BMI greater than 30 vary by ethnicity: non-Hispanic white women (31.3%), non-Hispanic black women (47.2%), and Hispanic women (37.6%).[10] This means that one-third to almost half of women between 20 and 39 years of age are at risk for obesity-related complications of pregnancy.

Complications of pregnancy increase as BMI increases. Maternal BMI of 50 or greater was positively associated with large-for-gestational-age (LGA) newborns, gestational diabetes (GDM), preeclampsia, cesarean delivery, and a

Table 3.1. Adverse Outcomes of Pregnancy Associated With Maternal Obesity Gestational Diabetes[3]
Hypertension[4]
Preeclampsia[4]
Eclampsia[4]
Infection[1]
Cesarean delivery[5]
Thromboembolic event[1]
Surgical complications[1]
Early miscarriage[6]
Induced preterm delivery[2]
Fetal/neonatal death[7]
Macrosomia[1]
Early neonatal death[1]
Suboptimal ultrasound visualization[8]
Maternal mortality[9]

5-minute Apgar score below 7.[11] The rates of cesarean section and induced preterm delivery also rise with increasing maternal BMI,[12,13] as does the rate of neonatal death (5.3/100,000 in nonobese women to 7.5/100,000 in women with morbid obesity).[11]

Maternal obesity results in altered infant body composition. Newborns of mothers with obesity have increased fat mass, body fat, and ponderal index (weight/height³) compared with newborns of nonobese mothers.[14] Newborns of mothers with obesity are more insulin-resistant than infants born to nonobese mothers. The degree of insulin resistance in an infant correlates with maternal insulin resistance and infant adiposity.[15]

Children of mothers who are obese in pregnancy are at increased risk of being obese in childhood and adolescence.[16,17] Overweight rates were even higher in offspring of mothers who were both overweight and had GDM.[4] One study reported that adequate treatment of GDM during pregnancy may attenuate this risk.[18] This increased risk may be attributable to the increased rates of prediabetes in this population.[19]

The incidence of GDM has increased in the general population, paralleling the increase in obesity.[20] The GDM rate for women with a BMI between 30 and 35 is 4.8%, and the rate is 11.5% for women with a BMI greater than 35 compared with 0.7% in women of normal weight.[21] Maternal diabetes alters the intrauterine environment. In a study of Pima Indians, siblings born after their mother developed type 2 diabetes were more likely to develop diabetes and obesity than those born before the onset of maternal diabetes.[22]

Mothers with obesity are also at an increased risk for hypertension, preeclampsia, and eclampsia during pregnancy. Risk of hypertension is 1.7% for women with a BMI between 25 and 29.9 and 2.2% for those with a BMI greater than 30 compared with women with a BMI less than 21.[23] The risk of preeclampsia doubles when a woman enters pregnancy overweight and triples when obese.[24]

The Institute of Medicine (IOM) recommends beginning pregnancy at a healthy weight and revised its pregnancy weight gain guidelines to improve pregnancy outcomes.[25]

In a study of 570,672 pregnancies of women 18 to 40 years of age between the years 2004 and 2007, 41.6% began pregnancy overweight or obese and 51.2% gained weight excessively during pregnancy according to 2009 IOM criteria. The proportions of LGA infants increased among obese women and increased with higher weight gain; conversely, small-for-gestational-age (SGA) newborns were less prevalent among obese women.[26] At 9 years of age, children of women who had gestational weight gain greater than the IOM recommendations had higher BMI, waist circumference, fat mass, systolic blood pressure, C-reactive protein, leptin, and interleukin-6 level and had lower high-density lipoprotein (HDL) cholesterol and apolipoprotein A1 levels, suggesting that maternal obesity and pregnancy weight gain alter the future health status of the offspring.[27]

3.2 How Can This Help Us?

Pediatricians are asked to attend to the health behaviors of the family because they are important mediators of child health.[28-30] In fact, the pediatrician's office may be one of the few places where families and children have the opportunity to spend time together focusing on individual health issues of the child in the context of the family. Thus, there is an opportunity to reinforce the family's impact of their own health and health behaviors on their children. Mothers may not be aware of pregnancy risks associated with obesity and may desire to adopt a healthier lifestyle before pregnancy.[31] Encouraging adoption of a healthy prepregnancy lifestyle and alerting prospective parents to the risks of maternal obesity in pregnancy can be included in obesity prevention for young families.

In addition, adolescent obesity has a high probability of continuing in adulthood and increasing risk for obesity in pregnancy. Risks of an obese pregnancy can be added to the many reasons to engage in prevention and treatment of obesity in adolescence. To prevent obesity, the expert committee recommends that BMI, nutrition, and activity counseling take place at all well visits.[28] There may also be additional opportunities to address obesity prevention with adolescents by using the opportunities presented at other visits. Longitudinal data suggest that high-risk health behaviors in teens may be linked and show an association between monthly alcohol consumption, weekly smoking, daily coffee consumption, and unhealthy food consumption. Counseling aimed at reducing high-risk health behaviors can include obesity prevention and risk assessment. Positive, healthy behaviors such as good oral hygiene, vitamin use, and regular physical activity are also associated with healthy food consumption and can be reinforced at every opportunity.[32] In addition, because both positive and negative health behaviors often cluster together,[32] a positive approach toward empowering adolescents to make a healthy lifestyle change may help break the intergenerational cycle of obesity.

References

1. Nohr EA, Timpson NJ, Andersen CS, Davey Smith G, Olsen J, Sørensen TI. Severe obesity in young women and reproductive health: the Danish National birth Cohort. *PLoS One.* 2009;4(12):e8444
2. Jarvie E, Ramsay JE. Obstetric management of obesity in pregnancy. *Semin Fetal Neonatal Med.* 2010;15(2):83–88. Epub 2009 Oct 31
3. Catalano PM, Roman NM, Tyzbir ED, Merritt AO, Driscoll P, Amini, SB. Weight gain in women with gestational diabetes. *Obstet Gynecol.* 1993;81(4):523–528
4. Lamb MM, Dabelea D, Yin X, et al. Early-life predictors of higher body mass index in healthy children. *Ann Nutr Metab.* 2010;56(1):16–22. Epub 2009 Nov 27
5. Poobalan AS, Aucott LS, Gurung T, Smith WC, Bhattacharya S. Obesity as an independent risk factor for elective and emergency caesarean delivery in nulliparous women-systematic review and meta analysis of cohort studies. *Obese Rev.* 2009; 10(1):28–35
6. Lashen H, Fear K, Sturdee DW. Obesity is associated with increased risk of first trimester and recurrent miscarriage: matched case-control study. *Hum Reprod.* 2004;19:1644–1646
7. Chen A, Feresu SA, Fernandez C, Rogan WJ. Maternal obesity and the risk of infant death in the United States Epidemiology. 2009;20(1): 74–81
8. Handler I, Blackwell SC, Bujold E, et al. The impact of maternal obesity on midtrimester sonographic visualization of fetal cardiac and craniospinal structures. *J Obes Relat Metab Disord.* 2004;28:1607–1611
9. Goffman D, Madden RC, Harrison EA, Merkatz IR, Chazotte C. Predictors of maternal mortality and near-miss maternal morbidity. *J Perinatol.* 2007;27(10):597–601. Epub 2007 Aug 16
10. Flegal KM, Carroll MD, Ogden CL, Curtin LR. Prevalence and trends in obesity among US adults 1999–2008. *JAMA* 2010;303:235–241. National Health and Nutrition Examination Survey, 2007–2008
11. Salihu HM, Alio AP, Wilson RE, Sharma PP, Kirby RS, Alexander GR. Obesity and extreme obesity: new insights into the black-white disparity in neonatal mortality. *Obstet Gynecol.* 2008;111(6):1410–1416
12. Nohr EA, Bech BH, Vaeth M, Rasmussen KM, Nenriksen TB, Olsen J. Obesity, gestational weight gain and preterm birth; a study within the Danish National Birth Cohort. *Paediatr Perinat Epidemiol.* 2007;21(10):5–14
13. Alanis MC, Goodnight WH, Hill EG, Robinson CJ, Villers MS, Johnson DD. Maternal super obesity (body mass index >/= 50) and adverse pregnancy outcomes. *Acta Obstet Gynecol Scand.* 2010;89(7):924–930
14. Sewell MF, Huston-Presley L, Super DM, Catalano P. Increased neonatal fat mass, not lean body mass is associated with maternal obesity. *Am J Obstet Gynecol.* 2006;195(4):1100–1103. Epub 2006 Jul 26
15. Catalano PM, Farrell K, Thomas A, et al. Perinatal risk factors for childhood obesity and metabolic dysregulation. *Am J Clin Nutr.* 2009;90(5):1303–1313. Epub 2009 Sep 16
16. Kuhle S, Allen AC, Veugelers PJ. Perinatal and childhood risk factors for overweight in a provincial sample of Canadian grade 5 students. *Int J Pediatr Obes.* 2010;5(1):88–96

17. Pirkola J, Pouta A, Bloigu A, et al. Risks of overweight and abdominal obesity at age 16 years associated with prenatal exposures to maternal prepregnancy overweight and gestational diabetes mellitus. *Diabetes Care.* 2010;33(5):1115–1121

18. Hillier TA, Pedula KL, Schmidt MM, Mullen JA, Charles MA, Pettitt DJ. Childhood obesity and metabolic imprinting: the ongoing effects of maternal hyperglycemia. *Diabetes Care.* 2007;30(9):2287–2292

19. Biggio JR Jr, Chapman V, Neely C, Cliver SP, Rouse DJ. Fetal anomalies in obese women: the contribution of diabetes. *Obstet Gynecol.* 2010;115(2 pt 1):290–296

20. Getahun D, Nath C, Ananth CV, Chavez MR, Smulian JC. Gestational diabetes in the United States: temporal trends 1989 through 2004. *Am J Obstet Gynecol.* 2008;198(5):525.e1–5

21. Kim SY, England L, Wilson HG, Bish C, Sastten GA, Dietz P. Percentage of gestational diabetes mellitus attributable to overweight and obesity. *Am J Public Health.* 2010;100(6):1047–1052

22. Dabelea D, Hanson RL, Lindsay RS, et al. Intrauterine exposure to diabetes conveys risks for type 2 diabetes and obesity: a study of discordant siblings. *Diabetes.* 2000;49(12):2208–2211

23. Thadhani R, Stampfer MJ, Hunter DJ, Manson JE, Solomon CG, Curhan GC. High body mass index and hypercholesterolemia: risk of hypertensive disorders of pregnancy. *Obstet Gynecol.* 1999;94(4):543–550

24. Sibai BM, Ewell M, Levine RJ, et al. Risk factors associated with preeclampsia in healthy nulliparous women. The Calcium for Preeclampsia Prevention (CPEP) Study Group. *Am J Obstet Gynecol.* 1997;177(5):1003–1010

25. Rasmussen KM, Yaktine AL, eds. Weight gain during pregnancy: reexamining the guidelines. Committee to Reexamine IOM Pregnancy Weight Guidelines Food and Nutrition Board and Board on Children, Youth, and Families. Institute of Medicine and National Research Council of the National Academies. National Academies Press. Washington, DC

26. Park S, Sappenfield WM, Bish C, Salihu H, Goodman D, Bensyl DM. Assessment of the Institute of Medicine Recommendations for Weight Gain During Pregnancy. Florida 2004-2007. *Matern Child Health J.* Epub 2010 Mar 20

27. Fraser A, Tilling K, Macdonald-Wallis C, et al. Association of Maternal Weight Gain in Pregnancy With Offspring Obesity and Metabolic and Vascular Traits in Childhood. Medical Research Council Centre for Causal Analyses in Translational Epidemiology, Department of Social Medicine, University of Bristol, Bristol, UK

28. Barlow SE. Expert committee recommendations regarding the prevention, assessment, and treatment of child and adolescent overweight and obesity: summary report. *Pediatrics.* 2007;120 (suppl 4):S164–192

29. Cohen RY, Felix, Brownell KD. The role of parents and older peers in school-based cardiovascular prevention programs: implications for program development. *Health Educ.* 1989;16:245–253

30. Black C, Ford-Gilboe M. Adolescent mothers; resilience, family health work and health promoting practices. *J Adv Nurs.* 2004;48:351–360

31. Kominiarek MA, Vonderheid S, Endres LK. Maternal obesity: do patients understand the risks? *J Perinatol.* Epub 2010 Apr 22

32. Nutbeam D, Aar L, Catford J. Understanding children's health behaviour: the implications for health promotion for young people. *Soc Sci Med.* 1989;29(3):317–325

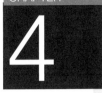

4

Before Birth: The Prenatal Visit

4.1 What Do We Know?

People often ask, "When should we begin to intervene in childhood obesity?" Surprisingly, the answer may be, "Before birth." Fetal life may be one of the critical times we can effectively focus a family's attention on genetic risk, parental influence, the intrauterine environment, and environmental factors that will make it more or less likely that their unborn baby will develop childhood obesity.

The impact of genetics on obesity has been known for a long time. Stunkard et al. determined that identical twins raised in different households had obesity rates that correlated closely with each other and with their biological family, independent of their adoptive families' weight status.[1] We know that there are a group of specific genetic deficits associated with obesity, such as Prader-Willi syndrome, Bardet-Biedl syndrome, Alström syndrome, and leptin deficiency, to name a few. These disorders account for only a small fraction of childhood obesity cases and are usually associated with other systemic signs, such as short stature and cognitive delay, but they have taught us a great deal about the fundamentals of energy regulation. The majority of our patients have an inherited predisposition toward obesity, which is polygenic and in some way triggered by interaction with an obesity-promoting environment.

4.2 How Can This Help Us?

A child with obesity as part of a syndrome needs to be identified, and genetic counseling is required. Tables 4.1 and 4.2 show a list of some of these syndromes associated with specific genetic defects.

In the case of most families, a clearer understanding of their own family history is in order when they are looking at obesity risk for their unborn baby. We know from work by Whitaker et al.[2] that parental obesity is a large and significant risk for the development of obesity in the offspring. In this study, children with 1 or 2 obese parents have a 90% chance of being obese by the time they are adolescents.

Further studies found an increased prevalence of congenital malformations associated with maternal morbid obesity

(BMI >40), including neural tube defects, cardiac defects, and orofacial clefts. Maternal obesity (BMI >30) significantly increased the risk of hydrocephaly, anal atresia, hypospadias, cystic kidney, pes equinovarus, omphalocele, and diaphragmatic hernia.[3]

The risk of congenital heart defects (atrial septal defects, hypoplastic left-sided heart syndrome, aortic stenosis, pulmonic stenosis, and tetralogy of Fallot) increases with increased maternal BMI.[4]

Parents with obesity need to be aware of these risks and work with their pediatrician to develop a plan to address feeding, activity, and inactivity changes as a family.

Taking a family history (Table 4.3) that focuses on obesity and obesity-related comorbidities could help the family understand the short- and long-term risks of obesity in their baby.

There is also growing evidence that "intrauterine life may be a critical period for the development of obesity."[5] It is known that infants of diabetic mothers have more adipose tissue than infants born to mothers without diabetes and are often large for gestational age (LGA). Even when macrosomia normalizes, these infants develop childhood obesity at higher rates than children born to mothers without diabetes.[6] Intrauterine exposure to hyperglycemia and resultant hyperinsulinemia may alter insulin receptor signaling in muscle and adipose tissue in utero.[7] There is also evidence that intrauterine exposure to diabetes is also associated with impaired glucose tolerance in adolescence[8] and a higher prevalence of type 2 diabetes.[9]

Alterations in the intrauterine environment during periods of maternal starvation are also thought to play a role in later obesity development. Male offspring of mothers subjected to famine from 1944 to 1945 during the first and second trimesters of pregnancy had a higher-than-expected incidence of obesity.[10] Barker, in an epidemiologic study of middle-aged adults, showed that small birth size conferred a risk for hypertension, glucose intolerance, and dyslipidemia in adulthood.[11] A study in children born small for gestational age (SGA) showed greater insulin resistance and higher BMIs

Table 4.1. Obesity Syndromes Associated With Developmental Abnormalities

Autosomal dominant	
Prader-Willi syndrome 15q11-q13	Short stature, hypotonia, excessive appetite, progressive obesity, hypogonadism, dysmorphic features, poor cognitive and language development, behavioral abnormalities, sleep disturbances, respiratory disease, impaired growth hormone secretion, low serum insulin-like growth factor-I
Albright hereditary osteodystrophy (AHO) 20q13.2	Short stature, brachydactyly, obesity, skull-facial deformities, short limbs or short metacarpal bones, subcutaneous calcinosis
Pseudohypoparathyroidism type Ia (PHP1A) 20q13.2	AHO phenotype plus multihormone resistance
BDNR (brain-derived neurotrophic factor); very rare	Hyperphagia, early-onset obesity, memory impairment
Autosomal recessive	
Bardet-Biedl syndrome BBS1/11q13, BBS2/16q21, BBS3/3p12-q13, BBS4/15q22.3, BBS5/2q31, BBS6/20p12, BBS7/4q27, BBS8/14q32.11, BBS9/7p14, BBS10/12q21.2, BBS11/9q33.1, BBS12/4q27, BBS13/17q23, and BBS14/12q21.3	Rod-cone dystrophy, central obesity, polydactyly, renal abnormalities, hypogonadism, learning disability
Alström syndrome 2p13.1	Obesity, short stature, progressive retinal dystrophy, sensorineural deafness
Carpenter syndrome 6p12.1-q12	Oxycephaly, facial deformities, craniosynostosis, polysyndactyly, obesity, cardiac defects
Cohen syndrome 8q22-q23	Mental retardation, microcephaly, typical facial features, progressive retinochoroidal dystrophy, obesity, short stature
X-linked	
Börjeson-Forssman-Lehman syndrome Xq26.3	Mental retardation, obesity, gynecomastia, hypogonadism, large thick ears
MEHMO syndrome Xp21.1-p22.13	Mental retardation, epileptic seizures, hypogonadism, microcephaly, obesity

Adapted from Kousta E, Hadjiathanasiou CG, Tolis G, et al. Pleiotropic genetic syndromes with developmental abnormalities associated with obesity. *J Pediatr Endocrinol Metab.* 2009;22(7):581–592

Table 4.2. Obesity Syndromes Associated With Early Onset Obesity

Leptin gene 7q31 Leptin receptor gene 1p31	Normal birth weight but exhibit rapid weight gain in the first few months of life, intense hyperphagia, food-seeking behavior, hypothalamic hypothyroidism and hypogonadotropic hypogonadism, T-cell abnormalities
PMC (proopiomelancortin deficiency) 2p23	Isolated adrenocorticotropic hormone deficiency, hyperphagia, and severe early-onset obesity; red hair in white children
MC4R (melanocortin 4 receptor) 18q21.3	Hyperphagia in first year of life, which may decrease with time; increased muscle mass; accelerated linear growth

Adapted from Farooqi IS, Matarese G, Lord GM, et al. Beneficial effects of leptin on obesity, T cell hyporesponsiveness, and neuroendocrine/metabolic dysfunction of human congenital leptin deficiency. *J Clin Invest.* 2002;110(8):1093–1103

Table 4.3. Family History, Before Birth

Complete the family history targeted toward obesity and related comorbidities.

	Mother	Father	Maternal Grandmother	Maternal Grandfather	Paternal Grandmother	Paternal Grandfather	Sibling 1	Sibling 2
Obesity	☐	☐	☐	☐	☐	☐	☐	☐
Bariatric surgery	☐	☐	☐	☐	☐	☐	☐	☐
Cardiovascular disease	☐	☐	☐	☐	☐	☐	☐	☐
High blood pressure	☐	☐	☐	☐	☐	☐	☐	☐
Stroke	☐	☐	☐	☐	☐	☐	☐	☐
High cholesterol	☐	☐	☐	☐	☐	☐	☐	☐
High triglyceride level	☐	☐	☐	☐	☐	☐	☐	☐
Type 1 or 2 diabetes	☐	☐	☐	☐	☐	☐	☐	☐
Polycystic ovarian syndrome	☐	☐	☐	☐	☐	☐	☐	☐
Liver disease (nonalcoholic steatohepatitis)	☐	☐	☐	☐	☐	☐	☐	☐
Sleep apnea	☐	☐	☐	☐	☐	☐	☐	☐

at 7 to 11 years of age than children born appropriate for gestational age (AGA) with equivalent family history, gestational ages, and gender.[12] Rapid postnatal weight gain in a child born SGA may increase risk for later obesity, cardiovascular disease, and impaired glucose metabolism.[13] One mechanism to explain this is that children born SGA who have rapid catch-up growth have higher rates of fat accumulation[14] combined with persistent deficits in lean body mass,[15] creating a scenario of increased insulin and leptin resistance.

Possibly related to the risk of impaired growth in utero as a result of obesity is a report that maternal smoking during pregnancy has a dose-response relationship to obesity at school entry.[16,17]

Therefore, it is critical to encourage mothers to access health care before and during pregnancy. Mothers who have diabetes, who are at risk for a baby with growth impairment, or who smoke need special attention when it comes to optimizing the intrauterine environment for their babies.

Pregnancy is also a time to plan for breastfeeding. Breastfeeding is recommended as the optimal nutrition source for an infant. Studies show that breastfed babies have a reduced incidence of obesity.[18,19]

There is a correlation between the amount of breastfeeding and the risk of obesity, with each month of breastfeeding up to 9 months conferring a 4% risk reduction for obesity.[20] There is also an association between excess weight in the second 6 months of life and receiving less than 80% of feedings from breast milk.[21]

The exact nature of this effect is unknown; however, breast milk contains both leptin and adiponectin, which are not in infant formula.[22,23] These hormones may enable breastfed babies to better regulate energy metabolism[21] intake and more precisely regulate satiety.[24]

Data exist that shows earlier cessation of breastfeeding in mothers who were obese before pregnancy.[25,26] Obesity may alter the hypothalamic pituitary gonadal axis and fat metabolism affecting milk production and composition.[27] However, mothers with obesity may need increased help in initiating and maintaining breastfeeding. A lactation consultant may provide helpful information and support for these families.

References

1. Stunkard AJ, Foch TT, Hrubec Z. A twin study of human obesity. *Am Med Assoc.* 1986;56:51–54

2. Whitaker RC, Wright JA, Pepe MS, Seidel KD, Dietz WH. Predicting obesity in young adulthood from childhood and parental obesity. *N Engl J Med.* 1997;337:869–873

3. Blomberg MI, Källén B. Maternal obesity and morbid obesity: the risk for birth defects in the offspring. *Birth Defects Res A Clin Mol Teratol.* 2010;88(1):35–40

4. Mills JL, Troendle J, Conley MR, Carter T, Druschel CM. Maternal obesity and congenital heart defects: a population-based study. *Am J Clin Nutr.* 2010;91(6):1543–1549. Epub 2010 Apr 7

5. Dietz WH. Critical periods in childhood for the development of obesity. *Am J Clin Nutr.* 1994;59:955–959

6. Plagemann A, Harder T, Kohlhoff R, Rhode W, Dorner G. Overweight and obesity in infants of mothers with long-term insulin dependent diabetes or gestational diabetes. *Int J Obes Relat Metab Disord.* 1997;21(6):451–456

7. Freinkel N. Banting lecture 1980. Of pregnancy and progeny. *Diabetes.* 1980;29:1023–1035

8. Silverman B, Metzger B, Cho N, Loeb C. Impaired glucose tolerance in adolescent offspring of diabetic mothers. Relationship to fetal hyperinsulinism. *Diabetes Care*. 1995;18:611–617

9. Pettitt D, Aleck K, Barrd H, Carraker M, Bennett P, Knowler WC. Congenital susceptibility to NIDDM: role of intrauterine environment. *Diabetes*. 1988;37:622–628

10. Ravelli G, Stern Z, Susser M. Obesity in young men after famine exposure in utero and early infancy. *N Engl J Med*. 1976;293:349–353

11. Barker DJ. The intrauterine origins of cardiovascular disease. *Acta Paetrica*. 1993;82(suppl 391):93–99

12. Veening M, Van Weissenbruch M, Delemarre-Van de Wall H. Glucose tolerance, insulin sensitivity and insulin secretion in children bore small for gestational age. *J Clin Endo Metab*. 2001;879(10):4657–4661

13. Ong KK, Ahmed ML, Emmett PM, Preece MA, Dunger DB. Association between postnatal catch-up growth and obesity in childhood: prospective cohort study. *BMJ*. 2000;320:967–971

14. Dulloo AG. Thrifty energy metabolism in catch-up growth trajectories to insulin and leptin resistance. *Best Pract Res Clin Endocrinol Metab*. 2008;22(1):155–171

15. Hediger ML, Overpeck MD, Kucamarski RJ, McGlynn A, Maurer KR, Davis WW. Muscularity and fatness of infants and young children born small or large for gestational age. *Pediatrics*. 1998;102(5):e60

16. Von Kreis R, Toschke A, Koletzko B, Slikker W. Maternal smoking during pregnancy and childhood obesity. *Am J Epidemiol*. 2002;156:954–961

17. Oken E, Levitan EB, Gillman MW. Maternal smoking during pregnancy and child overweight systematic review and meta analysis [review]. *Int J Obes (Lond)*. 2008;32(2):201–210. Epub 2007 Nov 27

18. Arenz S, Ruckerl R, Koletzko B, von Kries R. Breast-feeding and childhood obesity—a systematic review. *Int J Obes Relat Metab Disord*. 2004;28(10):1247–1256

19. Metzger MW, McDade TW. Breastfeeding as obesity prevention in the United States: a sibling difference model. *Am J Hum Biol*. 2010;22(3):291–296

20. Harder T, Bergmann R, Kallischnigg G, Plagemann A. Duration of breastfeeding and risk of overweight: a meta analysis. *Am J Epidemiol*. 2005;162(5):397–403

21. Li R, Fein SB, Grummer-Strawn LM. Association of breastfeeding intensity and bottle-emptying behaviors at early infancy with infants' risk for excess weight at late infancy. *Pediatrics*. 2008;122(suppl 2);S77–84

22. Houseknecht KI, McGuire MK, Portocarrero CP, McGuire MA, Beerman K. Leptin is present in human milk and is related to maternal plasma leptin concentrations and adiposity. *Biochem Biophy Res Commun*. 1997;240(3):742–747

23. Martin IJ, Woo JG, Geraghty SR, et al. Adiponectin is present in human milk and is associated with maternal factors. *Am J Clin Nutr*. 2006;83(5):1106–1111

24. WHO Working Group on Infant Growth. *An Evaluation of Infant Growth*. Geneva: World Health Organization; 1994

25. Chapman DJ, Perez-Escamille R. Identification of risk factors for delayed onset of lactation. *J Am Diet Assoc*. 1999;99:450–454

26. Li R, Jewell S, Gummer-Strawn L. Maternal obesity and breast feeding practices. *Am J Clin Nutr*. 2003;77:931–936

27. Rasmussen K, Hilson J, Kjohede C. Obesity may impair lactogenesis. *J Nutr*. 2001;131:3009S–3011S

5

Newborn and Infant

5.1 Background

At birth, newborns need to be ready to transition to extra-uterine sources of nutrition. Term neonates accumulate adipose tissue in the last trimester of pregnancy and in the early postnatal months. Fat stores are mobilized during infections and during transitions in sources of nutrition, which may explain the significantly greater amount of adiposity in human neonates compared to other mammals.[1] Nutrient composition and intake may influence later obesity, especially in genetically susceptible infants.

Evidence from multiple studies shows a relationship between breastfeeding and reduced risk of obesity.[2–4] Mixed breast and formula feeding is associated with higher weight and length for age z scores at 3 to 6 months, 6 to 9 months, and 9 to 12 months.[5] Infants frequently bottle-fed in early infancy were more likely to empty the milk from a bottle or cup in late infancy, indicating a possible effect on feeding self-regulation.[6]

Breastfed infants have a slightly decreased intake of energy and protein compared with formula-fed infants, and they gain more weight and lean body mass per gram of protein intake than formula-fed infants; this may indicate early differences in energy balance and body composition.[7] Leptin, a cytokine integral to energy regulation, is produced by mammary epithelial cells[8] and is found in breast milk.[9] Breast milk leptin levels vary with birth weight and rate of weight gain in small-for-gestational-age (SGA), average-for-gestational-age (AGA), and large-for-gestational-age (LGA) infants during the first month of life.[10] At 2 months of age, leptin levels were higher in breastfed infants than formula-fed infants independent of anthropometric measurements.[11]

Adiponectin is found in breast milk, and serum levels are inversely related to adiposity and inflammation. Children who were overweight at 2 years and breastfed for at least 6 months had elevated levels of adiponectin in maternal breast milk.[12,13] Ghrelin, a peptide associated with both short-term appetite regulation and long-term adiposity, is also found in breast milk and may serve to regulate energy balance and influence later adiposity.[14]

Feeding interactions may be important drivers of early weight gain. Mothers who breastfeed have less restrictive patterns of infant feeding at 1 year of age than mothers who formula-fed.[15] Timing of solid food introduction has been linked to type of feeding, with early introduction of solids among formula-fed infants being associated with higher body mass index (BMI) at age 3.[16–19]

Rate of weight gain in the first 4 months of life has been associated with risk of overweight at 7 years of age and may represent genetic influences on early energy balance and/or a vulnerable growth period that affects later energy balance.[20] Total energy intake and sucking behavior during a test meal rather than energy expenditure influence body weight of infants over the first 2 years of life.[21]

Studies also show an association even in early infancy between short sleep duration and increased weight gain.[22] The risk of overweight increases as more risk factors, such as maternal smoking during pregnancy, increased gestational weight gain, shortened breastfeeding duration, and decreased infant sleep duration, are added.[23]

5.2 Prevention: Talking to Parents (BALANCE)

Prevention touch points for parents include **belief, assessment, lifestyle, activity, nutrition, child,** and **environment** (BALANCE).

*B*elief

- Bringing home a new baby is a time of change in every family. This is a good time to help parents and families think about how their behavior will affect the baby in terms of eating, activity, and obesity prevention.
- Parents with obesity often have a heightened concern about obesity prevention and are actively looking at ways to begin these preventive efforts as early as possible.
- Maintaining optimal growth requires managing eating and activity behavior and helping families learn to interact with their baby around hunger and satiety (Box 5.1). Learning

to identify cues to hunger and satiety can help parents set the stage for an interactive approach to eating and feeding

Box 5.1. Signs of Satiety[24]

4–12 weeks

- Spontaneously releases nipple
- Moves head away from nipple
- Closes lips when nipple reinserted
- Slows sucking
- Falls asleep

16–24 weeks

- Bites nipple
- Blocks mouth with hands
- Turns away
- Cries or fusses if feeding persists
- Increases attention to surroundings
- Loses interest in feeding
- Releases nipple and withdraws head

28–36 weeks

- Changes posture
- Hands become more active
- Keeps mouth closed
- Plays with utensils
- Shakes head "no"

40–52 weeks

- Engages in the above
- Hands bottle back to parent
- Spits

Assessment

- Parents and grandparents have all kinds of ideas regarding what babies should look like and how much weight they should be gaining. This is a good time to explain growth- and weight-for-length charts and make sure families understand how to interpret them.
- Plotting the baby's height and weight and weight for length and sharing this with parents is a good way to highlight the importance of following the growth chart.

- Parents can identify with the goal of "keeping the baby on the chart." This can focus discussions on strategies to maintain energy balance, correct imbalances, and share strategies with other family members.

Lifestyle

- It is important to help new parents and families recognize the role of the family's lifestyle in supporting the proper nutrition and activity of the newborn.
- Encourage parents to communicate with the other members of the family about their plans and goals for feeding the baby and provide activity opportunities.
- Offering to have extended family members come to a doctor's visit if the parent wishes may also help get everyone on the same page.

Activity

- Encouraging parents to spend time in face-to-face interaction with their baby, making sounds, talking, and laughing, lays the groundwork for shared activity.
- Remind parents that "tummy time" in a safe and supervised setting is important not only for the baby's activity but for motor development as well.
- Taking the baby for a daily walk in a stroller helps establish outdoor time as a part of the routine.
- Parents should make sure their baby has safe and soft toys to play with. Remind them that the toys should be small enough for the baby to pick up but large enough that they cannot be put in the baby's mouth.
- Parents need to know that television watching is associated with obesity and overweight in children.
- The American Academy of Pediatrics (AAP) currently recommends that *TV should not be watched by children 2 years of age and younger.*

Nutrition

- Every effort should be made to encourage and support breastfeeding for all infants whenever possible.
- Parents who are overweight/obese or who have obesity in their families should be acquainted with the benefits of breastfeeding with regard to obesity prevention.
- Connections to lactation support may be especially helpful to overweight mothers.
- Parents who elect or need to formula-feed should be encouraged to use hunger and satiety cues rather than feeding strictly by volume.

Child

- Parents often respond to crying by feeding their infant. Help parents understand that crying is a baby's way of expressing needs, such as:
  - Hunger
  - Need for a diaper change
  - Gas pains
  - Need help from a caregiver (ie, wrapped in a blanket)
  - Illness
  - Need to be held
- Remind parents that feeding will quiet babies even if they are not hungry because sucking is comforting. However, food may become an inappropriate source of comfort if a baby learns to eat every time he or she has a problem.
- Reassure parents that although their baby's crying may be upsetting for them, learning to interpret particular cries is teaching the baby about communication.

Environment

- Work with parents on a safe home environment.
- Have parents find quiet spaces to play and read to their infant.
- Have families look in their neighborhood for safe and interesting places to walk with the baby.
- Remind parents that the AAP recommends that infants should not watch television.
- Watching television with the baby diverts people's attention away from one another and decreases face-to-face time, which can set up habits that contribute to obesity.
- Help parents assess their child care environment for healthy nutrition, no screen time, and age/developmentally appropriate safe activity.[25]

5.3 Intervention

Infancy is a time of feeding and eating transitions; paying careful attention to parent-child interactions can help smooth the way for healthy eating. Patterns of activity and inactivity also emerge; encourage families to take a close look at their own attitudes and behaviors about eating, activity, and inactivity. Families with parental obesity are at risk for an obese child and may need special attention regarding *energy balance, structure,* and *modeling healthy behavior* (discussed in the next sections).

Energy Balance

Every visit is an opportunity to monitor growth, review feeding practices, and encourage activity. Mothers with obesity have delayed lactogenesis and increased difficulty maintain-

ing breastfeeding.[26] Proactive and positive lactation support is important for all mothers, but especially for mothers with obesity. Mothers who are obese or who are worried about pregnancy weight gain should be encouraged to maintain an adequate and healthy diet with a wide variety of foods to optimize their own health, support breastfeeding, and avoid restrictive diets. Reinforce attention to hunger and satiety cues with families who choose to formula-feed.

Structure

As the immediate newborn period ends, families should be moving into a pattern of structured meals and activity. Parents may appreciate attention to time management and tips on balancing the needs of the newborn and other family members. Television time is not recommended for infants but may be the first thing parents think of when they need downtime. Active, supervised play may also get lost in the shuffle of day care, busy schedules, and siblings' activities and needs to be incorporated into the families' overall plan.

Modeling Healthy Behavior

Parents may think that their infant is too young to be affected by their own habits, but family eating and activity patterns may sneak into the infant's routine. There is ample evidence that infants transition to foods that the family is already consuming—this is the time to review the family's diet and nutritional patterns and eliminate high-calorie snacks and excess sugared beverages.

Consuming desserts, sweets, and juice may be second nature to the family and can roll right into the infant's diet. Other family members may have their own ideas of how and what to feed the infant, including larger-than-needed portion sizes and early solid foods. Parents need to start seeing themselves as being in charge of the infant's environment—at home, at child care, and when with extended family. Families can use this time to get into a routine of outdoor activity (stroller walks) and screen time reduction.

5.4 Treatment

Infants' weight trajectories can vary widely, but if an infant's weight for length is above the normal curve, then it is time to take a close look at both the medical condition of the infant and the eating and activity patterns of the infant and the family. If both parents are physically active, healthy eaters, and thin, logic and some studies show that the infant is less likely than average to become obese as an adult.[27] However, numerous studies show that infants who were classified as overweight in infancy were more likely to be children,[20] adolescents,[28] and adults[29] with obesity. It is important to review the issues discussed in the previous 2 sections because these are the building blocks of good nutrition and activity habits. However, you will also have to focus on the barriers to change, which may prevent parents and families from implementing these strategies. Rate of weight gain in infancy as early as 4 months predicts obesity risk in children and adults.[30] Rate of sucking rather than energy expenditure were linked to the risk of obesity later in life.[21]

5.5 Family History

A useful way to begin is to obtain a family history focused on obesity-related comorbidities. This can serve to emphasize the health risks involved and the necessity of taking early action once obesity is identified.

In Table 5.1, complete or update the family history targeted toward obesity and related comorbidities.

5.6 Review of Systems

The review of systems can also serve as a point of departure to discuss obesity-related comorbidities, pointing out particular risk factors as they relate to increasing BMI.

- LGA or SGA newborn, maternal diabetes, obesity or increased weight gain during pregnancy, maternal smoking, parental obesity
- Head, eyes, ears, nose, and throat (HEENT): Cataracts, deafness, orofacial cleft

- Cardiopulmonary: Murmur, cyanosis
- Gastrointestinal: Omphalocele and diaphragmatic hernia, anal atresia, hypospadias, cystic kidney
- Musculoskeletal: Infantile hypotonia and poor feeding followed by hyperphagia and weight gain, pes equinovarus
- Genitourinary: Hypogonadism, hypospadias, cystic kidney
- Neurologic: Neural tube defect, hydrocephaly
- Development: Delay in cognitive and/or motor development

5.7 Physical Examination

- Height % (World Health Organization [WHO] charts)
- Weight % (WHO charts)
- Weight for length (WHO charts)
- Blood pressure %
- General: Dysmorphic features, poor linear growth, developmental delay
- Skin: Dermatitis in skinfolds
- HEENT: Cataracts, deafness, orofacial cleft, cranio-synostosis, oxycephaly, facial dysmorphia, microcephaly
- Cardiopulmonary: Murmur, cyanosis
- Gastrointestinal: Omphalocele, and diaphragmatic hernia, anal atresia, hypospadias, cystic kidney
- Musculoskeletal: Hypotonia, pes equinovarus, polydactyly, short limbs
- Genitourinary: Hypogonadism, hypospadias, cystic kidney
- Neurologic: Neural tube defect, hydrocephaly

Table 5.1. Family History, Newborn and Infant

Complete the family history targeted toward obesity and related comorbidities.

	Mother	Father	Maternal Grandmother	Maternal Grandfather	Paternal Grandmother	Paternal Grandfather	Sibling 1	Sibling 2
Obesity	☐	☐	☐	☐	☐	☐	☐	☐
Bariatric surgery	☐	☐	☐	☐	☐	☐	☐	☐
Cardiovascular disease	☐	☐	☐	☐	☐	☐	☐	☐
High blood pressure	☐	☐	☐	☐	☐	☐	☐	☐
Stroke	☐	☐	☐	☐	☐	☐	☐	☐
High cholesterol	☐	☐	☐	☐	☐	☐	☐	☐
High triglyceride level	☐	☐	☐	☐	☐	☐	☐	☐
Type 1 or 2 diabetes	☐	☐	☐	☐	☐	☐	☐	☐
Polycystic ovarian syndrome	☐	☐	☐	☐	☐	☐	☐	☐
Liver disease (nonalcoholic steatohepatitis)	☐	☐	☐	☐	☐	☐	☐	☐
Sleep apnea	☐	☐	☐	☐	☐	☐	☐	☐
	☐	☐	☐	☐	☐	☐	☐	☐
	☐	☐	☐	☐	☐	☐	☐	☐

■ Development: Delay in cognitive and/or motor development

See the WHO weight-for-length growth charts for children 2 years of age and younger (see Appendix A.2).

5.8 Family Constellation and Social History

Information about the family can provide a starting point for discussing how nutrition and activity decisions are made and how changes might take place.

■ Who is living at home with the infant?
■ Who else feeds and cares for the infant?
■ Who decides what the infant will eat?
■ Do family members agree on how to feed the infant?

5.9 Parenting Questions

Parenting styles and skills are important when families are trying to make changes in lifestyle. The questions in Table 5.2 may help you focus on family factors that may either facilitate or hamper change.

5.10 Parenting Touch Points

Parenting touch points focus on helping families initiate and maintain change by helping them believe change can occur, identify the change needed, value the outcome of the change, know how to change, and have the energy to change and sustain the change.

■ *Value the outcome.* Infant weight and feeding are important to parents, and the measure of success may be the infant's weight gain, the time, or the amount of feeding. Working with families to have the infant's weight stay on the growth curve is important; to accomplish this, parents may need to expand their ideas of successful feeding. Focusing families on the dynamics of satiety and cued feeding to allow value for the interaction between parent and child to develop lays the groundwork for future eating behavior.

■ *Identify the change.* Parents base their feeding choices for their infants on their own knowledge of nutrition. This is the time to provide parents with information and an opportunity to explore and discuss their own choices and what they believe are the correct dietary choices for their infant. Juice is often seen as a healthy choice and should be virtually eliminated in the diet of an infant whose weight for length is greater than the 85th percentile. Parents may also see television time as being educational or allowing shared time with the family. Helping families regard nutrition and activity as health behaviors may help them evaluate their habits in a different light.

■ *Believe that change can occur.* Parents are the most important agents of change for the infant. Learning to assess the infant's nutrition and activity environment at home, in child care, and with other family members is a necessary skill if parents are to make the healthiest decisions for their infants.

■ *Know how to change.* Parents may believe that their infant is driving the changes. Reassurance that they are offering an appropriate amount and type of nutrition can be helpful to allay their anxiety that their infant is still hungry. Changing the nutrition and activity environment for their infant begins with the parents' own behavior change.

■ *Have the energy to change and sustain.* Positive support at each physician visit for healthy nutrition and activity helps sustain change. Involving the extended family members in visits to discuss nutrition and activity, when appropriate, may provide needed support for parents who are trying to effect family-based change.

5.11 Developmental Touch Point

Establishing communication is a critical step at this stage. Parents should be encouraged to have as much face-to-face interaction as possible with their infant, notice the infant's unique responses, and observe differences in cries. This interaction sets the stage for a responsive give and take.

Table 5.2. Parenting Questions, Newborn and Infant

	Never	Seldom	Sometimes	Often	Always
Parents agree on how to feed the child.	☐	☐	☐	☐	☐
Child and parent/parents fight about food.	☐	☐	☐	☐	☐
Parents set clear and simple expectations and limits.	☐	☐	☐	☐	☐
Parents understand child's developmental stage.	☐	☐	☐	☐	☐
Parents set boundaries and give child choice within them.	☐	☐	☐	☐	☐

5.12 Nutrition and Activity Questions and Approaches

Parents can answer the nutrition and activity questions in Tables 5.3 and 5.4, which can provide a focal point for targeted intervention (Tables 5.5 and 5.6) in a brief encounter. Questions answered "Often" or "Always" can be targeted first for change.

Table 5.3. Nutrition and Activity Questions, Newborn (0–6 Months)

These questions can be answered by the parents and provide a focal point for targeted intervention in a brief encounter. First have the parents answer these questions about the presence or absence of behaviors that promote weight gain; then refer to Table 5.5.

Please answer the following for the statements below: Does your infant…?

	Never	Seldom	Sometimes	Often	Always
1. Seem hungry all the time	☐	☐	☐	☐	☐
2. Spit up after meals	☐	☐	☐	☐	☐
3. "Watch" TV	☐	☐	☐	☐	☐
4. Eat without someone holding their bottle	☐	☐	☐	☐	☐
5. Need breast milk/formula in their bottle to go to sleep	☐	☐	☐	☐	☐
6. Have cereal in his/her bottle	☐	☐	☐	☐	☐
7. Have juice in his/her bottle	☐	☐	☐	☐	☐
8. Eat solid foods	☐	☐	☐	☐	☐
9. Have tummy time	☐	☐	☐	☐	☐
10. Finish an entire bottle	☐	☐	☐	☐	☐

Table 5.4. Nutrition and Activity Questions, Infant (6-12 Months)

These questions can be answered by the parents and provide a focal point for targeted intervention in a brief encounter. First have the parents answer these questions about the presence or absence of behaviors that promote weight gain, then refer to Table 5.6.

Please answer the following for the statements below: Does your infant…?

	Never	Seldom	Sometimes	Often	Always
1. Eat only small amounts of vegetables.	☐	☐	☐	☐	☐
2. Eat only small amounts of fruits.	☐	☐	☐	☐	☐
3. Seem hungry all the time.	☐	☐	☐	☐	☐
4. "Watch" TV.	☐	☐	☐	☐	☐
5. Need formula/breast milk in his or her bottle to go to sleep.	☐	☐	☐	☐	☐
6. Use a bottle.	☐	☐	☐	☐	☐
7. Have unscheduled meals and snacks throughout the day.	☐	☐	☐	☐	☐
8. Sleep less than 9–12 hours during the night and nap throughout the day.	☐	☐	☐	☐	☐
9. Eat meals without the rest of the family.	☐	☐	☐	☐	☐
10. Seldom use a spoon to feed self.	☐	☐	☐	☐	☐
11. Drink juice.	☐	☐	☐	☐	☐
12. Seldom have daily active play with you.	☐	☐	☐	☐	☐

Table 5.5. Nutrition and Activity Approaches, Newborn (0–6 Months)

Questions answered "Often" or "Always" in Table 5.3 can be targeted first for change. Using these specific questions, ask the parent, "How willing are you to…?"

Please answer the following for the statements below: How willing are you to…?

	Never	Seldom	Sometimes	Often	Always
1. Learn about and watch for signs of fullness.	☐	☐	☐	☐	☐
2. Find alternative play activities for your baby rather than watching TV.	☐	☐	☐	☐	☐
3. Hold your baby every time you feed him or her.	☐	☐	☐	☐	☐
4. Stop putting your baby to bed with a bottle.	☐	☐	☐	☐	☐
5. Limit food in your baby's bottle to only formula or breast milk.	☐	☐	☐	☐	☐
6. Change from juice to water between meals.	☐	☐	☐	☐	☐
7. Wait to start solids foods at 6 months.	☐	☐	☐	☐	☐
8. Schedule tummy time every day.	☐	☐	☐	☐	☐
9. Try ways other than feeding to comfort your baby.	☐	☐	☐	☐	☐

Table 5.6. Nutrition and Activity Approaches, Infant (6–12 Months)

Questions answered "Often" or "Always" in Table 5.4 can be targeted first for change. Using these specific questions, ask the parent, "How willing are you to…?"

Please answer the following for the statements below: How willing are you to…?

	Never	Seldom	Sometimes	Often	Always
1. Offer vegetables at meals and snacks.	☐	☐	☐	☐	☐
2. Offer fruits at meals and snacks.	☐	☐	☐	☐	☐
3. Learn about and watch for signs of fullness.	☐	☐	☐	☐	☐
4. Find alternative play activities for your baby rather than watching TV.	☐	☐	☐	☐	☐
5. Limit food in your baby's bottle to only formula or breast milk.	☐	☐	☐	☐	☐
6. Teach your baby how to hold and drink from a sippy cup.	☐	☐	☐	☐	☐
7. Schedule regular meals and snacks.	☐	☐	☐	☐	☐
8. Plan sleeping routine to ensure 9–10 hours of sleep at night and regular naps throughout the day.	☐	☐	☐	☐	☐
9. Eat meals together.	☐	☐	☐	☐	☐
10. Teach your baby to hold and use a spoon.	☐	☐	☐	☐	☐
11. Change from juice to water between meals.	☐	☐	☐	☐	☐
12. Schedule daily active play time.	☐	☐	☐	☐	☐
13. Try ways other than feeding to comfort your baby.	☐	☐	☐	☐	☐

5.13 A Case in Point: SC

SC is a newborn girl you are seeing in the nursery. Her birth weight was 9 lb 2 oz, and she is a healthy full-term baby. You meet her parents and note that both are significantly obese. SC is their first child, and as you ask about the family history, they note that SC's mother had gestational diabetes and that 2 of the grandparents developed type 2 diabetes in midlife. SC's mother wants to breastfeed but is having some difficulty and seems somewhat discouraged. Both parents are anxious to do the right thing for SC.

You note that SC's examination was normal and she seems to be a healthy and vigorous baby. You support the mother's desire to breastfeed and ask the nurse to support her efforts, showing her how to best hold SC and help with latching on. You schedule an office visit for 2 days later.

Second Visit

SC and Mom come to the office. Mom has had success initiating breastfeeding. Mom wonders if SC is getting enough to eat, and you reassure her after checking SC's weight and hydration. You offer her the number of a lactation support group and encourage her to continue breastfeeding. You mention SC's family history and the fact that she had gestational diabetes. You note that these are risk factors for obesity and diabetes and that breastfeeding can help reduce these risks. You also ask Mom to start noticing SC's hunger and satiety cues.

Ongoing Visits

As the visits progress, you plot SC's height, weight, and weight for height. You go over the growth charts with Mom with the goal of keeping SC "on the chart." You prepare Mom to start solid foods at 6 months and encourage her and Dad to take stock of their own diet and activity habits, noting the importance of parents modeling healthy behaviors. You remind SC's parents that television watching is not recommended for children younger than 2 years of age. You encourage SC's parents to find family activities that they can do together besides watch TV.

References

1. Kuzawa CW. Adipose tissue in human infancy and childhood: an evolutionary perspective. *Am J Phys Anthrop.* 1998;(suppl 27):177–209
2. Owen CG, Martin RM, Whincup PH, Smith GD, Cook DG. Effect of infant feeding on the risk of obesity across the life course: a quantitative review of published evidence. *Pediatrics.* 2005;115(5):1367–1377
3. Arenz S, Rückerl R, Koletzko B, von Kries R. Breast-feeding and childhood obesity—a systematic review. *Int J Obes.* 2004;28(10):1247–1256
4. Harder T, Bergmann R, Kallischnigg G, Plagemann A. Duration of breastfeeding and risk of overweight: a meta-analysis. *Am J Epidemiol.* 2005;162(5):397–403
5. Kramer MS, Guo T, Platt RW, et al. Promotion of Breastfeeding Intervention Trials Study Group. *J Pediatr.* 2004;145(50):600–605
6. Li R, Fein SB, Grummer–Strawn LM. Do infants fed from bottles lack self-regulation of milk intake compared with directly breastfed infants? *Pediatrics.* 2010;125(6):e1386–93. Epub 2010 May 10
7. Heinig MJ, Nommsen LA, Peerson JM, Lonnerdal B, Dewey KG. Energy and protein intakes of breast-fed and formula-fed infants during the first year of life and their association with growth velocity; the DARLING Study. *Am J Clin Nutr.* 1993;58(2):152–161
8. Smith-Kirwin SM, O'Connor DM, Johnston J, DeLancey ED, Hassink SG, Funange VL. Leptin expression in human mammary epithelial cells and breast milk. *J Clin Endocrinol Metab.* 1998;83(5):1810–1813
9. Houseknecht KL, McGuire MK, Portocarrero CP, McGuire MA, Beerman K. Leptin is present in human milk and is related to maternal plasma leptin concentration and adiposity. *Biochem Biophys Res Commun.* 1997;240(3):742–747
10. Dundar NO, Anal O, Dundar B, Ozkan H, Caliskan S, Buyukgebiz A. Longitudinal investigation of the relationship between breast milk leptin levels and growth in breast fed infants. *J Pediatr Endocrinol Metab.* 2005;18(2):181–187
11. Savino F, Nanni GE, Maccario S, Costamagna M, Oggero R, Silvestro L. Breast fed infants have higher leptin values than formula fed infants in the first four months of life. *J Pediatr Endocrinol Metab.* 2004;17(11):1527–1532
12. Newburg DS, Woo JG, Morrow AL. Characteristics and potential functions of human milk adiponectin. *J Pediatr.* 2010;156(2 suppl):S41–46
13. Weyermann M, Brenner H, Rothenbacher D. Adipokines in human milk and risk of overweight in early childhood: a prospective cohort study. *Epidemiology.* 2007;18(6):722–729
14. Savino F, Fissore MF, Grassino EC, Nanni GE, Oggero R, Silvestro L. Ghrelin, leptin and IGF-I levels in breast-fed and formula-fed infants in the first years of life. *Acta Paediatrica.* 2005;94(5):531–537
15. Taveras EM, Scanlon KS, Birch L, Rifas-Shiman SL, Rich-Edwards JW, Gillman MW. Association of breastfeeding with maternal control of infant feeding at age 1 year. *Pediatrics.* 2004;114(5):e577–583
16. Huh SY, Rifas-Shiman SL, Taveras EM, Oken E, Gillman MW. Timing of solid food introduction and risk of obesity in preschool-aged children. *Pediatrics.* 2011;127(3):e544–51. doi: 10.1542/peds.2010-0740. Epub 2011 Feb 7
17. Sievers E, Oldigs HD, Santer R, Schaub J. Feeding patterns in breast-fed and formula-fed infants. *Ann Nutr Metab.* 2002;46(6):243–248
18. Mathew OP, Bhatia J. Sucking and breathing patterns during breast- and bottle-feeding in term neonates. Effects of nutrient delivery and composition. *Am J Dis Child.* 1989;143(5):588–592
19. Mihrshahi S, Battistutta D, Magarey A, Daniels LA. Determinants of rapid weight gain during infancy: baseline results from the NOURISH randomised controlled trial. *BMC Pediatr.* 2011;11:99. doi: 10.1186/1471-2431-11-99

20. Stettler N, Zemel BS, Kumanyika S, Stallings VA. Infant Weight Gain and Childhood Overweight Status in a Multicenter, Cohort Study. *Pediatrics.* 2002;109(2):194–199

21. Stunkard AJ, Berkowitz RI, Scholeller D, Maislin G, Stallings VA. Predictors of body size in the first 2 y of life: a high-risk study of human obesity. *Int J Obes Relat Metab Disord.* 2004;28(4):503–13

22. Tikotzky L, DE Marcas G, Har-Toov J, Dollberg S, Bar-Haim Y, Sadeh A. Sleep and physical growth in infants during the first 6 months. *J Sleep Res.* 2010;19(1 pt 1):103–10. Epub 2009 Oct 14

23. Gillman MW, Rifas-Shiman SL, Kleinman K, Oken E, Rich-Edwards JW, Taveras EM. Developmental origins of childhood overweight: potential public health impact. *Obesity (Silver Spring).* 2008;16(7):1651–1656. Epub 2008 May 1

24. Trahms CM, Pipes PL. *Nutrition in Infancy and Childhood.* 6th ed. New York: WCB/McGraw-Hill; 1997

25. Healthy Child Care America Web site. http://www.healthychildcare.org/ResourcesHP.html

26. Lovelady CA. Is maternal obesity a cause of poor lactation performance? *Nutr Rev.* 2005;63(10):352–355

27. Whitaker RC, Wright JA, Pepe MS, Seidel KD, Dietz WH. Predicting obesity in young adulthood from childhood and parental obesity. *N Engl J Med.* 1997;337:869–873

28. Rolland-Cachera MR, Deheeger M, Guilloud-BatailleM, Avons P, Patois E, Sempe M. Tracking the development of adiposity from one month of age to adulthood. Ann *Human Biol.* 1987;14(3):219–229

29. He Q, Karlberg J. Prediction of adult overweight during the pediatric years. *Pediatr Res.* 1999;46:697–703

30. Ekelund U, Ong K, Linne Y, et al. Upward weight percentile crossing in infancy and early childhood independently predicts fat mass in young adults. The Stockholm Weight Development Study (SWEDES). *Am J Clin Nutr.* 2006;83(2):324–330

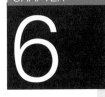

6 Toddler

6.1 Background

American babies born in the year 2000 have a 1 in 3 lifetime risk of developing diabetes[1]—a trend driven by escalating rates of obesity and inactivity. Prevention of obesity has never been more important, and the opportunity for prevention presents itself in the frequent contact these young children and their families have with their pediatricians.

Obesity is increasingly common in young children. The prevalence rates for children 2 to 5 years of age increased from 5% during the years 1971–1974 to 10.4% during 2007–2008.[2]

Early weight gain was found in 10.9% of children in a longitudinal study of childhood growth. Children with this weight gain pattern had obesity that persisted throughout childhood and were more likely to be African American, to be male, and to have higher birth weight. They were more likely to be born of mothers of older maternal age, mothers with a history of maternal overweight and obesity, and mothers with excess gestational weight gain. A late-onset pattern of weight gain observed in 5.2% of children was characterized by increasing rates of obesity after 8 years of age. Children with this pattern of weight gain had the same factors as the early-onset group with the exception of excess gestational weight gain and the inclusion of more firstborn children and more children whose mothers smoked cigarettes. Breastfeeding at 4 months of age was associated with a decreased risk of both early- and late-onset overweight.[3]

For good or ill, the toddler is a full participant in the family's nutritional environment. Food preferences develop early in childhood[4] and may predict eating preferences.[5] By 1 year of age children are eating an array of foods that usually reflects family preferences. A recent study of toddler diets found that the table foods to which they transitioned reflected the same problem areas seen in the diets of older children and adults, namely a high intake of sugar and fat.[6] For example, approximately 65% to 70% of 1- to 2-year-olds consumed dessert, ice cream, or candy once a day. From 30% to 50% of toddlers consumed sweetened beverages daily.[6] Sugared beverage consumption is higher in obese children than nonobese children.[7] Fruit and vegetable consumption did not fare much better; less than 10% of 1- to 2-year-olds consume a dark green vegetable a day,[6] with French fries and other potatoes accounting for the bulk of vegetable consumption.[6]

Because families have a tremendous influence on their children's food preferences, they should be encouraged to provide the appropriate amount of nutritious foods at meals and as snacks. Parental child feeding practices can also influence child excess weight gain. Three practices associated with excess weight gain include (1) feeding in response to emotional distress, (2) using food as a reward, and (3) prompting or encouraging excessively to eat.[8] Each of these practices provide the pediatrician with a good entry point for teaching prevention to a toddler's parents.

Sleep duration is also recognized as a potential modifier of childhood obesity. A study of preschool children found an increased rate of obesity in those who slept less than 11 hours per night, and the risk of obesity increased as sleep time decreased. Children who slept less than 9 hours a night had 1.5 times the risk of being obese compared with those who slept more than 11 hours a night.[9] A longitudinal study of more than 7,000 children 3 years of age found that sleep duration less than 10.5 hours a night at age 3 was associated with obesity at 7 years of age.[10] A meta-analysis of studies on the relationship of sleep and obesity found that for "each hour increase in sleep, the risk of overweight/obesity was reduced on average by 9% for children <10 years."[11]

Young children are not "automatically active." Studies show that 3- to 5-year-old children spend more than 30% of waking hours in sedentary activities.[12] Healthy routines are important; preschool children whose families routinely ate evening family meals together, limited screen time, and ensured adequate sleep had a 40% lower prevalence of obesity than preschoolers without these routines.[13]

6.2 Prevention: Talking to Parents (BALANCE)

Prevention touch points for parents include **belief, assessment, lifestyle, activity, nutrition, child,** and **environment** (BALANCE).

*B*elief

- Reviewing what constitutes a nutritionally adequate diet for a toddler is important because parents need to feel comfortable that they are providing adequate nutrition for their toddler in order to be willing to make changes in the child's diet.
- The maxim "Parents provide and the child decides" is important and can also be stated, "Your job (as a parent) is to provide optimal nutrition for your child. Your child's job is to decide how much of the correct portion to eat."
- Parents are the primary role models in developing good nutritional patterns for their child: "Good nutrition is a family affair."

*A*ssessment

- Growth charts are essential tools for helping families understand the trajectory of normal growth, and parents appreciate reviewing height, weight, and body mass index (BMI) charts with their child's pediatrician.
- The goal of keeping the child on the chart is one that can capture the purpose of discussing nutrition, activity, and lifestyle change.
- Normal growth trajectories are also valuable reassurance to parents whose child is a picky eater and reassure parents who are afraid the child is not getting enough to eat.

*L*ifestyle

- Children need structure, predictability, and limit setting from parents for eating and activity. This fosters a sense of security for the child.
- Parents should make sure that toddlers do not get their own food or snacks but that these are provided by parents and adult family members who can make healthy and appropriate choices.
- Parents may not realize that they carry over their own eating and activity patterns when interacting with their child and may need to reexamine their approach. For example:
  - Parents should exert control over meal timing, foods offered, and portion size but not the amount of food consumed by the child.
  - Parents should decide on the location and activity at meals, such as "no television while eating."

- Adequate sleep is part of a healthy lifestyle and parents may not realize the connection of sleep time to weight gain. Establishing a bedtime routine and keeping the child's bedroom television free can lay the groundwork for good sleep habits.

*A*ctivity

- It is important for parents to know what age-appropriate physical skills develop to provide safe and appropriate activity opportunities for their child.
- When planning family activities, parents should think about making them as active as possible.
- Strollers should be used sparingly.
- Television watching is not a health-promoting activity for children. The American Academy of Pediatrics currently recommends that children 2 years of age and younger not watch television.
- Children should not have televisions in their rooms or watch television during mealtime.
- For children older than 2 years of age, television watching (of educational, nonviolent programming) should be limited to no more than 1 to 2 hours a day.

*N*utrition

- Providing good food choices is important for parents; it may be helpful for them to think of the nutritional requirement of the toddler in terms of daily servings.[14]
  - Daily servings for toddlers (2–3 years old):
    - Fruit: 2 servings a day
    - Vegetables: 3 servings a day
    - Dairy: 4 to 5 servings a day
    - Protein: 2 servings a day
    - Grain products: 3 to 4 servings a day
- Serving size (portion) may be one of the most confusing aspects of nutrition for parents. Even preschool-aged children eat more when large portions of highly palatable foods are offered. Providing parents with some guidelines for age-appropriate portions may be helpful.
  - Serving sizes for 2- to 3-year-olds:
    - Fruit: Half to 1 small fruit, 2 to 4 tbsp canned fruit
    - Vegetables: 2 to 3 tbsp cooked vegetables
    - Dairy: ½ cup milk (whole milk for 2 years and younger) per serving or ½ cup yogurt
    - Protein: 1 to 2 oz meat, 1 egg per serving, or 4 to 5 tbsp cooked legumes
    - Grain products: Half to 1 slice of bread; ¼ to ½ cups rice or pasta; or ½ to 1 cup dry cereal, quarter to half bagel, half to 1 tortilla

Establishing family meals makes an important contribution to a healthy lifestyle and provides an opportunity for modeling healthy eating behavior.

Child

- A child's behavior can often drive food consumption. It is important for parents to understand and have support in changing these dynamics.
  - Picky eaters
    - Parents are often concerned about picky eaters. Providing reassurance about normal growth using the growth and BMI charts (or weight-for-height chart for children younger than 2 years) can help.
  - Food refusal
    - Children can gain control over their diets by refusing food.
    - Parents will often say the child does not like certain types of food and fall into a pattern of offering less nutritious alternative foods just because the child cries or whines, thereby allowing the child to direct the food selection.
    - In this situation parents should provide nutritious meals and appropriate snacks, let the child eat (or not eat) the amount of the food offered, and redirect the focus away from food.
  - Grazing
    - One to 2 planned snacks a day should be part of a toddler's diet, but grazing should be avoided.
    - Parents' recognition of this pattern often is enough to promote change, along with the reassurance that the child can get adequate nutrition from the 3 meals and 2 snacks the parents provide.
  - Food rewards
    - Families may not even realize that they are rewarding a child's behavior with food and may appreciate discussing alternative ways to give their child positive feedback.

Environment

- A safe and appropriate nutritional and activity environment is important.
  - How to prevent choking should be part of nutritional counseling.
  - Remind parents that children do not fully develop the grinding motion involved in chewing until they are about 4 years old.
  - Remind parents and family members to make sure to sit with their child when they are eating to prevent choking.

- Parents can view providing a "safe" nutritional environment as they do childproofing the house for safety. If junk foods are not purchased, parents will not need to worry about limiting or refusing to serve them. It is easier to promote eating healthy food if it is all that's available in the home.

6.3 Intervention

When a toddler has a BMI greater than 85% but less than 95% or is crossing growth percentiles in an upward direction, this is the time for a more in-depth look at eating and activity, family health history, and parental obesity—all of which can contribute to the risk of becoming an older child and young adult with obesity. In addition to reemphasizing concepts covered previously, parents and families may need to give increased attention to their ability to provide and influence nutrition and activity by focusing on *energy balance, structure,* and *modeling healthy behavior* (discussed next).

Energy Balance

Balancing energy intake for age and growth. Here is where many parents may need to be reminded of appropriate portion sizes for their toddler (see Nutrition in section 6.2) and that balancing food groups and providing the variety of recommended food group servings provides balanced vitamin, mineral, fat, protein, and carbohydrate intake for growth and activity.

Balancing activity and inactivity. This means limiting television time, encouraging supervised playtime, and changing family activities from sedentary to active.

Diet and activity records from parents, child care providers, and other family members can contain valuable information and serve as a tool for monitoring desired changes in eating and activity.

Structure

Planning meals and mealtime, organizing snacks and limiting grazing, and eating meals together are all important factors in moving toward a healthier lifestyle. Parents need to find out what the child's day is really like (What is the child eating at child care? Is the child going outdoors in nursery school? Is he watching television at Grandmother's house?). Taking time to organize meals and activities is one of the most important factors in maintaining a healthy lifestyle.

Modeling Healthy Behavior

Parents are the models for their children. Having parents reflect on their own eating and activity style as well as their hopes for their child and helping them recognize that they are the major influences on their toddler will help motivate them toward any changes that need to be made in the family's lifestyle. Parents also will need to reflect on their own parenting style and ability to help their family and child make necessary changes.

6.4 Treatment

It is time to initiate a focused treatment strategy when a child's BMI is greater than 95%, because you are usually dealing with excess adiposity or body fatness. It is important to review the issues discussed in the preceding 2 sections because these are the building blocks of good nutrition and activity habits. But you will also have to focus on the barriers to change that may have prevented parents and families from implementing these strategies.

Obtaining a family history focused on obesity-related comorbidities can serve to emphasize the health risks involved and the necessity of taking early action once obesity is identified.

6.5 Family History

The family history (Table 6.1) provides information on obesity and obesity-related comorbidity risk and serves as a starting point to discuss a child's BMI.

If parents are obese or have a history of obesity, they may want to relate their personal weight struggles. The desire to avoid these same struggles in their child often motivates parents to make family changes in nutrition and activity.

6.6 Review of Systems

The review of systems can also serve as a point of departure to discuss obesity-related comorbidities, pointing out particular risk factors as they relate to increasing BMI.

- Skin: Acanthosis nigricans, intertriginous dermatitis
- Head, eyes, ears, nose, and throat (HEENT): Headache, snoring, sleep disturbance
- Lungs: Asthma, shortness of breath during activity, cough at end of activity, decreased ability to keep up with other children at play
- Cardiac: History of congenital heart disease
- Abdomen: Gastroesophageal reflux, stomach pain before or after eating, chronic diarrhea or constipation, rapid eating
- Musculoskeletal: Limping, hip pain, knee pain
- Development: Delay, hypotonia, coordination difficulties, social interaction, poor height growth

Table 6.1. Family History, Toddler

Complete the family history targeted toward obesity and related comorbidities.

	Mother	Father	Maternal Grandmother	Maternal Grandfather	Paternal Grandmother	Paternal Grandfather	Sibling 1	Sibling 2
Obesity	☐	☐	☐	☐	☐	☐	☐	☐
Cardiovascular disease	☐	☐	☐	☐	☐	☐	☐	☐
High blood pressure	☐	☐	☐	☐	☐	☐	☐	☐
Stroke	☐	☐	☐	☐	☐	☐	☐	☐
High cholesterol	☐	☐	☐	☐	☐	☐	☐	☐
High triglyceride level	☐	☐	☐	☐	☐	☐	☐	☐
Type 1 or 2 diabetes	☐	☐	☐	☐	☐	☐	☐	☐
Liver disease (nonalcoholic steatohepatitis)	☐	☐	☐	☐	☐	☐	☐	☐
Bariatric surgery	☐	☐	☐	☐	☐	☐	☐	☐
Polycystic ovarian syndrome	☐	☐	☐	☐	☐	☐	☐	☐
Binge eating disorder	☐	☐	☐	☐	☐	☐	☐	☐
	☐	☐	☐	☐	☐	☐	☐	☐
	☐	☐	☐	☐	☐	☐	☐	☐

6.7 Physical Examination

- Height
- Weight
- BMI

Note: For children younger than 2 years of age, length should be measured and plotted on World Health Organization (WHO) weight-for-length percentiles charts (see Appendix A.2). For children 2 years of age and older, BMI should be plotted on the Centers for Disease Control and Prevention (CDC) BMI-for-age charts (see Appendix A.2).

- General: Dysmorphic features, poor linear growth, developmental delay
- Skin: Dermatitis in skinfolds, acanthosis nigricans
- HEENT: Funduscopic examination for papilledema, tonsillar hypertrophy
- Cardiopulmonary: Wheezing, poor ventilation, heart murmur
- Abdominal: Hepatomegaly
- Musculoskeletal: Range of motion, genu varum, limp, hip or knee pain
- Genitourinary: Undescended testicles, hidden penis

6.8 Family Constellation and Social History

Information about the family can provide a starting point for discussing how nutrition and activity decisions are made and how changes might take place.

- Who is living at home with the child?
- Who else feeds and cares for the child?
- Who decides what the child will eat?
- Who is in charge of the child's daily schedule?

6.9 Parenting Questions

Parenting styles and skills are important when families are trying to make changes in lifestyle. The questions in Table 6.2 may help you focus on family factors that may facilitate or hinder change.

6.10 Parenting Touch Points

Parenting touch points focus on helping families initiate and maintain change by helping them believe change can occur, identify the change needed, value the outcome of the change, know how to change, and have the energy to change and sustain the change.

- *Believe that change can occur.* Parents need to believe that change is possible. Setting realistic goals is important. For example, in the toddler age group, weight stability to allow the height to catch up is a realistic and healthy goal. Goals can be behavioral, keying on the attainment of a desired behavior change (ie, sitting at the table for meals and snacks), or incremental, starting with making diet records. It is important to demonstrate early on that realistic goals can be achieved.
- *Identify the change.* Parents need to have the necessary information to understand what change needs to occur.
- *This is often the area in which pediatricians feel most comfortable.* However, it is important to offer the family an array of possible changes and discuss what might be possible in their situation rather than simply telling them what to do.
  - For example, a toddler may be drinking too much juice, grazing, and getting snacks by refusing food at mealtimes. Parents may be ready to make a change and decide to first address juice drinking because changing grazing and food refusal requires also speaking to grandparents. It is best to start where the family is and continue to work over time on other changes that need to be made.
- *Value the outcome.* Parents need to believe that a healthy weight and healthy lifestyle is important for their child. Each parent and family is unique in their perspective about obesity. Reasons for managing a toddler's weight and lifestyle may range from "Doesn't look like his friends" to "Is hungry all the time" to "I don't want her to suffer like I did as an overweight child." It is important that parents be able to identify what they value and why, because this provides energy and motivation for change.

Table 6.2. Parenting Questions, Toddler	Never	Seldom	Sometimes	Often	Always
Parents agree on how to feed the child.	☐	☐	☐	☐	☐
Child and parents fight about food.	☐	☐	☐	☐	☐
Parents set clear and simple expectations and limits.	☐	☐	☐	☐	☐
Parents understand the child's developmental stage.	☐	☐	☐	☐	☐
Parents set boundaries and give child choice within them.	☐	☐	☐	☐	☐

■ *Know how to change.* Parents often need help devising concrete steps to make the desired change. This is a key step in the process of helping families change nutrition and activity patterns. Your knowledge of the family's circumstances, parenting attitudes and skills, and the child can all come into play as you help families implement the desired change. For example, in one family, eliminating sugared beverages may simply require a decision on the part of the parent to not buy them and the rest of the family will go along. In another family, a parent may believe that the thinner sibling "needs" juice and the decision to limit juice may require more extensive discussion about good family nutrition and parenting children with different body types.

■ *Have the energy to change and sustain.* Parents need resources and support to make the initial change, as well as to sustain the change. Maintaining any behavioral change is difficult. Engaging family support, making small incremental changes, and allowing the family to adjust to and feel good about the changes is important. Difficult behavior can also get in the way of sustaining change. For example, a 2-year-old throwing a tantrum can make even the most committed parent relent if a strategy is not in place.

6.11 Developmental Touch Point

At this stage of development children need confirmation of trust to know that a parent is nearby while they explore the world. Children are ambivalent, testing limits of authority. Food selection and inactivity (ie, television watching) may be a battleground for self-control. At this stage the child has an egocentric view of the world.

6.12 Nutrition and Activity Questions and Approaches

Parents can answer the nutrition and activity questions in Table 6.3, which can provide a focal point for targeted intervention (Table 6.4) in a brief encounter. Questions answered "Often" or "Always" can be targeted first for change.

These questions and the answers may provide targeted starting points that the parents feel they can tackle. For example, if the parents answered "Often" drinks juice or sugared beverages for question 17, and then answered that they thought they could change juice to water "Most of the time," this would be a good starting point for change. Even if the family believes that a change is doable, it is a good idea to explore with them exactly how they will make the change, what might make the desired change easier to implement, and what would make it more difficult. For example, if the mother thinks she would like to eliminate juice, she might also say that getting the grandmother to do this when the child is visiting might be difficult or that the child's older brother would object. Given this information, you can help her troubleshoot a solution.

In general, you should aim for weight stability with continued height growth in a toddler unless there is a medical morbidity, which has to be resolved quickly. Frequent visits to facilitate change are important, as is monitoring for nutritional adequacy and developmentally appropriate activity.

6.13 A Case in Point: LQ

LQ comes to your office at 2 years and 9 months of age for an upper respiratory infection. You note her height is 37″ (94 cm) (90% for age) and her weight is 58 lb (26.4 kg) (>95% for age). You calculate her BMI at 30, which is well above 95% for her age. You look in her chart and note that she gained 15 lb (6.8 kg) in the past 6 months. When you mention this to her parents, they say, "We're not concerned about her weight." They explain that her father's family was large and that he was chunky until 5 years of age. They also explain that LQ is very active, even in the house.

You ask about family history, and they note that a paternal grandfather had bypass surgery and a maternal grandmother and a maternal aunt have diabetes. At this point LQ's parents say that they have been concerned about the family history of diabetes. The mother is especially worried and says LQ looks "just like her aunt did as a child."

Your physical examination is unremarkable except for tibial torsion.

At the end of the examination, you review LQ's BMI chart and point out that her BMI places her at an increased risk for health problems, including diabetes. You ask her parents if they would like to discuss some ways to help keep LQ healthy, to which they agree. You ask them to fill out the first set of questions in Table 6.3, and they answer "Often" or "Always" to

1. Demand certain food or snacks.
   Mom thinks Dad is more likely to give in to LQ's demands but "could try," and Mom thinks that she could distract her "most of the time" when she demanded food.
2. Eat more than 2 snacks between meals a day.
   Parents think they could set times for meals and 2 snacks most of the time.
3. Drink juice or sugared beverages between meals.
   They think they could change juice to water most of the time.

4. Eat meals by themselves.
   Because Mom works at night, Dad says he will eat his dinner with LQ.
5. Eat as much as an older sibling or adult.
   They think it would be difficult to limit portions.

You ask them to try to change her juice to water and wean her from the bottle to a cup at night. You go over a schedule of meals and snacks, and Dad agrees to eat dinner with her.

You briefly discuss limiting portions as something to try and report back on.

In addition, you order laboratory work, which shows elevated cholesterol level of 194 mg/dL with normal triglyceride, glucose, insulin, and thyroid levels and normal liver function studies.

You ask the family to return in 3 weeks.

Table 6.3. Nutrition and Activity Questions, Toddler

These questions can be answered by the parents and provide a focal point for targeted intervention in a brief encounter. First have the parents answer these questions about the presence or absence of behaviors that promote weight gain; then refer to Table 6.4.

Please answer the following for the statements below: Does your toddler…?

	Never	Seldom	Sometimes	Often	Always
1. Have trouble getting a scheduled playtime each day.	☐	☐	☐	☐	☐
2. Play mostly indoors.	☐	☐	☐	☐	☐
3. Ride in a stroller.	☐	☐	☐	☐	☐
4. Sleep less than 11 hours a night.	☐	☐	☐	☐	☐
5. Watch television or play with computer/video games in his or her bedroom.	☐	☐	☐	☐	☐
6. Spend more than 2 hours watching television, playing video games, or using a computer each day.	☐	☐	☐	☐	☐
7. Ask for foods from commercials shown during his or her favorite cartoon or television show.	☐	☐	☐	☐	☐
8. Demand certain food or snacks.	☐	☐	☐	☐	☐
9. Eat in front of the television.	☐	☐	☐	☐	☐
10. Have unscheduled meals and snacks throughout the day.	☐	☐	☐	☐	☐
11. Skip meals.	☐	☐	☐	☐	☐
12. Eat more than 2 snacks between meals a day.	☐	☐	☐	☐	☐
13. Refuse to eat vegetables.	☐	☐	☐	☐	☐
14. Refuse to eat fruit.	☐	☐	☐	☐	☐
15. Refuse to eat dairy foods (yogurt, cheese, milk).	☐	☐	☐	☐	☐
16. Receive snacks from adults other than you (caregiver, child care, family member).	☐	☐	☐	☐	☐
17. Drink juice or sugared beverages between meals.	☐	☐	☐	☐	☐
18. Eat meals by themselves.	☐	☐	☐	☐	☐
19. Eat very fast.	☐	☐	☐	☐	☐
20. Eat as much as an older sibling or adult.	☐	☐	☐	☐	☐
21. Eat at fast-food restaurants.	☐	☐	☐	☐	☐
22. Eat in the car.	☐	☐	☐	☐	☐
23. Receive food as a reward or treat for good behavior.	☐	☐	☐	☐	☐

Table 6.4. Nutrition and Activity Approaches, Toddler

Questions answered "Often" or "Always" in Table 6.3 can be targeted first for change. Using these specific questions, ask the parent, "How willing are you to...?"

Please answer the following for the statements below: How willing are you to...?

	Impossible	Could Try	Could Do Sometimes	Could Do Often	Easy
1. Schedule time for active play with your child each day.	☐	☐	☐	☐	☐
2. Schedule time for supervised outdoor play.	☐	☐	☐	☐	☐
3. Encourage your child to walk rather than use the stroller.	☐	☐	☐	☐	☐
4. Plan bedtime to ensure 10–11 hours of sleep.	☐	☐	☐	☐	☐
5. Move television, computers, and video games out of your child's bedroom.	☐	☐	☐	☐	☐
6. Reduce time spent watching television, playing video games, or using the computer.	☐	☐	☐	☐	☐
7. Turn off the television during meals and snacks.	☐	☐	☐	☐	☐
8. Schedule regular meals and snacks.	☐	☐	☐	☐	☐
9. Reduce or eliminate extra snacks.	☐	☐	☐	☐	☐
10. Offer vegetables at meals or as snacks.	☐	☐	☐	☐	☐
11. Offer fruit at meals or as snacks.	☐	☐	☐	☐	☐
12. Offer dairy products at meals or as snacks.	☐	☐	☐	☐	☐
13. Learn what other people are feeding your child.	☐	☐	☐	☐	☐
14. Provide healthy snacks for your child to take to child care.	☐	☐	☐	☐	☐
15. Change from juice to water between meals.	☐	☐	☐	☐	☐
16. Eat meals together.	☐	☐	☐	☐	☐
17. Create a plan to slow down eating.	☐	☐	☐	☐	☐
18. Learn to serve appropriate portion sizes for your child.	☐	☐	☐	☐	☐
19. Limit how often you buy/serve fast food.	☐	☐	☐	☐	☐
20. Stop eating in the car.	☐	☐	☐	☐	☐
21. Reward your child with things other than food to encourage good behavior.	☐	☐	☐	☐	☐

Second Visit

LQ's weight upon return is 57 lb (26.0 kg), a decrease of 1 lb (0.4 kg). The parents report that they followed the previous instructions exactly. She is now drinking water between meals, her father is no longer giving her junk food for dinner, and mealtimes are now regular. You reinforce the changes and ask them to come back in 1 month.

Third Visit

Now LQ's weight has gone up to 60 lb (27.0 kg). Mom notes that Dad has changed his work schedule and is taking her outside less. Mom is also in the last part of her pregnancy and is less active with LQ. Review of the diet records you asked them to keep shows a slight increase in her portions. You raise the issue of activity. Mom says that there are no particular playgroups or outlets for LQ in their area. Dad said he would look into building a fenced-in area of the yard so that she can play outdoors. When she goes out now with Mom, she bolts and runs away, so outdoor safety is a priority.

Fourth Visit

You wanted to see LQ in 1 month, but because of the new baby, she comes back 3 months later. Her weight is still 60 lb (27.0 kg) and she has grown to 40″ (100.4 cm), lowering her BMI from 30 to 26.78. Dietary review notes that she is eating 3 meals and 2 snacks per day.

Fifth Visit

Two months later you see LQ again. Her weight is 55 lb (25.1 kg). Mom attributes this to increased activity ("She is running all the time"). Both parents are still structuring her meals and snacks; the quality of her diet is improved, with no junk or snack food. You repeat her cholesterol screening, and it is still elevated at 204 mg/dL. You give them specific dietary advice on lowering cholesterol.

Sixth Visit

LQ returns to your office 4 months later in midsummer with a weight of 50 lb (22.5 kg). Her height is 40″ (101.4 cm), and her BMI is 21.9. Her parents have maintained her dietary changes.

References

1. Narayan KM, Boyle JP, Thompson TJ, Sorensen SW, Williamson DF. Lifetime risk for diabetes mellitus in the United States. *JAMA.* 2003;290:1884–1890

2. Ogden C, Carroll M. Prevalence of obesity among children and adolescents: United States, trends 1963-1965 through 2007. http://www.cdc.gov/nchs/data/hestat/obesity_child_07_08/obesity_child_07_08.htm#table1

3. Li C, Goran M, Kaur H, Nollen N, Ahluwalia J. Developmental trajectories of overweight during childhood: role of early-life factors. *Obesity.* 2007;15:760–771

4. Birch LL. Development of food acceptance patterns in the first years of life. *Proc Nutr Soc.* 1998;57:617–624

5. Skinner JD, Carruth BR, Wendy B, Ziegler PJ. Children's food preferences: a longitudinal analysis. *J Am Diet Assoc.* 2002;102:1638–1647

6. Ludwig DS, Peterson KE, Gortmaker SL. Relation between consumption of sugar-sweetened drinks and childhood obesity: a prospective, observational analysis. *Lancet.* 2001;357:505–508

7. Fox MK, Pac S, Devaney B, Jankowski L. Feeding infants and toddlers study: what foods are infants and toddlers eating? *J Am Diet Assoc.* 2004;104(1 suppl 1):S22–S30

8. Wardle J, Sanderson S, Guthrie CA, Rapoport L, Plomin R. Parental feeding style and the intergenerational transmission of obesity risk. *Obes Res.* 2002;10:453–462

9. Sekine M, Yamagami T, Hamanishi S, et al. Parental obesity, lifestyle factors and obesity in preschool children: results of the Toyama Birth Cohort Study. *J Epidemiol.* 2002;12:33–39

10. Reilly JJ, Armstrong J, Dorosty AR, et al. Early life risk factors for obesity in childhood: cohort study. *BMJ.* 2005;330:1357

11. Chen X, Beydoun MA, Wang Y. Is sleep duration associated with childhood obesity? A systematic review and meta-analysis. *Obesity.* 2008;16:265–274

12. Montgomery C, Reilly JJ, Jackson DM, et al. Relationship between physical activity and energy expenditure in a representative sample of young children. *Am J Clin Nutr.* 2004;80:591–596

13. Anderson SE, Whitaker RC. Household routines and obesity in US preschool-aged children. *Pediatrics.* 2010;125:420–428

14. American Academy of Pediatrics. Kleinman RE, ed. *Pediatric Nutrition Handbook.* 5th ed. Elk Grove Village, IL: American Academy of Pediatrics; 2004

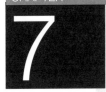

Preschool Age

7.1 Background

The preschool period is a time when children transition from a period of relatively slow weight gain to when many children accelerate their weight gain. Children who are overweight or obese at this age are at significant risk for becoming obese as adults. In one study, more than 50% of 3- to 6-year-olds with a body mass index (BMI) at or above 95% became obese adults.[1] The point when BMI reaches its nadir in early childhood is normally around 5 to 6 years of age (adiposity rebound).[2,3] Children who cross BMI percentiles younger than 4.8 years (early adiposity rebound) have a greater likelihood of becoming obese adults.[2,3]

Data from low-income preschool-age children participating in federally funded health and nutrition programs found that obesity increased from 12.4% in 1998 to 14.5% in 2003 and remained stable with a 14.6% prevalence in 2008. The prevalence was highest among Native American children (21.2%), followed by Hispanic children (18.5%), non-Hispanic white children (12.6%), Asian/Pacific Islander children (12.3%), and non-Hispanic black children (11.8%).[4]

Parental obesity continues to be a major influence on overweight and obesity in this age group; parents also exercise a tremendous influence over their preschooler's nutrition and activity environment. In a large nationally representative sample of 4-year-olds, 3 household routines were associated with a reduction in the risk of obesity: (1) eating the evening meal (dinner) as a family 6 to 7 times per week, (2) obtaining more than 10.5 hours of nighttime sleep, and (3) limiting screen viewing time (television/video/DVD) to 2 hours or less per day. Of the sample, 14.5% were exposed to all 3 routines and 12.4% had none of these routines. In children with all 3 routines, the prevalence of obesity was 14.3%, compared with 24.5% in children with none of the routines.[5]

Increased sweetened beverage consumption is a significant risk factor for obesity.[6] For children 2 to 3 years of age between 85% and 95%, as little as 1 additional sweetened drink a day (eg, juice, soda, fruit drink) doubled their risk of having a BMI greater than 95% in the following year.[6]

Accelerated weight gain in preschool children is associated with higher baseline fat intake[7] and inappropriately large portion sizes[8] that can negatively affect daily energy balance. A low level of physical activity in preschoolers is reported to be associated with an increased amount of subcutaneous fat in children by 1st grade.[9] The same study showed that preschool children with active parents were more likely to be active than those with sedentary parents.[9] The increase in stroller use and highly structured activity may also be limiting physical activity in this age group.

Time spent outdoors strongly correlates with physical activity in young children.[10] Time for free play dropped by 25% between the years 1981 and 1997. Free play in the preschool age group is composed of brief bouts of varied activity interspersed with frequent rest periods.[11] In a study of 1- to 5-year-old low-income children, 40% had a television in their room.[12] Time spent watching television has a direct positive relationship to overweight and obesity.[12] Children as young as 3 years of age watched an average of 1.7 hours per day, and each 1-hour increase in television viewing was associated with an increased intake of sugar-sweetened beverages, fast food, red and processed meat, total energy intake, and energy percent from trans-fats. Increased television time was also associated with lower intake of fruits and vegetables, calcium, and fiber.[13]

Type of early childhood care can also influence BMI status. A toddler cared for in someone else's home is more likely to have a higher BMI than a child cared for in a center or in his or her own home by a nonparent.[14]

Child temperament and behavior are also associated with a risk for overweight. In one study, young children with persistent tantrums over food and a highly emotional temperament were reported to be at increased risk for overweight.[15] Parenting skills that help deal with children's anger, temper tantrums, and emotions around boundary settings are crucial if they are to guide their preschoolers through challenges to healthy eating and activity.

It cannot be assumed that children with obesity are well nourished. Data from NHANES IV showed that iron deficiency was present in 20% of toddlers with obesity, 8% of toddlers who were overweight, and 7% of toddlers of normal weight; in a multivariable analysis, children with obesity and children who are not in child care had a greater risk of iron deficiency.[16]

High-risk nutritional behaviors for obesity can also pose a risk for dental caries; these behaviors include meal fragmentation, missed breakfast, low fruit consumption, and high carbohydrate intake.[17]

Parents of a preschool-age child are challenged to achieve consistency between spouses, family members, and caregivers in the nutritional choices offered to their child. Recognizing the importance of appropriate portion sizes, limiting sweetened beverages, and encouraging outdoor play need to become common themes among the adults who care for the overweight or obese child. Communication about the child's daily activities and eating is essential as the preschooler moves into environments outside the home. Small exceptions in portion sizes, treats, and snacks can add up to weight gain over time—as little as 150 kcal extra intake per day can become a 15-lb (6.8-kg) weight gain over the next year.

Because food and activity choices often become emotional for parents and children, it is important to have parents set the initial boundaries, such as what kinds of food will be in the house, how much television time the family will have, and what kind of activities are available to the child. Within these boundaries parents should provide the child with choices, such as a variety of possible healthy snacks and options for activities during outside play. This not only prevents every decision from becoming a battle but also encourages healthy decision making and avoids overrestriction.

7.2 Prevention: Talking to Parents (BALANCE)

Prevention touch points for parents include **belief, assessment, lifestyle, activity, nutrition, child,** and **environment** (BALANCE).

*B*elief

- Because preschool children are becoming more independent, parents and families may believe that they can make good food and activity decisions independently as well.
- At this point it is important to remind parents that they still need to be in charge of the nutrition and activity environment, allowing children to choose food and activities within the boundaries that they set.

*A*ssessment

- As eating patterns, eating venues, and caregivers change, it is important to review growth charts with parents and families. This helps them remain in charge of the child's daily activities and nutrition with the goal of staying on the chart.
- Parents may want to periodically assess diet and activity among all those who care for their child (grandparents, child care providers, preschool staff, friends) to "stay on top of" their child's daily routine.

*L*ifestyle

- Busy families frequently eat out, often leaving the decision about what to eat up to the preschool child. Remind parents it is important to limit eating out and to maintain oversight of their child's food choices when they do so.
- Parents are important role models for physical activity and inactivity and need to take stock of their own behavior to set healthy patterns for their child.

*A*ctivity

- During a child's preschool years, parents should encourage free play as much as possible to help develop motor skills.
- Outdoor time is the best way to encourage free play. Parents need to be reminded to avoid micromanaging their child's play. However, providing appropriate supervision is their job.
- It is appropriate for parents to provide their child with age-appropriate play equipment (ie, balls and plastic bats) to make exercise fun, but they should let the child choose exactly what to play with at any given time.
- The television should be off when the family is eating. This not only encourages conversation but also allows parents to model good eating behavior.
- If the child has a television in the bedroom, recommend that it be removed.
- The American Academy of Pediatrics advises a daily limit not to exceed 1 to 2 hours of television viewing; this includes time spent playing computer and video games.

*N*utrition

- Younger children should be served smaller portions than older siblings and parents.
- Parents and families still need to be reminded of the appropriate portion size and number of servings appropriate for the preschooler. Sometimes referring to a sample menu can help them calibrate the right amount of food to offer their child (Table 7.1).

- Sugar-sweetened beverages and juice creep in again at child care centers, preschools, and the homes of relatives and friends, and parents may want to provide milk or water or the occasional diet beverage as alternatives.

Child

- Parents need to understand that children as young as preschool age are a major target of food advertising.
- Parents may relent to requests for energy-dense or highly sugared foods when food shopping or eating out with their child.
- Dealing with a child's complaints of hunger between meals and snacks is often difficult for parents.
- Information about what constitutes an adequate diet and reassurance about other drivers for hunger such as visual cues, boredom, situational cues, and television advertising can help parents respond appropriately.
- Parents should observe the food advertising their child is exposed to with a critical eye and discuss with their child the untruths and exaggerations that are often present.

Environment

- Maintaining a structured eating environment is important. Predictable times for meals and snacks help children manage hunger and families deliver good nutrition instead of relying on filling in the gaps with snack food.
- Many parents assume that child care providers, preschool staff, and other caregivers are providing good nutrition and activity options for their child. It is important that families ask about these options and provide healthy alternatives as needed.

7.3 Intervention

When a preschool-age child has a BMI greater than 85% but less than 95% or is crossing growth percentiles in an upward direction, this is the time for a more in-depth look at eating and activity, family health history, and parental obesity—all of which can contribute to the risk of becoming an obese older child and young adult. In addition to reemphasizing concepts covered previously, parents and families may need to give increased attention to their ability to provide and influence nutrition and activity by focusing on *energy balance, structure,* and *modeling healthy behavior* (discussed next).

Energy Balance

Many factors can alter energy balance by disrupting nutrition or activity and begin an upward trend in a child's weight gain. Many of these have to do with increased family or child stress, including

- Parental divorce or separation
- Illness or death of a close family member
- Family move
- Birth of a sibling
- Physical illness or injury in the child
- Parental depression

If the causes of altered energy balance can be understood, many times a more effective intervention can be designed.

Table 7.1. Sample Menu and Serving Sizes for a 4-Year-Old Who Weighs About 36 lb (16.3 kg)	
Breakfast	– One-half cup of 1% milk – One-half cup of cereal – Four to 6 oz of 100% citrus or tomato juice or ½ cup of cantaloupe or strawberries
Snack	– One-half cup of 1% milk – One-half cup of banana – One slice of whole wheat bread – One teaspoon of margarine (or butter) – One teaspoon of jelly
Lunch	– One-half cup of 1% milk – One sandwich—2 slices of whole wheat bread, 1 teaspoon of mayonnaise or 2 teaspoons of salad dressing, and 1 oz of meat or cheese – One-fourth cup of dark-yellow or dark-green vegetables
Snack	– One teaspoon of peanut butter or 1 slice of low-fat cheese – One slice of whole wheat bread or 5 crackers
Dinner	– One-half cup of 1% milk – Two oz (slightly less than a deck of cards) or about ¼ cup of meat, fish, or chicken – One-half cup of pasta, rice, or potato – One-half cup of vegetables – One teaspoon of margarine (or butter) or 2 teaspoons of salad dressing

From American Academy of Pediatrics. The preschool years. In: Hassink SG, ed. *A Parent's Guide to Childhood Obesity: A Road Map to Health.* Elk Grove Village, IL: American Academy of Pediatrics; 2006:179

Parents of preschoolers can gradually reduce the energy imbalance by

- Switching from whole milk to skim, 1%, or 2% milk
- Selecting grilled or broiled fish or lean meats
- Serving cheese only in modest portions
- Serving whole fruit to meet recommended fruit intake
- Limiting fruit juice consumption to no more than 4 to 6 oz per day (from 1 to 6 years of age)—this should be 100% juice, not juice drinks
- Relying on low-fat snack choices, such as pretzels, fresh fruit, and fat-free yogurt
- Using cooking methods that do not require the use of fat during cooking, such as steaming, broiling, and roasting, or using only a small amount of olive oil or nonstick spray

Structure

Structured meals, snacks, and time for activity become more important as the family's time together decreases. Parents need to become acutely aware of what their preschooler is eating and what kind of activity is taking place at the child care center, preschool, or homes of extended family. A change in scheduling or the environment (eg, switch of child care provider, grandparents watching the child over vacation) can affect weight gain. It is equally important to review scheduling of television, computer, and outdoor time so that these activities become part of the family's health plan.

Modeling Healthy Behavior

Parents will need to work together and with other family members to help their preschooler. At this point a family meeting may be helpful to get all family members on the same page. At this meeting, it can be helpful to review growth rate, family history, age-appropriate activity, eating, and access to food. The family can also discuss ways to ensure other family members are on board with the strategy of offering healthy food choices to the child.

7.4 Treatment

When a child's BMI is greater than 95% and you are dealing with excess adiposity, it is time to initiate a focused treatment strategy. It is important to review the issues discussed in the previous 2 sections because these are the building blocks of good nutrition and activity habits. You will also have to focus on the barriers to change that may have prevented parents and families from implementing these strategies.

A useful way to begin is to obtain a family history focused on obesity-related comorbidities. This can serve to emphasize the health risks involved and the necessity of taking early action once obesity is identified.

7.5 Family History

The family history (Table 7.2) provides information on obesity and obesity-related comorbidity risk, as well as serves as a starting point to discuss the child's BMI.

Table 7.2. Family History, Preschool Age

Complete or update this family history targeted toward obesity and related comorbidities.

	Mother	Father	Maternal Grandmother	Maternal Grandfather	Paternal Grandmother	Paternal Grandfather	Sibling 1	Sibling 2
Obesity	☐	☐	☐	☐	☐	☐	☐	☐
Cardiovascular disease	☐	☐	☐	☐	☐	☐	☐	☐
High blood pressure	☐	☐	☐	☐	☐	☐	☐	☐
Stroke	☐	☐	☐	☐	☐	☐	☐	☐
High cholesterol	☐	☐	☐	☐	☐	☐	☐	☐
High triglyceride level	☐	☐	☐	☐	☐	☐	☐	☐
Type 1 or 2 diabetes	☐	☐	☐	☐	☐	☐	☐	☐
Liver disease	☐	☐	☐	☐	☐	☐	☐	☐
Bariatric surgery	☐	☐	☐	☐	☐	☐	☐	☐
Polycystic ovarian syndrome	☐	☐	☐	☐	☐	☐	☐	☐
Binge eating disorder	☐	☐	☐	☐	☐	☐	☐	☐
	☐	☐	☐	☐	☐	☐	☐	☐
	☐	☐	☐	☐	☐	☐	☐	☐

If parents are obese or have a history of obesity, they may want to relate their personal struggles with their weight. Often the desire to avoid these same struggles in their child motivates parents to make family changes in nutrition and activity.

7.6 Review of Systems

The review of systems can also serve as a point of departure to discuss obesity-related comorbidities, pointing out particular risk factors as they relate to increasing BMI.

- Skin: Acanthosis nigricans, striae, cervical fat pad, skin picking
- Head, eyes, ears, nose, and throat (HEENT): Headache, blurred vision
- Lungs: Snoring, sleep disturbance, sleep apnea, restless sleep, sleep position, daytime tiredness, napping, asthma, shortness of breath or subjective chest tightness during exercise, cough after exercise
- Cardiac: Murmur
- Abdomen: Gastroesophageal reflux, stomach pain, nausea or vomiting after eating
- Musculoskeletal: Limping, hip pain, knee pain, bowing
- Development: School problems, learning difficulties, attention problems
- Psychosocial: Depression, anxiety, behavior problems

7.7 Physical Examination

- Height
- Weight
- BMI + previous BMI measurements
- BMI %
- Blood pressure
- General: Dysmorphic features, poor linear growth, developmental delay
- Skin: Skin picking, acanthosis nigricans, dermatitis in skinfolds, striae, cervical fat pad
- HEENT: Funduscopic examination for papilledema, tonsillar hypertrophy
- Cardiopulmonary: Murmur, wheezing
- Abdominal: Hepatomegaly

- Musculoskeletal: Range of motion, genu varum, limp, hip or knee pain
- Genitourinary: Tanner stage

7.8 Family Constellation and Social History

Information about the family can provide a starting point for discussing how nutrition and activity decisions are made and how changes might take place.

- Who is living at home with the child?
- Who is with the child before school?
- Who is with the child after school?
- Who else besides the parents is responsible for the child's meals or snacks?

7.9 Parenting Questions

Parenting styles and skills are important when families are trying to make changes in lifestyle. The questions in Table 7.3 may help you focus on family factors that can facilitate or hamper change.

7.10 Parenting Touch Points

Parenting touch points focus on helping families initiate and maintain change by helping them believe change can occur, identify the change needed, value the outcome of the change, know how to change, and have the energy to change and sustain the change.

- ***Believe that change can occur.*** Parents need to believe that change is possible. Parents may start with the thought, "We are just a big family" or "My child isn't eating anything the other kids aren't eating." This is a good time to reinforce the individual factors that affect weight gain.
  - Family history
  - Parental obesity
  - Child's temperament
  - Family and cultural eating patterns

Parents may need to be encouraged to take charge of the nutrition and activity environment of their child and that this will make a difference if done consistently.

Table 7.3 Parenting Questions, Preschool Age	Never	Seldom	Sometimes	Often	Always
Parents set clear and simple expectations and limits.	☐	☐	☐	☐	☐
Parents set boundaries and give the child choice within them.	☐	☐	☐	☐	☐
Parents have developmentally appropriate goals for the child.	☐	☐	☐	☐	☐
Parents model healthy nutrition, activity, and inactivity behavior.	☐	☐	☐	☐	☐

■ *Identify the change.* Families may be concerned but not aware of what factors need to be changed. Asking families to go through their child's day often turns up unexpected problems, such as a child eating breakfast at home and again at preschool, not going outside at child care, or other caregivers rewarding the child with food. Families seeing this will often spontaneously change; other families will need help identifying possible changes from which to choose.

■ *Value the outcome.* At this point, parents may begin to worry about the child's constant hunger or the fact that he or she is being teased. Getting in touch with the family's worries and what they value (eg, good eating behavior, acceptance by other children, not fighting about food) is the first step toward helping them make necessary change. Each family will have a slightly different concern, and time spent articulating these concerns is well worth the effort.

■ *Know how to change.* Parents often need help devising concrete steps to make the desired change. Watchwords for parents of the preschooler are *consistency, appropriate choices, a calm approach to change,* and *patience.* Change is often best accomplished in small, measurable increments.

■ *Have the energy to change and sustain.* Parents need to have resources and support to make the initial change, as well as to sustain the change. Strong emotions are often at play, and parents need to be able to have a strategy to deal with anger and tantrums, whining, and pouting when the preschooler cannot get his or her way. Encouraging parents to discuss ways they will manage these situations and providing suggestions for time-outs, how to distract the child, and how to remain calm are all part of helping the family be able to implement the changes important to the child's health.

7.11 Developmental Touch Point

Children begin to develop impulse control, which leads to self-esteem. Social awareness of events outside the home and cultural norms leads to approval-seeking behavior. This is a good age to initiate time-outs to deal with inappropriate behavior.

7.12 Nutrition and Activity Questions and Approaches

Parents can answer the nutrition and activity questions in Table 7.4, which can provide a focal point for targeted intervention (Table 7.5) in a brief encounter. Questions answered "Often" or "Always" can be targeted first for change.

7.13 A Case in Point: OG

OG is a 5-year, 4-month-old boy who comes into your office because his mother is concerned about his constant hunger. She notes he is constantly bugging her for something to eat, even when he has just finished a meal. You look at his growth chart and note that he has gained 3 pounds in the past 6 weeks since he came in for an upper respiratory infection. His current height is 48″ (121.9 cm), and his weight is 65 lb (29.5 kg), giving him a BMI of 19.8 (>97% for age and gender). Mom also notes that she is worried about his weight because she and her husband have weight problems and she does not want OG to experience the same teasing they did as children.

Mom filled out the family history questionnaire in Table 7.2 in the waiting room, and you note that 3 of the 4 grandparents have hypertension, 2 are overweight, and 1 has type 2 diabetes. Dad has elevated blood pressure and sleep apnea and is overweight.

OG's review of systems reveals that he snores and is restless during sleep. His mom thinks he may have pauses in his breathing but is not sure. His physical examination shows a very active, overweight boy with no other abnormal physical findings except somewhat enlarged tonsils.

You review his family constellation and note that OG lives with his mother, father, older brother (10 years of age), and maternal grandparents. He attends half-day preschool, and his grandmother and grandfather look after him before and after school until his parents get home from work. His mom and grandmother share the cooking and shopping.

Mom answers "Always" or "Often" to spends more than 2 hours watching television, playing video games, or using a computer each day (question 6), becomes angry when demands for food are not met (question 11), complains constantly of being hungry (question 12), sneaks or hides food (question 13), and drinks juice or sugared beverages between meals (question 19).

On the second questionnaire she does not indicate that anything would be easy but notes that she could change from juice to water between meals most of the time, sometimes reduce television time, and use time-outs to help OG calm down.

Table 7.4. Nutrition and Activity Questions, Preschool Age

These questions can be answered by the parents and provide a focal point for targeted intervention in a brief encounter. First have the parents answer these questions about the presence or absence of behaviors that promote weight gain; then refer to Table 7.5.

Please answer the following for the statements below: Does your preschooler…?

	Never	Seldom	Sometimes	Often	Always
1. Have trouble getting a scheduled playtime each day.	☐	☐	☐	☐	☐
2. Prefer quiet activities.	☐	☐	☐	☐	☐
3. Prefer to ride in the stroller.	☐	☐	☐	☐	☐
4. Sleep less than 11 hours a night.	☐	☐	☐	☐	☐
5. Watch television or play with computer/video games in his or her bedroom.	☐	☐	☐	☐	☐
6. Spend more than 2 hours watching television, playing video games, or using a computer each day.	☐	☐	☐	☐	☐
7. Eat in front of the television.	☐	☐	☐	☐	☐
8. Have unscheduled meals and snacks throughout the day.	☐	☐	☐	☐	☐
9. Skip meals.	☐	☐	☐	☐	☐
10. Demand certain food or snacks.	☐	☐	☐	☐	☐
11. Become angry when demands for food are not met.	☐	☐	☐	☐	☐
12. Complain constantly about being hungry.	☐	☐	☐	☐	☐
13. Sneak or hide food.	☐	☐	☐	☐	☐
14. Refuse to eat vegetables.	☐	☐	☐	☐	☐
15. Refuse to eat fruit.	☐	☐	☐	☐	☐
16. Refuse to eat dairy foods (yogurt, milk, cheese).	☐	☐	☐	☐	☐
17. Eat more than 2 snacks between meals a day.	☐	☐	☐	☐	☐
18. Receive snacks from adults other than you (caregiver, child care provider, family member).	☐	☐	☐	☐	☐
19. Drink juice or sugared beverages between meals.	☐	☐	☐	☐	☐
20. Get his or her own snacks.	☐	☐	☐	☐	☐
21. Eat meals alone.	☐	☐	☐	☐	☐
22. Eat very fast.	☐	☐	☐	☐	☐
23. Eat as much as an older sibling or adult.	☐	☐	☐	☐	☐
24. Eat at fast-food restaurants.	☐	☐	☐	☐	☐
25. Eat in the car.	☐	☐	☐	☐	☐
26. Receive food as a reward or treat for good behavior.	☐	☐	☐	☐	☐

Problem #1: Obesity

You order laboratory studies to screen for obesity-related metabolic abnormalities and explain these to OG's mom.

Problem #2: Possible Sleep Apnea

Based on his obesity, enlarged tonsils, positive family history, snoring, restless sleep, and possible apnea, you arrange a sleep study.

Problem #3: Excess Consumption of Sweetened Beverages

From OG's diet history you estimate that he is drinking four to six 8-oz glasses of juice or soda a day.

- *Parenting dilemma: Changing family nutrition patterns*
  OG's mom agrees that she would like to get the juice and soda out of the house but is worried because her husband "needs his soda." She suggests she just ask Dad to hide it.

Table 7.5. Nutrition and Activity Approaches, Preschool Age

Questions answered "Often" or "Always" in Table 7.4 can be targeted first for change. Using these specific questions, ask the parent, "How willing are you to…?"

Please answer the following for the statements below: How willing are you to…?

	Impossible	Could Try	Could Do Sometimes	Could Do Often	Easy
1. Schedule time for active play with your child each day.	☐	☐	☐	☐	☐
2. Schedule time for your child to play outside.	☐	☐	☐	☐	☐
3. Encourage your child to walk rather than use the stroller.	☐	☐	☐	☐	☐
4. Plan bedtime to ensure 10–11 hours of sleep.	☐	☐	☐	☐	☐
5. Move television, computers, and video games out of your child's bedroom.	☐	☐	☐	☐	☐
6. Reduce time spent watching television, playing video games, and using 7. the computer.	☐	☐	☐	☐	☐
8. Turn off the television during meals and snacks.	☐	☐	☐	☐	☐
9. Schedule regular meals and snacks.	☐	☐	☐	☐	☐
10. Help your child find activities to do instead of munching.	☐	☐	☐	☐	☐
11. Work with your child on a plan to stop sneaking food.	☐	☐	☐	☐	☐
12. Offer vegetables at meals or as snacks.	☐	☐	☐	☐	☐
13. Offer fruit at meals or as snacks.	☐	☐	☐	☐	☐
14. Offer dairy products at meals or as snacks.	☐	☐	☐	☐	☐
15. Reduce or eliminate extra snacks.	☐	☐	☐	☐	☐
16. Learn what other people are feeding your child.	☐	☐	☐	☐	☐
17. Provide healthy snacks for your child to take to child care.	☐	☐	☐	☐	☐
18. Change from juice to water between meals.	☐	☐	☐	☐	☐
19. Keep only healthy snacks in the house.	☐	☐	☐	☐	☐
20. Eat meals together.	☐	☐	☐	☐	☐
21. Create a plan to slow down eating.	☐	☐	☐	☐	☐
22. Learn to serve appropriate portion sizes for your child.	☐	☐	☐	☐	☐
23. Limit how often you buy/serve fast food.	☐	☐	☐	☐	☐
24. Stop eating in the car.	☐	☐	☐	☐	☐
25. Reward your child with things other than food to encourage good behavior.	☐	☐	☐	☐	☐

■ *Strategy: Family-based change*

You ask mom to talk to Dad and try a soda- and juice-free house for 3 to 4 weeks. You explain that hiding foods and drinks may cause food seeking and sneaking and misses an opportunity for good role modeling. You ask them to come back to the office to recheck OG's weight and see how the family managed without these beverages in the house.

Problem #4: Too Much Screen Time

■ *Parenting dilemma: Background television*

Mom notes that the television is on all the time and OG is often watching it.

■ *Strategy: Creating routines*

You ask Mom if she can work with Dad and the grand-parents to get OG on a schedule in the afternoon after kindergarten. You ask if he could combine outdoor play with some small chores to reduce television time, turning on the television only when he is scheduled for a show. Mom is nervous about turning off the television, so you and she decide to try 30 minutes a day without television and move to 30 more minutes each week. You suggest that the family fill out a chart to detail their progress.

Problem #5: Constant Hunger

- *Parenting dilemma: Constant hunger*
  The mother feels constant hunger is OG's biggest problem, but she does not know what to do about it because he becomes very angry if denied food.
- *Strategy: Distraction*
  You introduce the concept of distraction. You ask OG, "What could you do besides eat when you are hungry?" Mom is surprised when he answers, "Go out and play." You encourage her to work with him to think about things he could do instead of eating, such as play with toys.

  You schedule a return appointment for OG, Mom, and Dad in 3 to 4 weeks to check on OG's progress and see how the family has done with beginning to make changes.

Second Visit

One month later, OG, Mom, and Dad return. His weight is 64 lb (29.0 kg), a decrease of 1 lb (0.5 kg).

- *Problem #1: Obesity.* You review his laboratory studies, all of which are within the normal range.
- *Problem #2: Possible sleep apnea.* Mom reports that his sleep study is scheduled for next week.
- *Problem #3: Excess consumption of sweetened beverages.* Mom and Dad report that except for a few times when they ate out, they were able to limit OG's and the family's beverage consumption to milk with meals and diet beverages or water between meals. OG accepts this fairly well, especially because Dad is doing the same thing.

- *Problem #4: Too much screen time.* Reducing screen time is more difficult, especially because all family members are big television watchers. They are able to turn the television off during dinner and keep it off for about an hour every day. Mom notes that they frequently play a board game after dinner to accomplish this. They feel they can keep trying to reduce television time and note that as the weather gets nicer, it will be easier because OG likes being outside.
- *Problem #5: Constant hunger.* Mom wants to work on OG's complaints of constant hunger; she notes that it is very hard distracting him but did try it a few times.
  - Strategy: Structured activity
  - Mom says that she thinks OG sometimes eats because he is bored. You and Mom talk about enrolling him in an after-school activity 1 to 2 days a week, possibly a karate class or swimming at the YMCA; she thinks this is a good idea. You reinforce her attempts distraction, rewarding him with a sticker if he can transition to another activity. You also give her a list of healthy snacks to use if she cannot distract him (Table 7.6).

You schedule OG for a return appointment in 1 month to check his progress and the results of the sleep study.

Third Visit

This time the grandmother brings in OG because Mom and Dad are working. You received the sleep study results; he is having some apneic episodes, and you recommend that he see the pediatric otolaryngologist to inquire about a tonsillectomy.

His weight on this visit is 62 lb (28.1 kg), and his height is 49″ (124.5 cm). His BMI is 18.2, just at 95% (down 1.6 since his first visit). You show his grandmother the plot and praise the family's efforts.

Table 7.6. Examples of Healthy Snacks

– Fruit	– Bran muffins	– Sugar-free cereals
– Low-fat/frozen yogurt	– Fresh strawberries	– Unsalted pretzels
– Celery stalks	– Air-popped popcorn	– Dried raisins or apricots
– Low-fat oatmeal cookies	– Low-fat cheeses	
– Cucumber slices	– Frozen juice bars (without added sugar)	
– Frozen bananas	– Crackers	
– Baked potato chips		

Adapted from American Academy of Pediatrics. *A Parent's Guide to Childhood Obesity: A Road Map to Health.* Hassink SG, ed. Elk Grove Village, IL: American Academy of Pediatrics; 2006:39

- **Problem #3: Excess consumption of sweetened beverages.** The family is now very well adjusted to drinking water or diet drinks between meals. The grandmother notes that parties and extended family get-togethers are still a problem; you suggest offering to bring along a diet drink.

- **Problem #4: Too much screen time.** The grandmother notes that OG is watching about 2 hours of television a day and going outside more and that the family is getting better at helping him think of other things to do instead of watching television. For example, they bought an outdoor basketball hoop.

- **Problem #5: Constant hunger.** OG seems less hungry; he is enjoying his karate class and spends some time at home practicing his moves. They substituted low-calorie snacks for the chips and ice cream he used to have, which he does not seem to mind.

You reschedule him for a 2-month visit.

References

1. Whitaker RC, Wright JA, Pepe MS, Seidel KD, Dietz WH. Predicting obesity in young adulthood from childhood and parental obesity. *N Engl J Med.* 1997;337:869–873

2. Rolland-Cachera MF, Deheeger M, Bellisle F, Sempe M, Guillound-Bataille M, Patois E. Adiposity rebound in children: a simple indicator for predicting obesity. *Am J Clin Nutr.* 1984;39:129–135

3. Whitaker RC, Pepe MS, Wright JA, Seidel KD, Dietz WH. Early adiposity rebound and the risk of adult obesity. *Pediatrics.* 1998;101:e5

4. Centers for Disease Control and Prevention. Obesity prevalence among low-income, preschool-aged children—United States, 1998-2008. *MMWR Morb Mortal Wkly Rep.* 2009;58(28):769–773

5. Anderson SE, Whitaker RC. Household routines and obesity in US preschool-aged children. *Pediatrics.* 2010;125(3):420–428

6. Welsh JA, Cogswell ME, Rogers S, Rockett H, Mei Z, Grummer-Strawn LM. Overweight among low-income preschool children associated with the consumption of soft drinks: Missouri, 1999-2002. *Pediatrics.* 2005;115:e223–e229

7. Klesges RC, Klesges LM, Eck LH, Shelton ML. A longitudinal analysis of accelerated weight gain in preschool children. *Pediatrics.* 1995;95:126–130

8. Orlet Fisher J, Rolls BJ, Birch LL. Children's bite size and intake of an entrée are greater with large portions than with age-appropriate or self-selected portions. *Am J Clin Nutr.* 2003;77:1164–1170

9. Moore LL, Lombardi DA, White MJ, Campbell JL, Oliveria SA, Ellison RC. Influence of parents' physical activity levels on activity levels of young children. *J Pediatr.* 1991;118:215–219

10. Burdette HL, Whitaker RC, Daniels SR. Parental report of outdoor playtime as a measure of physical activity in preschool-aged children. *Arch Pediatr Adolesc Med.* 2004;158:353–357

11. Burdette HL, Whitaker RC. Resurrecting free play in young children: looking beyond fitness and fatness to attention, affiliation, and affect. *Arch Pediatr Adolesc Med.* 2005;159:46–50

12. Dennison BA, Erb TA, Jenkins PL. Television viewing and television in bedroom associated with overweight risk among low-income preschool children. *Pediatrics.* 2002;109:1028–1035

13. Miller SA, Taveras EM, Rifas-Shiman SL, Gillman MW. Association between television viewing and poor diet quality in young children. *Int J Pediatr Obes.* 2008;3(3):168–176

14. Benjamin SE, Rifas-Shiman SL, Taveras EM, et al. Early child care and adiposity at ages 1 and 3 years. Pediatrics. 2009;124:555–562

15. Agras WS, Hammer LD, McNicholas F, Kraemer HC. Risk factors for child-hood overweight: a prospective study from birth to 9.5 years. *J Pediatr.* 2004;145:20–25

16. Brotanek JM. Iron deficiency in early childhood in the United States: risk factors and racial/ethnic disparities. *Pediatrics.* 2007;120(3):568–567

17. Dye BA, Shenkin JD, Ogden CL, Marshall TA, Levy SM, Kanellis MJ. The relationship between healthful eating practices and dental caries in children aged 2-5 years in the United States. 1988-1994. *J Am Dent Assoc.* 2004;135:55–66

8 School Age

8.1 Background

Over the past 3 decades, the percentage of 6- to 11-year-olds with weights greater than 95% for age has more than tripled, from 6% to 19.6%.[1,2] Of children entering kindergarten, 11% are already overweight.[3] A study of predictors of overweight in children found that 20% of obese boys younger than 8 years became obese adults.[4]

Elementary school enrollment characterizes this age group, and factors in the school environment add to family and environmental factors in promoting obesity. Families need skills and information to assess and structure their children's nutrition and activity as time demands shift upon school entry.

Physical activity tends to decrease with age. In 1 meta-analysis, 6- to 7-year-olds engaged in 46 minutes per day of moderate to vigorous activity, compared with 10- to 16-year-olds, who had only 16 to 45 minutes per day. Mean activity levels decreased with age by 2.7% per year in boys and 7.4% per year in girls.[5]

Physical education (PE) is not uniform across schools. In a national study of 1,000 schools, approximately 65% of 1st graders had PE 1 to 2 times a week, 16.2% had PE 2 to 3 times a week, and only 12.5% had daily PE.[6]

Time previously spent on physical activity is often taken up with academic subjects in school and homework after school. Parents are increasingly challenged to create activity opportunities for their children at home, find opportunities in the community, and encourage schools to increase PE and recess. It is important to remember that incremental increases or decreases in regular activity can have a major effect over time. It has been predicted that adding 30 minutes a week to PE time could decrease the prevalence of obesity among girls by 5% and the prevalence of overweight among girls by 10%.[7]

Schools can also be the site of exposure to increased amounts of sweetened beverages and snack foods. Such foods are called *competitive foods* and are sold as à la carte items in school cafeterias, vending machines, school stores, and snack bars and are often used in fund-raisers.[8]

Exposure to competitive foods begins in elementary school and escalates through high school. Vending machines can be found in 17% of elementary schools and fund-raisers using competitive foods in 37%. The third School Nutrition and Dietary Assessment study (SNDAIII) requires the US Department of Agriculture (USDA) to establish national nutrition standards for all food sold and served in schools at any time during the school day.[9]

Sugar-sweetened beverages can add to total energy consumption and enhance weight gain.[10] A 12-oz sugar-sweetened drink consumed daily is associated with an 0.18% increase in a child's body mass index (BMI).[11] Soft drinks and other beverages sold in vending machines are often provided under an exclusive beverage contract. From 2003 to 2004, nearly 75% of high schools, 65% of middle schools, and 30% of elementary schools had exclusive beverage contracts. Such contracts, which grant a company the exclusive right to sell beverages in a school, may provide incentives to these schools based on the amount of beverages students consume.[12] More than 12 oz of juice consumption of per day is also linked to overweight.[13] The American Academy of Pediatrics recommends that children 7 to 18 years of age limit their juice consumption to 8 to 12 oz per day and that children 6 years and younger limit juice to 4 to 6 oz per day.[14]

Pediatricians are encouraged to work to eliminate sweetened drinks and competitive foods in schools; this involves educating parents, families, and patients, as well as school authorities, about the health effects of soft drink consumption[15] and energy-dense snack food.[16]

Parents may be unaware of exactly what kind of foods their children are purchasing at school. In addition to sweetened beverages, many children are exposed to snack foods offered in vending machines, school stores, and the cafeteria. These items are available and often purchased with a food credit card funded by monthly allotments from parents.

In addition to lunch, many children are also eating breakfast at school. School breakfast and lunch choices may be limited in elementary school to 1 high-calorie offering. In its 2009 report, *School Meals: Building Blocks for Healthy Children,* the committee recommends that the USDA adopt standards for menu planning, including increasing the amount and variety of fruits, vegetables, and whole grains; setting a minimum and maximum level of calories; and focusing more on reducing saturated fat and sodium.[17] In 2012, the USDA unveiled its new standards for school meals, which focus on

- Ensuring students are offered both fruits and vegetables every day of the week
- Increasing offerings of whole grain–rich foods
- Offering only fat-free or low-fat milk varieties
- Limiting calories based on the age of children being served to ensure proper portion size
- Increasing the focus on reducing the amounts of saturated fat, trans-fats, and sodium[18]

Mid-morning snacks are often encouraged, and after-school programs usually provide a snack, which means that the bulk of a child's caloric intake may occur outside the home, making it difficult for parents to know the quality or quantity of food their child consumes. Parents need to be knowledgeable about what is being offered at each meal so that they can adjust eating patterns at home as needed. In a study of 8- to 10-year-old African American girls, greater low-fat food preparation at home was related to lower consumption of total fat.[19] Children may occasionally eat breakfast at home or a child care center and again at school, or they may add on to a packed lunch from home with lunch or snacks at school.

Parents need to assess their child's level of daily physical activity. Most PE occurs only 1 to 2 times a week, and children may not be active for the entire class. Recess may or may not be outside, and after-school programs or child care centers may not offer extended periods of free play.

After-school time can be problematic for many overweight children, because this is a time when hunger and access to food at home, combined with unstructured time and boredom, can give rise to excess caloric intake. Parents often view after-school time, once homework is complete, as a time for the child to wind down. Although true, this may take the form of watching television or using the computer and can take up all of the child's free time. In a study of 5- to 9-year-old girls, those who watched more television consumed more snacks in front of the television, and those from families in which one or both parents were overweight had more frequent higher-fat snacks.[20] Parents need to be encouraged to structure after-school and evening time to include a regular mealtime, screen time limited to less than 2 hours a day, homework time, and time for free play. Parents and families may believe that structure precludes free time or playtime,

but the message these days is clear that unless parents create an opportunity for activity, screen time tends to take over.

Planning skills for parents have become increasingly important as they help their child juggle the increased time demands of school. Planning ahead for school events, visits to friends, and parties at which children will be exposed to different nutritional environments becomes important for children who are overweight.

Elementary school entry provides an opportunity to discuss with parents their role in planning, assessing, and structuring their child's activity and nutritional environment.

8.2 Prevention: Talking to Parents (BALANCE)

Prevention touch points for parents include **belief, assessment, lifestyle, activity, nutrition, child,** and **environment** (BALANCE).

*B*elief

- Parents may believe that a child's weight will take care of itself as the child grows. Although this may be true in an environment of optimal activity and nutrition, it is clear that parents and families will have to participate in the effort to achieve energy balance and optimal weight.
- Parents may also assume, without checking, that healthy snacks and time for activity are being provided at school, at after-school care, and during extracurricular activities.
- It may help to alert parents to the fact that their role in helping to oversee their child's nutrition and activity environment outside of the home is part of helping their child achieve optimal energy balance.

*A*ssessment

- It is important to help keep parents focused on assessing their child's dietary and exercise habits while health professionals are attending to ongoing changes in energy balance and BMI.
- As the child begins school, assessing the school's nutrition and activity environment and advocating for needed change are important skills for parents.
- Helping parents and families monitor shifts in the nutrition and activity environment over time is also important. Weekends, vacations, summers, and seasonal changes in activity may require different decisions to balance nutrition and activity and do not necessarily happen automatically.

Lifestyle

- These are very important years for helping a child adopt healthy eating and activity habits that last a lifetime.
- Parents should continue to focus on a wholesome lifestyle for everyone in the family.
  - Develop a structured family meal and snack schedule (3 well-thought-out meals and 2 snacks a day).
  - Minimize junk food consumption.
  - Eliminate sugared beverages such as soft drinks.
  - Pay attention to portion sizes.
  - Add some physical activity to the mix.
- A reasonable approach for parents at this age is to frame the changes in eating and nutrition in terms of "health decisions" for the family.
- Suboptimal sleep is correlated with obesity in childhood. Average sleep for the early school-age child ranges from 8 to 11 hours per night. Parents can check to see if they:
  - Established healthy sleep routines
  - Removed the television from the bedroom

Activity

- Free play is still important at this age.
- Parents will need to start striking a balance between unstructured outdoor time and entry-level sports such as baseball and soccer.
- Children still have short attention spans but are improving their reaction times and directionality. Fundamental skill development is the main task with minimal competition and flexible rules.
- Organized and spontaneous activity should focus on fun and participation.
- Television and computer use may start to increase; parents need to keep in mind that no more than 2 hours of screen time daily is recommended. Limiting television and computer time is usually best accomplished by
  - Not having a television or computer in a child's bedroom
  - Not watching television during meals
  - Having the whole family limit television use
  - Not being outnumbered by the number of televisions in the house
  - Helping the child and other family members find other indoor activity options

Nutrition

- Nutritional choices begin at the grocery store. Parents who buy a few pieces of fruit and a selection of high-fat or high-sugar snacks have inadvertently set up their families for difficult choices. Providing larger amounts of fruits and vegetables than was previously the case and avoiding other snack food purchases paves the way for easier choices for all family members.
- Family meals are important and can be planned around selections such as
  - Fresh fruits and vegetables
  - Whole-grain cereals and breads
  - Low-fat or nonfat dairy products, such as milk, yogurt, and cheese
  - Lean and skinless meats, including chicken, turkey, fish, and lean hamburger
- Portion sizes should be less than an adult-sized serving.
- If the school cafeteria does not offer many healthy choices, parents can pack a healthy lunch each day; some ideas include:
  - Preparing a turkey sandwich on multigrain or pita bread (a peanut butter and jelly sandwich is fine, too)
  - Adding a piece of fruit or perhaps a bag of pretzels
  - Packing a small water bottle or encouraging the child to buy low-fat milk in the cafeteria
  - Avoiding pastrami, salami, and other high-fat lunch meats
  - Packing a healthy snack for after-school care or activities if one is not offered
  - Checking the school or child care breakfast menu's offerings too (if applicable). If selections revolve around items such as Pop-Tarts, breakfast pizza, or sausage sticks, they may want to pack some nonsugared cereal and fruit as an alternative.

Child

- Although children at this age are becoming increasingly independent, they still need structure and support of nutrition and activity by the family.
- After-school time can be problematic for children and parents.
  - Children tend to be hungry when they get home and are not in a position to make good nutritional choices.
  - Parents can help by preparing a snack to have ready for the child.
  - Children may not automatically ask to go outside after school. Parents may need to plan this time into the after-school schedule, reserving television and computer time for later in the evening.

Environment

- Managing the child's nutrition and activity environment takes on an expanded dimension when home, school, after-school care, and activities all have their own balance of activity, inactivity, and eating.

- Parents may need to have an active role in promoting change. For example, parents can advocate for more PE in school, promote healthier snacking in after-school care, and ask if teachers can offer healthier snacks for class rewards and parties.
- Extended family members may need to be reminded about providing healthy after-school snacks, encouraging activity, and helping limit television and computer time.

8.3 Intervention

When a school-age child has a BMI greater than 85% but less than 95% or is crossing growth percentiles in an upward direction, this is the time for a more in-depth look at eating and activity, family health history, and parental obesity—all of which can contribute to the risk of becoming an older child and young adult with obesity. In addition to reemphasizing concepts covered previously, parents and families may need to give increased attention to their ability to provide and influence nutrition and activity by focusing on *energy balance, structure,* and *modeling healthy behavior* (discussed next).

Energy Balance

As children move out into the environment, the challenges to staying in optimal energy balance increase. When a child starts to cross percentiles or is in the at-risk range of BMI between 85% and 95%, an examination of the daily nutrition and activity routine is in order. In an otherwise reasonable diet, an increase in snacks and portion sizes are ways in which energy balance can shift, often without parents noticing. Once recognized, parents can initiate changes by preparing healthy snacks for their children and preventing them from going right to the refrigerator or cabinets after coming home from school. Parents can also continue to serve meals restaurant style (portioning out food onto plates) instead of family style (everyone helping themselves to the food on the table).

Structure

Planning and time management become increasingly important, particularly when the actual amount of time the family has to manage homework, dinner, bedtime routines, and free time shrinks because of school and work. A reasonable look at the flow of after-school time is in order, and often parents can restructure this time to include a snack, outdoor time,

dinner, homework, and free time, in that order. When a child is in after-school care, activity time may be squeezed out and parents must be creative in finding indoor activities and limiting television and computer time. Weekends can also be challenging because, unless parents plan the time, children may go to the television or computer as the activity that is most available.

Modeling Healthy Behavior

Children at this age are quick to detect and point out discrepancies in what a parent is asking them to do and what the parent is actually doing for them. They are also sensitive to what other children are doing and are aware of fairness issues in relation to siblings and friends. This may cycle into resistance to change and cause parents to give in to demands for snacking and television time more than they realize. This is a good time to establish positive lifestyle changes as a household with boundaries set by parents and input from the child on how to limit television watching, get the family to become more active, and eliminate junk food. Parents, however, need to stay in the role of setting overall boundaries for healthy eating and activity.

8.4 Treatment

When a child's BMI is greater than 95% and you are dealing with excess adiposity, it is time to initiate a focused treatment strategy. It is important to review the issues discussed in the previous 2 sections because these are the building blocks of good nutrition and activity habits. But you will also have to focus on the barriers to change that may have prevented parents and families from implementing these strategies.

A useful way to begin is to obtain a family history focused on obesity-related comorbidities. This can serve to emphasize the health risks involved and the necessity of taking early action once obesity is identified.

8.5 Family History

The family history (Table 8.1) provides information on obesity and obesity-related comorbidity risk and serves as a starting point to discuss the child's BMI.

If parents are obese or have a history of obesity, they may want to relate their personal struggles with their weight. Often the desire to avoid these same struggles in their child motivates parents to make family changes in nutrition and activity.

Table 8.1. Family History, School Age

Complete or update this family history targeted toward obesity and related comorbidities.

	Mother	Father	Maternal Grandmother	Maternal Grandfather	Paternal Grandmother	Paternal Grandfather	Sibling 1	Sibling 2
Obesity	☐	☐	☐	☐	☐	☐	☐	☐
Cardiovascular disease	☐	☐	☐	☐	☐	☐	☐	☐
High blood pressure	☐	☐	☐	☐	☐	☐	☐	☐
Stroke	☐	☐	☐	☐	☐	☐	☐	☐
High cholesterol	☐	☐	☐	☐	☐	☐	☐	☐
High triglyceride level	☐	☐	☐	☐	☐	☐	☐	☐
Type 1 or 2 diabetes	☐	☐	☐	☐	☐	☐	☐	☐
Liver disease	☐	☐	☐	☐	☐	☐	☐	☐
Bariatric surgery	☐	☐	☐	☐	☐	☐	☐	☐
Polycystic ovarian syndrome	☐	☐	☐	☐	☐	☐	☐	☐
Binge eating disorder	☐	☐	☐	☐	☐	☐	☐	☐
	☐	☐	☐	☐	☐	☐	☐	☐
	☐	☐	☐	☐	☐	☐	☐	☐

8.6 Review of Systems

The review of systems can also serve as a point of departure to discuss obesity-related comorbidities, pointing out particular risk factors as they relate to increasing BMI.

- Skin: Acanthosis nigricans, striae, cervical fat pad, skin picking
- Head, eyes, ears, nose, and throat (HEENT): Headache, blurred vision
- Lungs: Snoring, sleep disturbance, sleep apnea, restless sleep, sleep position, daytime tiredness, napping, asthma, shortness of breath or subjective chest tightness when exercising, cough after exercising
- Cardiac: Murmur
- Abdomen: Gastroesophageal reflux, stomach pain, nausea or vomiting after eating
- Musculoskeletal: Limping, hip pain, knee pain
- Development: School problems, learning difficulties, attention problems
- Psychosocial: Depression, anxiety, behavior problems

8.7 Physical Examination

- Height
- Weight
- BMI + previous BMI measurements
- BMI %
- Blood pressure

- General: Dysmorphic features, poor linear growth, developmental delay
- Skin: Skin picking, acanthosis nigricans, dermatitis in skinfolds, striae, cervical fat pad
- HEENT: Funduscopic examination for papilledema, tonsillar hypertrophy
- Cardiopulmonary: Murmur, wheezing
- Abdominal: Hepatomegaly
- Musculoskeletal: Range of motion, genu varum, limp, hip or knee pain
- Genitourinary: Tanner stage

8.8 Family Constellation and Social History

Information about the family can provide a starting point for discussing how nutrition and activity decisions are made and how changes might take place.

- Who is living at home with the child?
- Who is with the child before school?
- Who is with the child after school?
- Who else besides parents is responsible for the child's meals or snacks?

8.9 Parenting Questions

Parenting styles and skills are important when families are trying to make changes in lifestyle. The questions in Table 8.2 may help you focus on family factors to facilitate or hinder change.

8.10 Parenting Touch Points

Parenting touch points focus on helping families initiate and maintain change by helping them believe change can occur, identify the change needed, value the outcome of the change, know how to change, and have the energy to change and sustain the change.

- **Believe that change can occur.** Parents may believe that the pressure of school, homework, and activity, as well as their jobs and responsibilities, do not allow for any changes. The idea of incremental changes being effective and important is crucial to allowing families to attempt to change behavior. Helping parents pick a feasible and measurable change to tackle, such as packing a lunch, taking a daily walk, or enrolling the child in an activity, will help encourage parents that change is possible.

- **Identify the change.** After-school time is a major area of focus when it comes to looking at ways to improve nutrition and activity. Helping parents identify alternatives to watching television, using the computer, and snacking will be useful. Some options might include:
  - Creating a schedule for after-school time, allowing for snack, outdoor, dinner, homework, and television or computer time
  - Enrolling the child in an after-school program or activity
  - Choosing extracurricular activities that emphasize participation and skill building
  - For children who are reluctant to participate, choosing an activity such as karate or dance rather than a team sport

  - Choosing activities involving peers and participation, such as scouts, church groups, or school clubs, which can be very important for structuring time, relieving boredom, decreasing screen time, and enhancing social skills
  - For a reluctant child, providing 2 or 3 activities from which the child can choose rather than requiring a "yes" or "no" to a specific activity.

- **Value the outcome.** Screening for obesity-related comorbidities is always important and becomes increasingly more so as children get older. Health outcomes and the future of childhood obesity can be powerful motivators for families. The family history and laboratory and physical assessments of the child can be focused on obesity-related outcomes.

For many families, the link between health, weight, and behavior will be enough to help them initiate change. Psychosocial issues such as teasing and lowered self-esteem may also motivate families to change.

When a family seems unable to initiate change, it may be useful to explore barriers to change with them, such as

- Parents may have a history of failed attempts to change their own weight and feel discouraged.
- Other family issues may become overwhelming and prevent the family from focusing their energy on making a change.
- Parents may think that it is up to the child to make change.
- External factors, such as an unsafe community, other caregivers, or lack of money, may be operative.
- Families that are able to change their lifestyle but are unable to improve BMI may become discouraged. It is important to point out that healthier diet and physical activity habits are predictors of longer lives, independent of weight or BMI.

Table 8.2. Parenting Questions, School Age	Never	Seldom	Sometimes	Often	Always
Parents set clear and simple expectations and limits.	☐	☐	☐	☐	☐
Parents set boundaries and give the child choice within them.	☐	☐	☐	☐	☐
Parents have developmentally appropriate goals for the child.	☐	☐	☐	☐	☐
Parents model healthy nutrition, activity, and inactivity behavior.	☐	☐	☐	☐	☐
Parents limit the availability of high-sugar or high-fat snacks in the home.	☐	☐	☐	☐	☐
Parents maintain an abundant supply of fruits and vegetables in the home.	☐	☐	☐	☐	☐

- *Know how to change.* It is important for the family to work together to make change. It is equally important that parents be on the same page regarding the changes they want to make. Extended families and parents who are separated or divorced face special challenges that make communication even more important. Talking about family goals and ways to implement them are an integral part of moving forward. For example, asking a child, "How many hours of television or computer time do you need?" will be enlightening and can start the discussion of how to decrease television time. Another question worth asking the child is, "What can you do when you're not watching TV?" Frequently, it is evident that the child does not have any alternative plans in mind and the family can then help design some activities to fill the time.
- *Have the energy to change and sustain.* As families become busier, it is important that parents take time to be with their child—just hanging out together. These special times can energize the parent-child relationship and fuel the changes in nutrition and activity that the family is trying to make. If appropriate, parents and extended family members may need to frequently communicate how things are going and support one another in their efforts to sustain the desired changes.

8.11 Developmental Touch Point

School-age children balance between tuning into their parents and peer group. Structure and negotiation are effective tools in modifying behavior. This may be a good time for families to initiate family meetings to establish house rules, vent feelings and thoughts, and make positive lifestyle changes. Input from the children gives them a sense of control and engages them in following through on changes discussed. Topics can include how to limit television watching, get the family more active, and eliminate junk food from the house.

8.12 Nutrition and Activity Questions and Approaches

Parents can answer the nutrition and activity questions in Table 8.3, which can provide a focal point for targeted intervention (Table 8.4) in a brief encounter. Questions answered "Often" or "Always" can be targeted first for change.

8.13 A Case in Point: SB

SB is a 6-year, 10-month-old boy who has been followed in your practice for several years. On his recent checkup, you ordered a lipid panel because of a family history of hyperlipidemia. SB's cholesterol level was elevated at 200 mg/dL, and his low-density lipoprotein (LDL) cholesterol level was 143 mg/dL. You note that his weight gain has been steadily accelerating and his parents are concerned because of his preoccupation with food.

They note that he tends to argue with them a lot, especially about food, and they are worried about his self-esteem. They answer "Always" to eats more than 1 snack between meals each day (question 20), requests second helpings (question 28), and is a fast eater (question 25). They also answer "Often" to seems unmotivated to play (question 3). The family already made numerous dietary changes and answers "Never" to drinks juice or sugared beverages between meals (question 21) and eats at fast-food restaurants (question 26), having eliminated juice, junk food, and fast food from their diet.

SB is in good health, with no problems except for an occasional ear infection and complaints of stomach pain after eating, which was mentioned during the review of systems. He is in 1st grade and doing well.

Family history is positive for high cholesterol (in 3 of 4 grandparents) and negative for diabetes, hypertension, and obesity.

The results of the physical examination show that his height is 50″ (125.9 cm) and his weight is 91 lb (41.4 kg), with a BMI of 26.2 (>97% for his age and gender). His blood pressure is 111/67 mm Hg, with systolic and diastolic pressure at 90%. Physical examination is essentially normal, with no positive findings.

All laboratory values are normal with the exception of the total and LDL cholesterol levels.

Problem #1: Snacking

Based on the family's answers to your questionnaire, you ask the family how they view SB's snacking. They say they know he is eating too many snacks between meals and would like to change this but have found it difficult to do in the past.

- *Parenting dilemma: Fairness*
  The parents want to be fair and avoid SB's angry outbursts if they limit snacks. They are concerned because his 13-year-old (thin) brother "needs" snacks and SB always wants whatever he sees his brother eating. SB becomes upset if he cannot eat, too.

Table 8.3. Nutrition and Activity Questions, School Age

These questions can be answered by the parents and provide a focal point for targeted intervention in a brief encounter. First have the parents answer these questions about the presence or absence of behaviors that promote weight gain; then refer to Table 8.4.

Please answer the following for the statements below: Does your school age child...?

	Never	Seldom	Sometimes	Often	Always
1. Spend after-school time indoors.	☐	☐	☐	☐	☐
2. Prefer quiet activities.	☐	☐	☐	☐	☐
3. Seem unmotivated to play.	☐	☐	☐	☐	☐
4. Lack interest in activities with friends.	☐	☐	☐	☐	☐
5. Sleep less than 8 hours a night.	☐	☐	☐	☐	☐
6. Watch television or play with computer/video games in his or her bedroom.	☐	☐	☐	☐	☐
7. Spend more than 2 hours watching television, playing video games, or using a computer each day.	☐	☐	☐	☐	☐
8. Eat in front of the television.	☐	☐	☐	☐	☐
9. Skip meals.	☐	☐	☐	☐	☐
10. Demand certain food or snacks.	☐	☐	☐	☐	☐
11. Become angry when demands for food are not met.	☐	☐	☐	☐	☐
12. Eat when bored.	☐	☐	☐	☐	☐
13. Sneak or hide food.	☐	☐	☐	☐	☐
14. Refuse to eat vegetables.	☐	☐	☐	☐	☐
15. Refuse to eat fruit.	☐	☐	☐	☐	☐
16. Refuse to eat dairy foods (yogurt, cheese, milk).	☐	☐	☐	☐	☐
17. Skip breakfast.	☐	☐	☐	☐	☐
18. Have trouble eating healthy lunches and snacks at school.	☐	☐	☐	☐	☐
19. Get his or her own snacks.	☐	☐	☐	☐	☐
20. Eat more than 1 snack between meals a day.	☐	☐	☐	☐	☐
21. Drink juice or sugared beverages between meals.	☐	☐	☐	☐	☐
22. Drink flavored milk.	☐	☐	☐	☐	☐
23. Eat as much as an older sibling or adult.	☐	☐	☐	☐	☐
24. Eat meals alone.	☐	☐	☐	☐	☐
25. Eat very fast.	☐	☐	☐	☐	☐
26. Eat at fast-food restaurants.	☐	☐	☐	☐	☐
27. Receive food as a reward or treat for good behavior.	☐	☐	☐	☐	☐
28. Request second helpings.	☐	☐	☐	☐	☐

Table 8.4. Nutrition and Activity Approaches, School Age

Questions answered "Often" or "Always" in Table 8.3 can be targeted first for change. Using these specific questions, ask the parent, "How willing are you to…?"

Please answer the following for the statements below: How willing are you to…?

	Impossible	Could Try	Could Do Sometimes	Could Do Often	Easy
1. Schedule time for active play with your child each day.	☐	☐	☐	☐	☐
2. Schedule time for your child to play outside.	☐	☐	☐	☐	☐
3. Plan healthy activities to do with your child.	☐	☐	☐	☐	☐
4. Make a peer group activity part of after-school time.	☐	☐	☐	☐	☐
5. Plan bedtime to ensure 8–10 hours of sleep.	☐	☐	☐	☐	☐
6. Move television, computers, and video games out of your child's bedroom.	☐	☐	☐	☐	☐
7. Reduce time spent watching television, playing video games, and using the computer.	☐	☐	☐	☐	☐
8. Turn off the television during meals and snacks.	☐	☐	☐	☐	☐
9. Schedule regular meals and snacks.	☐	☐	☐	☐	☐
10. Help your child find activities to do instead of munching.	☐	☐	☐	☐	☐
11. Work with your child on a plan to stop sneaking food.	☐	☐	☐	☐	☐
12. Offer vegetables at meals or as snacks.	☐	☐	☐	☐	☐
13. Offer fruit at meals or as snacks.	☐	☐	☐	☐	☐
14. Offer dairy products at meals or as snacks.	☐	☐	☐	☐	☐
15. Schedule time for breakfast each day.	☐	☐	☐	☐	☐
16. Pack healthier school snacks.	☐	☐	☐	☐	☐
17. Reduce or eliminate extra snacks.	☐	☐	☐	☐	☐
18. Change from juice or soda to water between meals.	☐	☐	☐	☐	☐
19. Serve unflavored milk at meals and snacks.	☐	☐	☐	☐	☐
20. Keep only healthy snacks in the house.	☐	☐	☐	☐	☐
21. Learn to serve appropriate serving sizes for your child.	☐	☐	☐	☐	☐
22. Eat meals together.	☐	☐	☐	☐	☐
23. Create a plan to slow down eating.	☐	☐	☐	☐	☐
24. Limit how often you buy/serve fast food.	☐	☐	☐	☐	☐
25. Reward your child with things other than food to encourage good behavior.	☐	☐	☐	☐	☐
26. Offer second helpings of vegetables.	☐	☐	☐	☐	☐

Strategy: Family-based change

You take care of their older son and note that he is growing along his weight and height curves and is not underweight. You ask about his eating and his parents note that he is picky, often eating very little at meals and then asking for snacks.

You note that fairness is not necessarily equality. Meeting each child's needs is the goal and each child's nutritional and activity needs may vary.

You also note that grazing or frequent snacking is not a recommended eating behavior at any weight because snacks tend to be less nutritious than food offered at a well-balanced family meal and that eating 3 meals and 1 snack per day is a goal for the whole family.

The parents feel somewhat encouraged and are ready to try to structure eating times to 3 meals and 1 snack per day for everyone.

Problem #2: Rapid Eating

The parents note that SB eats rapidly, gets done eating before anyone else, and always asks for a second helping.

Parenting dilemma: Need for a new approach

SB's parents have tried telling him to slow down but to no avail. They tell you that they are not sure what to do next.

Strategy: Splitting portions

You ask them to offer a salad or vegetables as an appetizer before the meal with a small glass of water. You then ask them to portion out his dinner on a plate, divide the portion, and place half on another plate. They are to give the first plate with a half portion and then offer the second plate. If SB is still hungry, he can have extra salad or vegetables.

Problem #3: Unmotivated to Get Active

The parents are very aware that SB needs to increase his activity; in fact, they are active themselves.

Parenting dilemma: Dealing with resistance

When they ask him if he wants to join a sport, he always says "no," and when they try to get him outside, he resists and they get worn out.

Strategy: Partnering

One-on-one time with parents can be an important motivator for children. SB's father offers to walk with him after dinner. He says they could take a ball along and toss it, and this would be their special time together. Hearing this, SB brightens and says he thinks this would be OK.

Problem #4: Hypercholesterolemia

To address his hypercholesterolemia, you ask the parents to keep detailed diet records for a few days for review during SB's next visit.

Second Visit

For his second visit 1 month later, his weight decreased by 4 lb (1.9 kg).

Problem #1: Snacking

SB's parents believe that the diet records they were asked to keep actually helped them keep on track with the scheduled snacking. After a few weeks, SB and his brother seemed to adjust to the new routine and the parents feel things are going OK except for a few complaints.

Problem #2: Rapid eating

The parents think the technique of splitting portions has worked; SB now seems to feel full after the meal.

Problem #3: Unmotivated to get active

SB has been walking every day, rain or shine, and he and his father are now up to 25 minutes a day. They take a football with them and toss it during their walk, and SB seems to enjoy this.

Problem #4: Hypercholesterolemia

You review his diet and ask the family to pack a lunch to lower saturated fat (eg, skip the cheese on the sandwich; use light mayo or try mustard; pack fruit instead of chips or cookies; include 1% milk, skim milk, or water to drink). His review of systems and physical examination are normal.

New Problem #5: Eating at parties

The parents have questions about parties, and you ask them to talk to SB before parties and ask him to take only one helping of food, praising him for making good decisions.

Third Visit

Six weeks later, his weight is down 4 lb (1.7 kg) from the previous visit. The family is now taking walks together. They say it is harder to get him outside when the weather is not so good, but they are persevering. They are concerned that he will not eat the carrots or other vegetables they pack in his lunch.

His repeated cholesterol is now 159 mg/dL; you reinforce the positive changes the family made.

Fourth Visit

SB returns with a weight loss of 5 lb (2.2 kg) over the 11 weeks since his last visit. His BMI decreased from 26.2 to 22.2, which places his BMI at 97%. He is eating a well-balanced diet and is walking daily. His family notes he is increasingly more active and that his endurance is increasing as well.

His review of systems and physical examination continue to be normal. The family has now established a solid family-based approach to eating and activity. SB is more positive about himself and is willing to try new activities. You ask the family to return in 6 months and to feel free to check in with you if they have any difficulties.

References

1. Ogden CL, Carroll MD, Curtin LR, Lamb MM, Flegal KM. Prevalence of high body mass index in US children and adolescents, 2007-2008. *JAMA.* 2010;303(3):242–249

2. Ogden CL, Carroll MD, Curtin LR, McDowell MA, Tabak CJ, Flegal KM. Prevalence of overweight and obesity in the United States, 1999-2004. *JAMA.* 2006;295:1549–1555

3. Datar A, Sturm R, Magnabosco JL. Childhood overweight and academic performance: national study of kindergartners and first-graders. *Obes Res.* 2004;12:58–68

4. Guo SS, Wu W, Chumlea WC, Roche AF. Predicting overweight and obesity in adulthood from body mass index values in childhood and adolescence. *Am J Clin Nutr.* 2002;76:653–658

5. Sallis JF. Epidemiology of physical activity and fitness in children and adolescents. *Crit Rev Food Sci Nutr.* 1993;33:403–408

6. Datar A, Sturm R. Physical education in elementary schools and body mass index: evidence from the early childhood longitudinal study. *Am J Public Health.* 2004;94:1501–1506

7. National Institute for Health Care Management. Obesity in young children: impact and intervention. *Research brief.* August 2004. www.nihcm.org/OYCbrief.pdf. Accessed May 25, 2006

8. Story M, Nanney MS, Schwartz MB. Schools and obesity prevention: creating school environments and policies to promote healthy eating and physical activity. *Milbank Q.* 2009;87(1):71–10

9. Finkelstein DM, Hill EL, Whitaker RC. School food environments and policies in US public schools. *Pediatrics.* 2008;122(1):e251–e259

10. Berkey CS, Rockett HR, Field AE, Gillman MW, Colditz GA. Sugar-added beverages and adolescent weight change. *Obes Res.* 2004;12:778–788

11. Ludwig DS, Peterson KE, Gortmaker SL. Relation between consumption of sugar-sweetened drinks and childhood obesity: a prospective, observational analysis. *Lancet.* 2001;357:505–508

12. United States Government Accountability Office. School meal programs: competitive foods are widely available and generate substantial revenues for schools. 2005;GAO-05-563.4

13. Dennison BA, Rockwell HL, Baker SL. Excess fruit juice consumption by preschool-aged children is associated with short stature and obesity. *Pediatrics.* 1997;99:15–22

14. American Academy of Pediatrics Committee on Nutrition. The use and misuse of fruit juice in pediatrics. *Pediatrics.* 2001;107:1210–1213

15. American Academy of Pediatrics Committee on School Health. Soft drinks in schools. *Pediatrics.* 2004;113:152–154

16. Centers for Disease Control and Prevention. Low-energy-dense foods and weight management: cutting calories while controlling hunger. Research to Practice Series, No. 5. http://www.cdc.gov/nccdphp/dnpa/nutrition/pdf/r2p_energy_density.pdf

17. Institute of Medicine. School meals: building blocks for healthy children. National Academy of Sciences. 2009

18. Nutrition Standards in the National School Lunch and School Breakfast Programs; Final Rule, Food and Nutrition Service (FNS), USDA. *Federal Register.* 2012;77(17):4088-4167. http://www.gpo.gov/fdsys/pkg/FR-2012-01-26/pdf/2012-1010.pdf

19. Cullen KW, Baranowski T, Klesges LM, et al. Anthropometric, parental, and psychosocial correlates of dietary intake of African-American girls. *Obes Res.* 2004;12:20S–31S

20. Francis LA, Lee Y, Birsch LL. Parental weight status and girls' television viewing, snacking, and body mass indexes. *Obes Res.* 2003;11:143–151

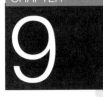

9 Early Adolescent

9.1 Background

Body size, shape, and composition change dramatically during puberty: adolescent females increase deposition of body fat; regional deposition of adipose tissue changes in boys and girls; and concerns about body image may heighten. At the hormonal level, gonadotropins, leptin, sex steroids, and growth hormone interact to produce and complete the pubertal transition.[1]

The increase in insulin resistance that occurs with the onset of puberty[2] may accentuate the risk for obesity and obesity-related comorbidities. Several studies report that children entering puberty are at increased risk for developing impaired glucose tolerance.[3,4] Pubertal transition from Tanner stage 1 to Tanner stage 3 is associated with a 32% reduction in insulin sensitivity and increases in fasting glucose, insulin, and insulin resistance. These changes were similar across gender, ethnicity, and obesity and were not associated with changes in body fat, visceral fat, insulin-like growth factor-1, androgens, or estradiol.[5]

Timing of menarche can also affect factors such as insulin, glucose, blood pressure, fat-free mass, and peripheral body fat levels. Girls with early menarche have higher glucose, insulin, and blood pressure measurements than girls with an average or late menses onset. These changes were independent of age and changes in fat-free mass or peripheral body fat.[6] Early maturity differs in effect between boys and girls. In one study, body mass index (BMI) and skinfold thickness were associated with early sexual maturity stages in boys and girls, but early-maturing boys were leaner than their counterparts, whereas early-maturing girls had increased adiposity compared with girls maturing at average ages or later.[7]

Physical activity in children is important for the maintenance of metabolic control. In a study of 589 Danish children with an average age of 9.7 years, a strong relationship was found between insulin resistance and physical activity.[8] There is an inverse relationship between physical activity and increasing age in boys and girls.[9] Decreases in physical education classes and participation in extracurricular activities may play a role.

Only 7.9% of middle schools have daily physical education, and 22% of schools do not require students to take any physical education.[10] Of children 9 to 13 years of age, 62% do not spend any time outside of school hours in organized physical activities such as sports.[11] There is a strong correlation between fitness and academic performance.[12] A study of children examining the link between childhood obesity, activity, and screen time found that heavier children spend more time in sedentary activities than those with a lower BMI.[13] Physical activity behaviors track from early to middle childhood[14] and from adolescence to adulthood.[15]

Insulin resistance is more common in children with obesity and is important in the etiology of cardiovascular disease.[16] These risk factors have been referred to as components of the metabolic syndrome and include[17,18]:

1. Abdominal obesity
2. Elevated triglyceride levels (>150 mg/dL)
3. Low high-density lipoprotein (HDL) cholesterol levels (<40 mg/dL)
4. Increased low-density lipoprotein (LDL) cholesterol levels (>130 mg/dL)
5. Increased blood pressure (systolic or diastolic blood pressure >90% for age and gender)
6. Impaired fasting glucose[19] (fasting glucose ≥100 mg/dL; random glucose >200 mg/dL)

Other components of increased cardiometabolic risk include a prothrombotic and proinflammatory state and hyperuricemia.[17] These indicators have been demonstrated to be stable from childhood and adolescence to young adulthood.[20]

Hyperinsulinemia and insulin resistance are already present in prepubertal children with obesity. Because hyperinsulinemia is a potentially reversible condition and the complications related to it may be prevented, early assessment should be undertaken so that children with obesity lose body weight before the onset of puberty.[5]

9.2 Prevention: Talking to Parents and Teens (BALANCE)

Prevention touch points for parents and teens include **belief, assessment, lifestyle, activity, nutrition, child/young adolescent,** and **environment** (BALANCE).

*B*elief

- Parents may see the middle school child as being able to negotiate food and activity choices independently. Although it is true that the child will push to have choices, he or she still needs and desires decision support.
- Parents partnering in a healthy change, whether taking a daily walk together, shooting hoops, or making a healthy snack choice, is a powerful way for parents to help their adolescent without a "battle of words."
- As the peer group becomes more of an influence on the middle school child, the drive to fit in may become more important in determining nutrition and activity choices.
- Food choices, packed lunches, and family activities that were taken for granted by the younger child may become areas of conflict.
- Early adolescents may think it is unfair that they have to follow a nutrition and activity plan while their friends do not.
- This is a time when parents need to be encouraged to maintain a calm, supportive, and communicative environment when encouraging change and to avoid "going negative."

*A*ssessment

- Self-assessment is still important, but this can be shared. For example, talking over situations that may arise, such as making healthy food choices at an upcoming family gathering, sets the stage for two-way communication and avoids the potential power struggle when parents try for complete control.
- Parents and their child can participate in setting goals together by jointly setting the goal (eg, getting outside every day) and communicating about exactly how the goal will be achieved.

*L*ifestyle

- Caregivers can be reminded that modeling the behavior they desire is a powerful way to stay believable.
- Family meals continue to be important anchors of the day for providing good nutrition and enhancing communication.

- It is tempting for parents to have televisions and computers in their child's room, but they may need to be reminded that this not only increases sedentary time but also decreases parent-child communication and increases unhealthy marketing to teens.

*A*ctivity

- Unfortunately, middle school can be a time of dramatic decreases in activity for many children. Demands of schoolwork and increased competitiveness of sports teams, as well as elimination of recess, can dramatically shift energy balance.
- Parents can emphasize the value of participation versus competition in activities. Clubs, volunteer groups, and church groups can all be valuable activities for this age group, getting them away from "screen and snack" mode after school.
- Total screen time should continue to have a 2-hour limit.
- Parents and children are often surprised at the energy cost of snacks and drinks. For example, 12 oz of a fruit drink can be 180 kcal (>1 hour of outdoor activity) and a large order of French fries from a fast-food restaurant can be 430 kcal (1 hour of karate).
- Helping parents and children understand the energy output required to balance snacks, fast food, and sugared beverages can affect their motivation to change.
- In addition, the time it takes to consume 250 kcal can be very short (5–10 minutes), whereas the time it takes to expend 250 kcal can be up to 1 hour of activity. A child can literally run out of time in the day to exercise (Table 9.1).

Table 9.1. One Hour of Activity for a 100-lb. Child	
Outdoor cycling, exercise of moderate intensity	160 kcal
Basketball	270 kcal
Dancing	216 kcal
Martial arts	450 kcal
Soccer	325 kcal

*N*utrition

- Many children come home from school "starving"; if they have unlimited access to food, they will often eat a high-calorie snack or even a small meal.
- Although young adolescents have greater freedom to purchase their choice of foods outside of the home, the home is still where good nutrition habits are formed. Parents establish the food choices a child has at home when they shop at the grocery store. Growing appetites should be

satisfied with fruits and vegetables instead of snack food. It is unfair to expect children at this age to resist temptation when they are hungry at home if the parent purchasing the products cannot resist those temptations when shopping.

- Early lunch periods, eating to unwind, or boredom if there is nothing to do after school can all contribute to oversnacking. Parents still need to oversee the young adolescent's selections of snacks.
- Packing a snack eliminates the child's decision making at a time when the child is feeling too hungry to choose well.
- Stopping at a neighborhood store after school may also be an issue. Limiting snack money and discussing choices may help.

Child/Young Adolescent

- The physical changes of puberty may lead young adolescents to feel unsure and critical about their bodies.
- Parents need to educate their child about the normal diversity of body types at this age and discuss individual differences.
- Puberty may also trigger increased expectations from parents and disappointment if these expectations are not met.[21]
- Parents need to be encouraged to continue supporting their child in terms of nutrition and activity while encouraging the development of independent decision making.

Environment

- Finding venues for activity may be more challenging at this age.
- Safety issues that are important to parents may cause early adolescents to complain about undue restriction.
- Parents continue to need to provide transportation and financing for extracurricular activities.
- Computer and television time can creep upward rapidly at this age. Parents need to continue limiting screen time and explore alternatives for activity with their child.
- It is probably not enough to assume that the child will automatically find something to replace screen time without ideas and opportunities offered by the parents and family.

9.3 Intervention

When an early adolescent has a BMI greater than 85% and less than 95% or is crossing growth percentiles in an upward direction, it is time for a more in-depth look at eating and activity. This is especially true in relation to emotional eating,

increases in sedentary time, and poor food choices—all of which can contribute to the risk of becoming a young adult with obesity. In addition to reemphasizing concepts covered previously, parents and families may need to give increased attention to their ability to provide and influence nutrition and activity by focusing on *energy balance, structure,* and *modeling healthy behavior* (discussed next).

Energy Balance

- Ask the question, "How has the energy balance shifted?" (eg, increased snacking after school, more screen time, late-night eating).
- The question "Why has it shifted?" may be even more important.
- After-school eating may become an increasing problem when young adolescents are not participating in after-school activities.
- Sports participation may fall off as a result of increased team competitiveness or the adolescent's self-consciousness about skill level or body image.
- Increased eating linked to boredom, stress, anxiety, or depression may also occur.
- Shifts in meal patterns, with breakfast skipping and late-night eating, may have altered calorie balance.
- Activity may be harder to sustain with increased demands of homework and less spontaneous activity opportunities.
- Identifying the reasons for the shift in energy balance can help parents and families target areas for change.

Structure

- Meal timing and structure can become more difficult at this age because of breakfast skipping, early school lunches, and late-night eating.
- Because of a shift in sleep schedule, adolescents may find it difficult to get up, get ready for school, and eat a meal. Simplifying breakfast may help. Prefilling a bowl with cereal or putting cereal in a plastic bag for eating on the go may make eating breakfast easy enough for the young adolescent to accomplish.
- It is important to have a plan for the after-school snack. Preparing a snack in advance that the child and parents agree on may limit the foraging that can occur.
- Predictable family meals are still important; it is hard for the teen to manage hunger if dinner can occur unpredictably, for example, at 5:00 pm one day and 8:00 pm the next.
- It is important to carry meal and activity structure through the weekend and on vacations. These times are often seen as downtimes when the rigor of school schedules can

be loosened; however, meal and activity structure often become disorganized, and this can lead to overeating and underactivity.

Modeling Healthy Behavior

- Modeling healthy behavior takes on a new twist—parents are still major influences on their adolescents, but peer groups and media are also giving these children messages about eating and activity that may be unhealthy.
- Fad diets are appealing to young teens concerned about their weight. Parents need to be on the lookout for these and emphasize healthy approaches to weight control.
- It is important that parents stay positive and supportive as they try helping their teen with weight issues and continue to take a family-based approach to healthy nutrition and activity without targeting the teen as the only one who has to change.
- Parents can also help with some media education for teens concerning food advertisements and how eating and activity are portrayed in the media.
- Helping teens look their best and strengthening their competencies, whether academic achievement, club participation, individual hobbies, or positive personality traits, are important buffers for the negative self-image that can develop when a young teen is struggling with weight.

9.4 Treatment

When an early adolescent's BMI is greater than 95% and you are dealing with excess adiposity, it is time to initiate a focused treatment strategy. It is important to review the issues discussed in the previous 2 sections because these are the building blocks of good nutrition and activity habits. But you will also have to focus on the barriers to change that may have prevented parents, families, and teens from implementing these strategies.

A useful way to begin is to obtain a family history focused on obesity and obesity-related comorbidities. This can serve to emphasize the health risks involved and the necessity of taking early action once obesity is identified.

9.5 Family History

The family history (Table 9.2) provides information on obesity and obesity-related comorbidity risk and serves as a starting point to discuss the child's BMI.

If parents are obese or have a history of obesity, they may want to relate their personal struggles. Often the desire to avoid these same struggles in their child motivates parents to make family changes in nutrition and activity.

Table 9.2. Family History, Early Adolescent

Complete or update this family history targeted toward obesity and related comorbidities.

	Mother	Father	Maternal Grandmother	Maternal Grandfather	Paternal Grandmother	Paternal Grandfather	Sibling 1	Sibling 2
Obesity	☐	☐	☐	☐	☐	☐	☐	☐
Cardiovascular disease	☐	☐	☐	☐	☐	☐	☐	☐
High blood pressure	☐	☐	☐	☐	☐	☐	☐	☐
Stroke	☐	☐	☐	☐	☐	☐	☐	☐
High cholesterol	☐	☐	☐	☐	☐	☐	☐	☐
High triglyceride level	☐	☐	☐	☐	☐	☐	☐	☐
Type 1 or 2 diabetes	☐	☐	☐	☐	☐	☐	☐	☐
Liver disease	☐	☐	☐	☐	☐	☐	☐	☐
Bariatric surgery	☐	☐	☐	☐	☐	☐	☐	☐
Polycystic ovarian syndrome	☐	☐	☐	☐	☐	☐	☐	☐
Binge eating disorder	☐	☐	☐	☐	☐	☐	☐	☐
	☐	☐	☐	☐	☐	☐	☐	☐
	☐	☐	☐	☐	☐	☐	☐	☐

9.6 Review of Systems

The review of systems can also serve as a point of departure to discuss obesity-related comorbidities, pointing out particular risk factors as they relate to increasing BMI.

- Skin: Acanthosis nigricans, striae, cervical fat pad
- Head, eyes, ears, nose, and throat (HEENT): Headache, blurred vision
- Lungs: Snoring, sleep disturbance, sleep apnea, restless sleep, sleep position, daytime tiredness, napping, asthma, shortness of breath or subjective chest tightness during exercise, cough after exercise
- Cardiac: Murmur
- Abdomen: Gastroesophageal reflux, stomach pain, nausea or vomiting after eating
- Musculoskeletal: Limping, hip pain, knee pain
- Development: School problems, learning difficulties, attention problems
- Psychosocial: Depression, anxiety, behavior problems

9.7 Physical Examination

- Height
- Weight
- BMI + previous BMI measurements
- BMI %
- Blood pressure
- General: Dysmorphic features, poor linear growth, developmental delay
- Skin: Skin picking, acanthosis nigricans, dermatitis in skinfolds, striae, cervical fat pad
- HEENT: Funduscopic examination for papilledema, tonsillar hypertrophy
- Cardiopulmonary: Murmur, wheezing
- Abdominal: Hepatomegaly
- Musculoskeletal: Range of motion, genu varum, limp, hip or knee pain
- Genitourinary: Tanner stage

9.8 Family Constellation and Social History

Information about the family can provide a starting point for discussing how nutrition and activity decisions are made and how changes might take place.

- Who is living at home with the early adolescent?
- How is the early adolescent spending time before and after school?
- Is someone other than the early adolescent responsible for meal or snack preparation?

9.9 Parenting Questions

Parenting styles and skills are important when families are trying to make changes in lifestyle. The questions in Table 9.3 may help you focus on family factors that can facilitate or hinder change.

9.10 Parenting and Teen Touch Points

Parenting touch points focus on helping families initiate and maintain change by helping them believe change can occur, identify the change needed, value the outcome of the change, know how to change, and have the energy to change and sustain the change.

- ***Believe that change can occur.*** Early teens may believe that change is too hard; they are often very aware that not everyone in their peer group needs to focus so acutely on eating and activity patterns. Acknowledging the difficulties and staying positive about what change can accomplish is important for parents. Bringing up areas in the teen's life where he or she is successful, such as doing well academically, having a musical talent, or being a good friend, can help the teen focus on what he or she can do.

Table 9.3. Parenting Questions, Early Adolescent

	Never	Seldom	Sometimes	Often	Always
Parents set clear and simple expectations and limits.	☐	☐	☐	☐	☐
Parents set boundaries and give their young teen choices within those boundaries.	☐	☐	☐	☐	☐
Parents have developmentally appropriate goals for the young teen.	☐	☐	☐	☐	☐
Parents model healthy nutrition and activity.	☐	☐	☐	☐	☐
Parents limit the availability of high-sugar or high-fat snacks in the home.	☐	☐	☐	☐	☐
Parents maintain an abundant supply of fruits and vegetables in the home.	☐	☐	☐	☐	☐

- *Identify the change.* Parents may be concerned and very explicit about eating behaviors and attitudes they want to see their young teen change. It is important to provide background and education to parents and young teens about the etiology of obesity and factors that affect energy balance. Identifying needed changes can lead to a discussion of what is possible in the current family setting. Parents and teens frequently want to attempt to change everything at once, and it is worth emphasizing the incremental nature of lifestyle change and the importance of choosing achievable goals.

- *Value the outcome.* Issues of health, family history of obesity-related comorbidities, and their teen's declining self-esteem are often uppermost in parents' minds. Young teens may be much more concerned about fitting in with their peers in terms of body type, eating style, and clothing selections. It is important to take some time and let the parents and teens share each other's concerns. Parents can be reassured that they have legitimate interests in and responsibility for their teen's health. However, the teen's concerns also need to be validated and seen as developmentally appropriate.

- *Know how to change.* The techniques of establishing structure, such as helping the teen organize after-school time, planning ahead for family and social events, and helping create activity opportunities, are important. At this age parents can provide the structure and encouragement for change. Communicating how to make the desired change and troubleshooting when things do not go as expected are keys to supporting the young teen. Structured times for parents and the teen to touch base can be important. This is a good time to initiate family meetings to establish house rules, express feelings and thoughts, and make positive lifestyle changes. Parents need to maintain and help teenagers follow through on a schedule of meals, activity, homework, and chores. Input from the teen gives him or her a sense of control and engages him or her in following through on discussed changes.

- *Have the energy to change and sustain.* Time with parents is still important, and shared activities, family meals, and car rides can be venues for sharing thoughts and feelings on how things are going. Parents need to be alert for the times when teens want to talk as well. When setbacks occur (eg, eating more than intended at a party), it helps if parents discuss these calmly and ask what different choices the young teen might have made, how the parent could help, and what to do next time.

9.11 Developmental Touch Point

In this age group, children strive to fit in with defined peer groups through cooperation and competition. They are absorbed in their bodily changes as they approach puberty. Concern about being different from their peers can be a painful topic, and parents need to help the early adolescent understand the concept of individual nutrition and activity needs.

During early to mid-adolescence, more formal thought processes with the ability to evaluate logic with deductive reasoning appear. Teens grow more emancipated from the adults in their lives and follow their peer groups.

9.12 Nutrition and Activity Questions and Approaches

Parents can answer the nutrition and activity questions in Table 9.4, which can provide a focal point for targeted intervention (Table 9.5) in a brief encounter. Questions answered "Often" or "Always" can be targeted first for change.

9.13 A Case in Point: AN

AN is an 11-year-old African American boy who comes to you for his yearly school physical. He is being raised by his maternal grandparents, and his grandmother says she has no specific health concerns about AN but notes that his grandfather has diabetes and hypertension, as do several of his great aunts and uncles.

The grandmother answers "Often" to feels bad about self (question 28), "Always" to chooses unhealthy snacks (question 24), "Often" or "Always" to eats in front of the television or computer (question 10), "Often" to prefers quiet activities and seems unmotivated to get active (questions 3 and 4).

During the review of systems, AN notes that he cannot keep up with his peers when playing, but other than that he has no physical complaints. He had a tonsillectomy and adenoidectomy at 8 years of age and no longer snores. He is having some difficulty in the 6th grade with math and reading. He also gets teased and occasionally bullied by classmates.

His weight is 145 lb (65.8 kg), and his height is 4′10″ (147.3 cm), giving him a BMI of 30.3 (>95%). His blood pressure is elevated at 124/78 mm Hg. Upon physical examination you note mild acanthosis nigricans of his neck and axilla. His Tanner stage is 2. His waist circumference is 30″ (76.2 cm).

His laboratory studies show that his triglyceride level is elevated at 185 mg/dL, his insulin level is 2.5 times the laboratory normal at 45 μU/L, and his HDL cholesterol is low (30 mg/dL).

His combination of abdominal obesity, elevated triglyceride levels, low HDL cholesterol levels, and increased blood pressure meet the criteria for metabolic syndrome. His elevated insulin and family history of type 2 diabetes and acanthosis nigricans further raise your concerns about associated abnormalities, such as impaired glucose tolerance or diabetes and nonalcoholic steatohepatitis.

You order a 2-hour glucose tolerance test (GTT) and find that his glucose at 2 hours is 155 mg/dL, which indicates impaired glucose tolerance. His liver function studies are within normal limits.

Table 9.4. Nutrition and Activity Questions, Early Adolescent

These questions can be answered by the parents and provide a focal point for targeted intervention in a brief encounter. First have the parents answer these questions about the presence or absence of behaviors that promote weight gain; then refer to Table 9.5.

Please answer the following for the statements below: Does your adolescent …?

	Never	Seldom	Sometimes	Often	Always
1. Not have time to participate in physical activity every day.	☐	☐	☐	☐	☐
2. Not have a favorite way to be active (ie, sports team, riding bikes, etc).	☐	☐	☐	☐	☐
3. Prefer quiet activities.	☐	☐	☐	☐	☐
4. Seem unmotivated to get active.	☐	☐	☐	☐	☐
5. Lack interest in activities with friends or extracurricular activities.	☐	☐	☐	☐	☐
6. Stay indoors after school.	☐	☐	☐	☐	☐
7. Sleep less than 8 or more than 11 hours a night.	☐	☐	☐	☐	☐
8. Watch television or play with computer/video games in his or her bedroom.	☐	☐	☐	☐	☐
9. Spend more than 2 hours watching television, playing video games, or using a computer each day.	☐	☐	☐	☐	☐
10. Eat in front of the television or computer.	☐	☐	☐	☐	☐
11. Eat late at night or right before bed.	☐	☐	☐	☐	☐
12. Eat when bored.	☐	☐	☐	☐	☐
13. Demand certain food or snacks.	☐	☐	☐	☐	☐
14. Become angry when demands for food are not met.	☐	☐	☐	☐	☐
15. Sneak or hide food.	☐	☐	☐	☐	☐
16. Refuse to eat any vegetables.	☐	☐	☐	☐	☐
17. Refuse to eat any fruits.	☐	☐	☐	☐	☐
18. Refuse to eat any dairy foods (yogurt, cheese, milk).	☐	☐	☐	☐	☐
19. Skip breakfast.	☐	☐	☐	☐	☐
20. Have trouble eating a healthy lunch and snacks at school.	☐	☐	☐	☐	☐
21. Frequent the school vending machines for snacks and drinks.	☐	☐	☐	☐	☐
22. Eat more than 1 snack between meals a day.	☐	☐	☐	☐	☐
23. Graze between meals.	☐	☐	☐	☐	☐
24. Choose unhealthy snacks.	☐	☐	☐	☐	☐
25. Overeat after school.	☐	☐	☐	☐	☐
26. Drink juice or sugared beverages between meals.	☐	☐	☐	☐	☐
27. Eat meals alone.	☐	☐	☐	☐	☐
28. Feel bad about himself or herself.	☐	☐	☐	☐	☐
29. Eat at fast-food restaurants.	☐	☐	☐	☐	☐

Table 9.5. Nutrition and Activity Approaches, Early Adolescent

Questions answered "Often" or "Always" in Table 9.4 can be targeted first for change. Using these specific questions, ask the parent, "How willing are you to…?"

Please answer the following for the statements below: How willing are you to…?

	Impossible	Could Try	Could Do Sometimes	Could Do Often	Easy
1. Schedule time for your teen to be active every day.	☐	☐	☐	☐	☐
2. Find extracurricular activities your teen will enjoy and add activity to his or her lifestyle.	☐	☐	☐	☐	☐
3. Plan an activity you can do with your teen.	☐	☐	☐	☐	☐
4. Have your teen partner with a family member or friend in a physical activity.	☐	☐	☐	☐	☐
5. Encourage a peer group activity to be part of after-school time.	☐	☐	☐	☐	☐
6. Develop a plan to increase sleep for your teen.	☐	☐	☐	☐	☐
7. Move televisions, computers, and video games out of your teen's bedroom.	☐	☐	☐	☐	☐
8. Reduce time spent watching television, playing video games, and using the computer.	☐	☐	☐	☐	☐
9. Encourage activities other than screen time, such as playing board games, reading, and doing chores.	☐	☐	☐	☐	☐
10. Turn off the television during meals and snacks.	☐	☐	☐	☐	☐
11. Help your teen find activities to do instead of munching.	☐	☐	☐	☐	☐
12. Work with your teen on a plan to stop sneaking food.	☐	☐	☐	☐	☐
13. Offer vegetables at meals and as snacks.	☐	☐	☐	☐	☐
14. Offer fruit at meals and as snacks.	☐	☐	☐	☐	☐
15. Offer dairy products at meals and as snacks.	☐	☐	☐	☐	☐
16. Schedule time for breakfast each day.	☐	☐	☐	☐	☐
17. Help your teen prepare healthier school snacks ahead of time.	☐	☐	☐	☐	☐
18. Pack a school lunch and snacks; limit extra money for vending machines.	☐	☐	☐	☐	☐
19. Schedule regular meals.	☐	☐	☐	☐	☐
20. Keep only healthy snacks in the house.	☐	☐	☐	☐	☐
21. Change from juice or soda to water between meals.	☐	☐	☐	☐	☐
22. Eat meals together.	☐	☐	☐	☐	☐
23. Limit how often you buy/serve fast food.	☐	☐	☐	☐	☐

Problem #1: Metabolic Syndrome, Increased Risk for Type 2 Diabetes

This increases the emphasis that needs to be placed on diet and activity management for weight loss and will intensify your behavioral intervention.

Problem #2: Inactivity

- **Parenting dilemma: Lack of motivation**
  The grandmother understands that AN needs to increase his activity but worries about the neighborhood's safety.

She also notes that although he seems to love basketball, he refuses to try out for the community center basketball team.

- **Strategy: Create boundaries and allow choice**
  You explore community and family resources with the grandmother to evaluate activity options. She notes that a Boys & Girls Clubs of America location is close by and that she is willing to take him after school and pick him up. She also says that his 13-year-old cousin lives nearby and he could come over and shoot baskets with AN. There is also a Boy Scout troop at their church that has activities

every weekend. You encourage the grandmother to let AN know that activity is not optional but that he can choose among these possibilities.

Problem #3: Snacking

- #### Parenting dilemma: Snacking

  The grandparents want to treat AN to snacks because he is a good kid and does well at school and sometimes feels bad about himself. The grandmother is glad AN is doing well in school and not getting in any trouble. She likes to have snacks around that AN enjoys.

- #### Strategy: Substitutions and positive reinforcement

  You give the grandmother a list of low-calorie snacks she can have at home (see Table 7.6 on page 49). You also explore with the grandmother and AN other ways she can reinforce AN's good behavior and school achievements. Praise, one-on-one time with her, and increased privileges, such as a later bedtime on weekends, are some suggestions.

Problem #4: Low Self-esteem

- #### Parenting dilemma: Peer teasing

  The grandmother is worried about AN. She wants him to feel better but does not know exactly how to help him. She suspects he is being teased, but he will not talk about what is going on at school.

- #### Strategy: New activities and alternative peer groups

  You ask AN if he is being teased, and he says that he is. His usual response to teasing is to ignore it, but you can tell it really bothers him. You reinforce ignoring the teasing and ask specifically about any physical pushing or hitting. He denies any fighting.

  You begin to explore AN's interests and competencies. You encourage his grandmother to pursue the activities you discussed previously to give him an alternative peer group. You ask the grandmother to check in with AN's teacher about the teasing. You encourage AN to try something new and ask him to report back at his next visit.

Second Visit

AN returns to a scheduled visit in 1 month. His weight is down 2 lb (0.9 kg). His height is unchanged. His blood pressure decreased to 120/75 mm Hg, and he lost 1″ (2.54 cm) from his waist circumference. The grandmother provides him with lower-calorie snacks, which he accepts. He reports that he goes to the Boys & Girls Clubs of America and plays basketball after school. The grandmother notes that he seems happier and more cooperative at home.

You congratulate AN and the grandmother on the changes they made and schedule him for another visit in a month.

Third Visit

AN lost another 2.5 lb (1.1 kg) and 2″ (5.08 cm) from his waist, and his blood pressure is down to 118/68 mm Hg. He is more talkative and is telling you about his basketball buddies. You order a fasting glucose, insulin, and lipid profile.

When laboratory results come back, his insulin is 25 µU/L (mildly elevated), his triglyceride level is 150 mg/dL, and his HDL is 35 mg/dL.

You schedule him to come back in 1 month and plan to repeat his 2-hour GTT at that visit.

References

1. Rogol AD, Roemmich JN, Clark PA. Growth at puberty. *J Adolesc Health.* 2002;31(suppl 6):192–200
2. Hannon TS, Janosky J, Arslanian SA. Longitudinal study of physiologic insulin resistance and metabolic changes of puberty. *Pediatr Res.* 2006;60(6):759–763. Epub 2006 Oct 25
3. Dolan LM, Bean J, D'Alessio D, et al. Frequency of abnormal carbohydrate metabolism and diabetes in a population-based screening of adolescents. *J Pediatr.* 2005;146:751–758
4. Reinehr T, Wabitsch M, Kleber M, de Sousa G, Denzer C. Parental diabetes, pubertal stage, and extreme obesity are the main risk factors for prediabetes in children and adolescents: a simple risk score to identify children at risk for prediabetes. *Diabetes.* 2009;10:395–400
5. Goran MI, Gower BA. Longitudinal study on pubertal insulin resistance. *Diabetes.* 2001;50:2444–2450
6. Remsberg KE, Demerath EW, Schubert CM, Chumlea WC, Sun SS, Siervogel RM. Early menarche and the development of cardiovascular disease risk factors in adolescent girls: the Fels Longitudinal Study. *J Clin Endocrinol Metab.* 2005;90:2718–2724
7. Wang Y. Is obesity associated with early sexual maturation? A comparison of the association in American boys versus girls. *Pediatrics.* 2002;110:903–910
8. Brage S, Wedderkopp N, Ekelund U, et al. Objectively measured physical activity correlates with indices of insulin resistance in Danish children. The European Youth Heart Study (EYHS). *Int J Obes Relat Metab Disord.* 2004;28:1503–1508
9. Thompson AM, Baxter-Jones AD, Mirwald RL, Bailey DA. Comparison of physical activity in male and female children: does maturation matter? *Med Sci Sports Exerc.* 2003;35:1684–1690
10. Centers for Disease Control and Prevention. School Health Policies and Programs Study (SHPPS) 2006. *J Sch Health.* 2007;27(8)
11. Trager S. Preventing weight problems before they become too hard to solve. *The State Education Standard.* 2004;5:13–20
12. Rauner RR, Walters RW, Avery M, Wanser TJ. Evidence that aerobic fitness is more salient than weight status in predicting standardized math and reading outcomes in fourth- through eighth-grade students. *J Pediatr.* Epub 2013 Mar 1
13. Vandewater EA, Shim MS, Caplovitz AG. Linking obesity and activity level with children's television and video game use. *J Adolesc.* 2004;27:71–85

14. Pate RR, Baranowski T, Dowda M, Trost SG. Tracking of physical activity in young children. *Med Sci Sports Exerc.* 1996;28:92–96

15. Kvaavik E, Tell GS, Klepp KI. Predictors and tracking of body mass index from adolescence into adulthood: follow-up of 18 to 20 years in the Oslo Youth Study. *Arch Pediatr Adolesc Med.* 2003;157:1212–1218

16. Kohen-Avramoglu R, Theriault A, Adeli K. Emergence of the metabolic syndrome in childhood: an epidemiological overview and mechanistic link to dyslipidemia. *Clin Biochem.* 2003;36:413–420

17. Hauner H. Insulin resistance and the metabolic syndrome— a challenge of the new millennium. *Eur J Clin Nutr.* 2002;56 (suppl 1):S25–S29

18. Sinaiko AR, Donahue RP, Jacobs DR, Prineas RJ. Relation of weight and rate of increase in weight during childhood and adolescence to body size, blood pressure, fasting insulin, and lipids in young adults. The Minneapolis Children's Blood Pressure Study. *Circulation.* 1999;99:1471–1476

19. Sinha R, Fisch G, Teague B, et al. Prevalence of impaired glucose tolerance among children and adolescents with marked obesity. *N Engl J Med.* 2002;346:802–810

20. Eisenmann JC, Welk GJ, Wickel EE, Blair SN, Aerobics Center Longitudinal Study. Stability of variables associated with the metabolic syndrome from adolescence to adulthood: the Aerobics Center Longitudinal Study. *Am J Hum Biol.* 2004;16:690–696

21. D'Angelo SL, Omar HA. Parenting adolescents. *Int J Adoles Med Health.* 2003;15:11–19

10 Middle Adolescent

10.1 Background

Obesity-related comorbidities increase as obesity persists into adolescence. Sleep apnea and hypertension are commonly diagnosed and are linked to body mass index (BMI). Features of the metabolic syndrome, such as hyperinsulinemia, obesity, hypertension, hyperlipidemia, and dyslipidemia are much more common in adolescents who are overweight.[1] Type 2 diabetes is also increased in obese adolescents with rates exceeding those of type 1 diabetes in this population. There is a normal increase in insulin resistance at the onset of puberty (Tanner stages 1-2), reaching a peak mid-puberty (Tanner stage 3) that coincides with peak height velocity and returns to almost prepubertal levels at the completion of puberty (Tanner stage 5). A strong correlation with insulin resistance and BMI persists throughout puberty.[2,3] In one study, up to 21% of obese adolescents had impaired glucose tolerance,[4] and in another, impaired glucose tolerance was identified in 35% of adolescents with both obesity and a positive family history of type 2 diabetes.[5] Obesity is clearly a risk factor for type 2 diabetes in childhood,[6] paralleling the increasing incidence in adults[7]; therefore, a focus on obesity treatment in this age group is prevention of obesity-related comorbidities.

Elevated BMI in adolescence, even with normalization of weight as an adult had an independent association with the onset of coronary artery disease in young adulthood.[8]

Elevated BMI is also related to depression; adolescents with obesity who have the highest depression scores had the greatest increase in BMI.[9] Unhealthy weight control behaviors are associated with obesity in both boys and girls. Low life satisfaction for both genders and negative affect and body size dissatisfaction in boys were associated with unhealthy weight control behaviors.[10]

Energy balance continues to be problematic in the mid-adolescent age group. Although recommendations for exercise include 60 minutes of exercise a day,[11] some measures suggest that as few as 30% of teens are meeting this goal.[9] Girls, older adolescents, minority adolescents, and disad-

vantaged teens are less likely to meet this baseline requirement. Healthy People 2010 set a goal that the proportion of adolescents who watch television for less than 2 hours per day would be 75%, but as of 1999, only 57% of adolescents met this goal.[11] Adolescents with obesity have been found to have limited exercise tolerance because of the greater oxygen demand of their excess mass.[12] Exercise recommendations for these adolescents should be tailored to allow for activities that can be sustained without causing fatigue caused by lactate accumulation.[12]

10.2 Prevention: Talking to Parents and Teens (BALANCE)

Prevention touch points for parents and teens include **belief, assessment, lifestyle, activity, nutrition, child/adolescent,** and **environment** (BALANCE).

*B*elief

- Parents of middle adolescents often believe that their teens are old enough to take charge of their own nutrition and activity and conversely may complain that their teens are unmotivated to do so. However, people of all ages do better with family support, and nutrition and activity should continue to be discussed openly within the family.

- In enlisting family support, teens and parents often respond to the idea of the parent as coach, and parents need to be encouraged to provide support and positive role modeling of good decision making when it comes to eating and activity.

- Parents may tend to generalize from one set of behaviors to another; for example, if the child is a good student, parents may assume that it should be easy for the teen to take charge of making healthy nutrition and activity decisions. Parents may need to be reminded that maintaining a healthy lifestyle is tough even for adults and that a family-based approach has the best chance of success.

Assessment

- Going over normal growth and development and sharing height, weight, and BMI measurements are important ways of normalizing the changes the teen is experiencing.
- Providing a short list of some problem behaviors that can interfere with healthy eating and activity can be helpful to introduce the concept of self-assessment (Table 10.1). Focusing on healthy lifestyle behavior rather than "weight loss" can help the adolescent and family avoid a sense of blame and/or guilt.

Lifestyle

- It may be helpful at this point to have the teen help with an environmental assessment of nutrition and activity. Going through a kitchen inventory with parents and discussing healthy and unhealthy choices can foster communication and dialogue.
- In the same way, getting together and evaluating what is available inside and outside the home to support activity and what gets in the way of being active can create dialogue and lead to healthier changes.
- Activity alternatives in the community can also be explored together. Parents can partner with their teens as they choose among activities that are within the family's financial and time constraints. This keeps the focus on family partnership in determining healthy eating and activity.

Activity

- At this point in their school and social lives, physical activity often is on the decline for most adolescents, with options for participation in sports giving way to competitive activities in which relatively few teens can take an active role.
- Screen time may correspondingly increase, and many teens are at a loss to come up with alternative activities. This is where parents and families can try to offer creative alternatives to electronic media. Sports that the teen may not have tried before, such as tennis, golf, karate, or swimming, can be offered. Part-time jobs, volunteer work, hobbies, and clubs are good alternatives to screen time.

Nutrition

Breakfast is a meal that is often omitted during the teen years. In a study of adolescent eating patterns, the 26% of adolescents classified as inconsistent breakfast consumers had significantly higher BMIs and lower iron intake relative to consistent breakfast consumers.[13]

- Lack of time, not being hungry, and an early lunch period are frequently cited reasons to skip breakfast. Troubleshoot possible breakfast options together, such as
  - Portioning out cereal in a small plastic bag in the evening to be readily available while getting ready for school
  - If healthy choices are available, taking advantage of the school breakfast program
  - Setting up a breakfast bar with fruit and a glass of milk as a way to transition to a more standard breakfast
  - Providing low-fat yogurt with fruit
  - Avoiding toaster pastries, liquid breakfasts, leftovers, and fast-food breakfasts

Child/Adolescent

- Most adolescents move through the teen years without major difficulties[14] and are engaged in the process of negotiating more independent relationships with their parents.
- Parental warmth and involvement are found to increase adolescents' response to parental influence. When these parental traits are combined with structure and support, the transition to self-regulation occurs more smoothly.[15]

Environment

- Teens' nutrition and activity environments expand beyond home and school to include social gatherings, workplaces, and community settings.
- Teens need to continue to develop assessment and decision-making skills that will allow them to make healthy choices as they move outside the more or less controlled environments of the family and school.
- Providing information about nutritional content of fast foods, discussing how to handle eating at buffets and social events, and helping the teen look for opportunities to increase physical activity as part of a daily routine are all issues that foster critical thinking about eating and activity.

Table 10.1. Self-assessment Questions for Teens		
I eat in front of the television or computer.	☐ Yes	☐ No
There are times when I skip meals.	☐ Yes	☐ No
I snack at night before bedtime.	☐ Yes	☐ No
I watch television or use the computer more than 2 hours each day.	☐ Yes	☐ No
I find it hard to exercise daily.	☐ Yes	☐ No

10.3 Intervention

When an adolescent has a BMI greater than the 85% but less than 95% or is crossing growth percentiles in an upward direction, this is the time for a more in-depth look at eating and activity, especially related to unregulated eating, increased sedentary time, and poor food choices—all of which can contribute to the risk of becoming an adult with obesity. In addition to reemphasizing concepts covered previously, parents and families may need to give increased attention to their ability to provide and influence nutrition and activity by focusing on *energy balance, structure,* and *modeling healthy behavior* (discussed next).

Energy Balance

Unregulated eating and activity can quickly undermine energy balance at a time when the growth spurt peak may be waning. Overdoing screen time, snacking late at night, and skipping meals all can contribute to weight gain. It is important to grasp the teen's daily diet and activity, which may or may not correspond to the rest of the family's routine. Many adolescents get up to one-third of their calories from snacks, which add calories and compromise nutritious eating at meals. Grazing after school until after dinner is frequently a cause of increased weight gain. Eating from boredom, stress, or depression is also a cause weight gain. Late-night eating, usually associated with screen time, can also lead to decreased hunger in the morning and further disrupt eating patterns. Unregulated eating can veer into binging and feelings of loss of control over eating, leading to low self-esteem.

Structure

Structured eating and activity continue to be important. At this point parents can support the adolescent by picking out a few areas to focus on to reinstitute healthy eating and activity. Family dinners, an after-school snack prepared in advance, and exercise equipment at home are some ways parents can support their adolescent's efforts. Working with their teen on decision making, creating a schedule for free time, and working on ideas for healthy meals can help create positive communication about food and exercise. Part-time jobs, volunteer work, clubs, and activities are also ways of adding structure to the teen's after-school time and mitigate prolonged screen time with its attendant eating.

Modeling Healthy Behavior

Adolescents may get quite a bit of information about diet and exercise from their peers. Dietary routines that may seem like they make sense, such as skipping meals or using dietary supplements, are common. Helping adolescents sift through information about diets and drugs is one of the important components of enhancing decision making.

10.4 Treatment

When a teen's BMI is greater than the 95% and you are dealing with excess adiposity, it is time to initiate a focused treatment strategy. It is important to review the issues discussed in the previous 2 sections because these are the building blocks of good nutrition and activity habits. But you will also have to focus on the barriers to change that may have prevented parents, families, and teens from implementing these strategies. Many obese adolescents experience obesity-related comorbidities, and screening for these becomes even more crucial.

A useful way to begin is to obtain a family history focused on obesity-related comorbidities. This can serve to emphasize the health risks involved and the necessity of taking early action once obesity is identified.

10.5 Family History

Family history (Table 10.2) should be updated at this time, with attention to obesity-related comorbidities, the family weight trajectory, eating behaviors, and a mental health diagnosis.

10.6 Review of Systems

The review of systems can also serve as a point of departure to discuss obesity-related comorbidities, pointing out particular risk factors as they relate to increasing BMI.

- Skin: Acanthosis nigricans, striae, acne, hirsutism
- Head, eyes, ears, nose, and throat (HEENT): Headache, snoring, sleep disturbance, daytime napping, attention problems, poor school functioning, irritability, visual disturbance
- Lungs: Asthma, shortness of breath during exercise, cough at end of exercise, decreased exercise tolerance
- Cardiac: Hypertension, hyperlipidemia, chest pain, dizziness or shortness of breath during exercise
- Abdomen: Gastroesophageal reflux, stomach pain before or after eating, chronic diarrhea or constipation, morning anorexia, right upper quadrant discomfort or pain
- Musculoskeletal: Limping, hip pain or decreased motion, knee pain, bowing, ankle pain

Table 10.2. Family History, Middle Adolescent

Complete or update this family history targeted toward obesity and related comorbidities.

	Mother	Father	Maternal Grandmother	Maternal Grandfather	Paternal Grandmother	Paternal Grandfather	Sibling 1	Sibling 2
Obesity	☐	☐	☐	☐	☐	☐	☐	☐
Cardiovascular disease	☐	☐	☐	☐	☐	☐	☐	☐
High blood pressure	☐	☐	☐	☐	☐	☐	☐	☐
Stroke	☐	☐	☐	☐	☐	☐	☐	☐
High cholesterol	☐	☐	☐	☐	☐	☐	☐	☐
High triglyceride level	☐	☐	☐	☐	☐	☐	☐	☐
Type 1 or 2 diabetes	☐	☐	☐	☐	☐	☐	☐	☐
Liver disease	☐	☐	☐	☐	☐	☐	☐	☐
Bariatric surgery	☐	☐	☐	☐	☐	☐	☐	☐
Polycystic ovarian syndrome	☐	☐	☐	☐	☐	☐	☐	☐
Binge eating disorder	☐	☐	☐	☐	☐	☐	☐	☐
	☐	☐	☐	☐	☐	☐	☐	☐
	☐	☐	☐	☐	☐	☐	☐	☐

- Genitourinary: Enuresis, delayed pubertal development, vaginal infections, irregular or absent menses
- Psychological: Symptoms of depression, anxiety, low self-esteem, self-injury or suicidal ideation, sleep disturbance

10.7 Physical Examination

- Height
- Weight
- BMI + previous BMI measurements
- Blood pressure
- General: Height deceleration or poor linear growth, centripetal or visceral fat distribution
- Skin: Acanthosis nigricans (neck, axilla, groin), acne, cervical fat pad, striae, hirsutism
- HEENT: Funduscopic examination for papilledema, tonsillar hypertrophy, thyroid enlargement
- Cardiopulmonary: Wheezing, poor ventilation, heart murmur
- Abdominal: Hepatomegaly
- Musculoskeletal: Range of motion, genu varum, limp, hip or knee pain, ankle pain
- Genitourinary: Tanner stage

10.8 Family Constellation and Social History

Information about the family can provide a starting point for discussing how nutrition and activity decisions are made and how changes might take place.

- Who is living at home with the adolescent?
- Who is providing the adolescent with meals and snacks?
- Who is purchasing food for meals and snacks?
- Who is eating with the adolescent at meals?

10.9 Parenting Questions

Parenting styles and skills are important when families are trying to make lifestyle changes. The questions in Table 10.3 may help you focus on family factors that may facilitate or hinder change.

10.10 Parenting and Teen Touch Points

Parenting and teen touch points focus on helping families initiate and maintain change by helping them believe change can occur, identify the change needed, value the outcome of the change, know how to change, and have the energy to change and sustain the change.

- *Believe that change can occur.* Adolescents who have been struggling with their weight are often discouraged about their ability to make change. Starting slowly, being consis-

Table 10.3. Parenting Questions, Middle Adolescent

	Never	Seldom	Sometimes	Often	Always
Parents set clear expectations and limits.	☐	☐	☐	☐	☐
Parents set boundaries that are consistent and appropriate for an adolescent's development.	☐	☐	☐	☐	☐
Parents provide opportunities for healthy nutrition and activity.	☐	☐	☐	☐	☐

tent, and having a strategy for dealing with setbacks are all important for ensuring success that will contribute to further change. It is important to help dispel negative attitudes in the teen and family that may have been fostered by failed attempts in the past.

■ *Identify the change.* An important component of making change is identifying possibilities for change with the teen and parents, for example, eliminating juice and soda, going to the YMCA after school, or cutting down on screen time. Equally important is identifying which change or changes the teen thinks is doable. Parental support is still crucial. Changes that depend on the adolescent alone have less chance of success than ones that the parents support.

■ *Value the outcome.* It is more important than ever to include the adolescent in discussions of the value of change. Reasons for working on weight can vary from "my parents want me to" to "the prom is coming up" to worry about decreased ability to participate in physical activities. Worry about family history and obesity-related comorbidities might not be uppermost in the minds of adolescents. Reducing the effects of obesity-related comorbidities, such as diabetes or sleep apnea, might also have value if the teen believes that he or she will be directly affected. Validating the teen's concerns as well as those of the parents is helpful. Teens may also be concerned about feelings of their eating being out of control and making bad decisions about food. It is important to start wherever the teen is and use this as the fulcrum for making change.

■ *Know how to change.* Goal setting is important. Clear goals such as eating breakfast every day or walking home from school are important. It is more important to focus on the behaviors that need to change as goals rather than weight loss only. The concept of consistency is very important because adolescents will often discount exceptions, and the extra snack or hour of screen time will be enough to positively shift energy balance. Remind the teen that an extra 150 kcal a day over a year can result in a 15-lb (6.8-kg) weight gain. Persistence is also important, and the concept of permanent change rather than a temporary diet should be addressed.

■ *Have the energy to change and sustain.* Parents are perhaps most important in helping to provide the emotional energy and support for teens to stick to the changes they are trying to make. Providing healthy foods at home, as well as opportunities for activity, such as partnering in a walking program, are some concrete ways parents can help. Other family members can be very important contributors to supporting the teen.

10.11 Developmental Touch Point

Striving for independence and a separate identity from parents is a normal process of adolescence. Adolescents may resist limit setting but respond to mutual goal setting in the family.

10.12 Nutrition and Activity Questions and Approaches

Parents can answer the nutrition and activity questions in Table 10.4, which can provide a focal point for targeted intervention (Table 10.5) in a brief encounter. Questions answered "Often" or "Always" can be targeted first for change.

10.13 A Case in Point: BT

BT is a 13-year-old African American girl whose parents scheduled an appointment with you so that you can talk to BT about her weight and eating. BT's parents are concerned about her weight because of a family history of obesity and diabetes in 3 of the 4 grandparents and BT's father. They are frustrated with BT because she will not listen to what they say.

At the visit, BT's weight is 230 lb (104.3 kg), and her height is 5′4″ (162.6 cm), giving her a BMI of 39.5 (>95%). You ask BT if she is worried about her health, and she says, "No, but my parents are."

On the initial questionnaire, the parents noted that BT always drinks soda between meals (question 23), grazes between meals (question 20), seems depressed (question 28),

Table 10.4. Nutrition and Activity Questions, Middle Adolescent

These questions can be answered by the parents and provide a focal point for targeted intervention in a brief encounter. First have the parents answer these questions about the presence or absence of behaviors that promote weight gain; then refer to Table 10.5.

Please answer the following for the statements below: Does your adolescent…?

	Never	Seldom	Sometimes	Often	Always
1. Not have time to participate in physical activity every day.	☐	☐	☐	☐	☐
2. Not have a favorite way to be active (ie, sports team, riding bikes, etc).	☐	☐	☐	☐	☐
3. Prefer quiet activities.	☐	☐	☐	☐	☐
4. Seem unmotivated to get active.	☐	☐	☐	☐	☐
5. Lack interest in activities with friends or extracurricular activities.	☐	☐	☐	☐	☐
6. Stay indoors after school.	☐	☐	☐	☐	☐
7. Sleep less than 8 or more than 11 hours a night.	☐	☐	☐	☐	☐
8. Watch television or play with computer/video games in his or her bedroom.	☐	☐	☐	☐	☐
9. Spend more than 2 hours watching television, playing video games, or using a computer each day.	☐	☐	☐	☐	☐
10. Eat in front of the television or computer.	☐	☐	☐	☐	☐
11. Eat late at night or right before bed.	☐	☐	☐	☐	☐
12. Eat when bored.	☐	☐	☐	☐	☐
13. Refuse to eat any vegetables.	☐	☐	☐	☐	☐
14. Refuse to eat any fruits.	☐	☐	☐	☐	☐
15. Refuse to eat any dairy foods (yogurt, cheese, milk).	☐	☐	☐	☐	☐
16. Skip breakfast.	☐	☐	☐	☐	☐
17. Have trouble eating a healthy lunch and snacks at school.	☐	☐	☐	☐	☐
18. Frequent the school vending machines for snacks and drinks.	☐	☐	☐	☐	☐
19. Eat more than 1 snack between meals a day.	☐	☐	☐	☐	☐
20. Graze between meals.	☐	☐	☐	☐	☐
21. Choose unhealthy snacks.	☐	☐	☐	☐	☐
22. Overeat after school.	☐	☐	☐	☐	☐
23. Drink juice or sugared beverages between meals.	☐	☐	☐	☐	☐
24. Eat meals alone.	☐	☐	☐	☐	☐
25. Feel bad about himself or herself.	☐	☐	☐	☐	☐
26. Eat at fast-food restaurants.	☐	☐	☐	☐	☐
27. Choose unhealthy foods when eating at restaurants.	☐	☐	☐	☐	☐
28. Seem depressed.	☐	☐	☐	☐	☐

eats at late at night or before bed (question 11), and seems unmotivated to get active (question 4).

Her parents indicate that they "could try" to change from soda or juice to water or diet drinks (approach 20), could "sometimes" provide BT with healthy snack options (approach 19), could "easily" have BT evaluated for depression (approach 24), feel it would be "impossible" to keep BT from eating at night (approach 11), and that it would be "impossible" to motivate BT to get active (approach 1).

During the review of systems, it is learned that BT has acanthosis nigricans and irregular periods and, despite being a very good student, seems unmotivated and depressed to her parents. BT herself says that she frequently feels sad and frustrated about her weight and expresses some anger at her parents for not helping her.

Table 10.5. Nutrition and Activity Approaches, Middle Ado

Questions answered "Often" or "Always" in Table 10.4 can be targeted first for change. Using these specific questions, ask the parent, "How willing are you to…?"

Please answer the following for the statements below: How willing are you to…?

	Impossible	Could Try	Could Do Sometimes	Could Do Often	Easy
1. Schedule time for your teen to be active every day.	☐	☐	☐	☐	☐
2. Find extracurricular activities your teen will enjoy and add activity to his or her lifestyle.	☐	☐	☐	☐	☐
3. Plan an activity you can do with your teen.	☐	☐	☐	☐	☐
4. Have your teen partner with a family member/friend in a physical activity.	☐	☐	☐	☐	☐
5. Encourage a peer group activity to be a part of after-school time.	☐	☐	☐	☐	☐
6. Develop a plan to increase sleep for your teen.	☐	☐	☐	☐	☐
7. Move televisions, video games, and computers out of your teen's bedroom.	☐	☐	☐	☐	☐
8. Reduce time spent watching television, playing video games, and using the computer.	☐	☐	☐	☐	☐
9. Encourage activities other than screen time, such as playing board games, reading, and doing chores.	☐	☐	☐	☐	☐
10. Turn off the television during meals and snacks.	☐	☐	☐	☐	☐
11. Help your teen find activities to do instead of munching.	☐	☐	☐	☐	☐
12. Offer vegetables at meals and as snacks.	☐	☐	☐	☐	☐
13. Offer fruits at meals and as snacks.	☐	☐	☐	☐	☐
14. Offer dairy products at meals and as snacks.	☐	☐	☐	☐	☐
15. Schedule time for breakfast each day.	☐	☐	☐	☐	☐
16. Help your teen prepare healthier school snacks ahead of time.	☐	☐	☐	☐	☐
17. Pack a school lunch and snack; limit extra money for vending machines.	☐	☐	☐	☐	☐
18. Schedule regular meals.	☐	☐	☐	☐	☐
19. Keep only healthy snacks in the house.	☐	☐	☐	☐	☐
20. Change from juice or soda to water between meals.	☐	☐	☐	☐	☐
21. Eat meals together.	☐	☐	☐	☐	☐
22. Limit how often you buy/serve fast food.	☐	☐	☐	☐	☐
23. Learn how to choose healthier options when dining out.	☐	☐	☐	☐	☐
24. Have a pediatrician, counselor, or therapist evaluate for depression.	☐	☐	☐	☐	☐

On physical examination you note that her blood pressure is 130/82 mm Hg and that she has acanthosis nigricans not only of her neck creases but also in her axillae and groin area. The rest of her physical examination is unremarkable.

When her parents initially scheduled her appointment, you ordered laboratory studies. These show an elevated triglyceride level of 215 mg/dL, high-density lipoprotein (HDL) cholesterol at a low level of 30 mg/dL, and an elevated insulin level of 73 µU/dL, with a normal fasting glucose of 85 mg/dL and a hemoglobin A_{1C} of 5.9%. Total cholesterol and liver enzymes are normal.

You note that the combination of elevated blood pressure, increased triglyceride levels, low HDL cholesterol, and high insulin would make the diagnosis of metabolic syndrome. This constellation of signs in addition to the positive family history place her at risk for type 2 diabetes. In addition, the constellation of acanthosis nigricans, insulin resistance, and irregular periods indicate possible polycystic ovary syndrome (PCOS). You order free and total testosterone, dehydroepiandrosterone levels, and sex hormone binding globulin. Her testosterone is elevated at 80 ng/dL, with a normal range of less than 50 mg/dL; her sex hormone binding globulin is decreased; and her dehydroepiandrosterone level is slightly elevated. Her luteinizing hormone level is low, and her follicle-stimulating hormone level is high, strongly indicating the diagnosis of PCOS. You refer her to the endocrinologist for hormonal treatment and possible treatment with metformin hydrochloride and/or hormonal birth control.

Problem #1: Metabolic Syndrome and Polycystic Ovary Syndrome

BT already has both risk factors and comorbidity associated with obesity. You emphasize the health issues to the family (who are already concerned) and BT and offer to work intensely with them to reduce the risk of diabetes and treat the PCOS.

Problem #2: Consumption of Soft Drinks

- **Parenting dilemma: BT won't listen**
  When this issue is mentioned, BT immediately says to her mother, "You keep buying regular soda at the store for yourself and hide it in your room." BT's parents say she is old enough to listen and drink the diet soda they provide for her.

- **Strategy:** Modeling healthy lifestyle
  You go over the family history of diabetes, the parents' concern about BT developing diabetes, and the need for BT's father to follow a diabetic nutrition plan as well. You point out that adolescents do better with their dietary changes if the whole family works with them. BT's mother notes that she can try diet drinks in an effort to help BT.

Problem #3: Possible Depression

- **Parenting dilemma: Possible depression**
  The parents have been worried about BT and wondered if she was depressed. They say she won't talk about it. Their concern is increased because her mother and grandmother have a history of depression and treatment.

- **Strategy: Depression screening and counseling options**

- **You ask the parents to find out what counseling options exist in their medical plan.** You also perform a brief depression inventory and note that currently BT is feeling sad but is not depressed or suicidal. BT's parents agree to counseling and were relieved to have a pathway to address BT's depression.

Problem #4: Grazing Between Meals

- **Parenting dilemma: Out-of-control eating**
  The parents believe BT should be able to control her eating between meals. They are frustrated because she often reaches for snacks while watching television and becomes very irritable and angry when they try to interfere.

- **Strategy: Family-based lifestyle change**
  You explain the high-calorie, sugar, and fat content of most snack foods. You also acknowledge that emotions can be a trigger for snacking. You offer the family a list of lower-calorie snack options to have available for BT and ask her if she would consider trying these. BT says she would if everyone else would have to eat them, too.

  You acknowledge to the family that BT's eating at night and lack of motivation to exercise are very important but that these issues will be tackled at the next visits as the family moves through making healthy lifestyle changes.

  You ask the family to try these strategies and return in 3 to 4 weeks.

Second Visit

BT returns having gained only 0.44 lb (0.2 kg) in 1 month, compared with her previous rate of weight gain of 3.3 lb (1.5 kg) per month. Her blood pressure is 126/80 mm Hg.

- **Problem #1: Metabolic syndrome and PCOS**
  BT saw the endocrinologist, was prescribed birth control pills, and was encouraged in her lifestyle changes with a revisit in 3 months. So far she has not had any problems.

- **Problem #2: Consumption of soft drinks**
  The family successfully converted to drinking water or diet drinks between meals. There is no regular soda at home, and BT offers that when she is out with her friends, she orders a diet soda instead of a regular one.

- **Problem #3: Possible depression**
  The parents found a counselor for BT, and she had 1 visit. When asked about how the session went, BT replies, "OK, I guess." She does say she is willing to go again.

- **Problem #4: Grazing between meals**
  The parents have provided healthy snacks, which BT is eating at home, but she is having trouble making good choices when she is out with friends and at family gatherings.

  You reinforce the good choices she is able to make, noting her slowed weight gain, and you go over strategies to handle exposure to snacks and treats socially.

Problem #5: Lack of Motivation to Be Active

- **Parenting dilemma: Not listening**

  The parents have become very tired of nagging BT to go out and get involved with no results.

- **Strategy: Partnering**

  You ask the parents to start by partnering BT in a family activity such as walking, biking, or bowling once a week.

  You schedule another visit in 4 weeks and order insulin, glucose, and hemoglobin A_{1C} level tests.

Third Visit

BT's weight on this visit is 227 lb (103.0 kg), and her blood pressure is 122/78 mm Hg. She seems happier and is pleased she has lost weight. Her fasting insulin is 40 μU/mL, and her hemoglobin A_{1C} is 5.6%.

- **Problem #1: Metabolic syndrome and PCOS**

  Her insulin is starting to come down, as are her hemoglobin A_{1C} and blood pressure. She continues taking birth control pills and has an endocrinology revisit appointment in the next month.

- **Problem #2: Consumption of soft drinks**

  The consumption of water or diet drinks is now part of the family's routine. BT's father even says he believes his blood sugar levels have improved because of it. BT says she is choosing nonsugared beverages in almost all social situations.

- **Problem #3: Possible depression**

  BT had her second counseling visit and feels things are going OK. She reports decreased feelings of sadness, and her parents feel her mood is improved.

- **Problem #4: Grazing between meals**

  BT seems to be making healthier choices. She noted that one day when she was really upset, she bought candy at the local store but was able to stay with the healthy snacks the rest of the time. You spend a little time talking about the link between emotions and eating, and BT is starting to recognize this connection. You encourage BT to continue making good choices.

- **Problem #5: Lack of motivation to be active**

  BT and her parents report that they enjoy their family activities and actually look forward to them. You explore with the parents and BT what other possible extracurricular activities are available and encourage them to pick several possibilities and see if BT will try one of them.

  You schedule a return visit in 1 month.

References

1. Cook S, Weitzman M, Auinger P, Nguyen M, Dietz WH. Prevalence of a metabolic syndrome phenotype in adolescents: findings from the third National Health and Nutrition Examination Survey, 1988-1994. *Arch Pediatr Adolesc Med.* 2003;157:821–827

2. Moran A, Jacobs DR, Steinberger J, et al. Insulin resistance during puberty. Results from clamp studies in 357 children. *Diabetes.* 1999;48:2039–2044

3. Li C, Ford ES, Zhao G, Mokdad AH. Prevalence of pre-diabetes and its association with clustering of cardiometabolic risk factors and hyperinsulinemia among US adolescents: NHANES 2005–2006. *Diabetes Care.* 2009;32:342–347

4. Sinha R, Fisch G, Teague B, et al. Prevalence of impaired glucose tolerance among children and adolescents with marked obesity. *N Engl J Med.* 2002;346:802–810

5. Wiegand S, Maikowski U, Blankenstein O, Biebermann H, Tarnow P, Gruters A. Type 2 diabetes and impaired glucose tolerance in European children and adolescents with obesity—a problem that is no longer restricted to minority groups. *Eur J Endocrinol.* 2004;151:199–206

6. Centers for Disease Control and Prevention. National diabetes fact sheet: national estimates and general information on diabetes and prediabetes in the United States. Atlanta, GA: US Department of Health and Human Services; 2011

7. Rosenbloom AL, Joe JR, Young RS, Winter WE. Emerging epidemic of type 2 diabetes in youth. *Diabetes Care.* 1999;22(2):345–354

8. Tirosh A, Shai I, Afek A, et al. Adolescent BMI trajectory and risk of diabetes versus coronary disease. *N Engl J Med.* 2011;364(14): 1315–1325

9. Pate RR, Freedson PS, Sallis JF, et al. Compliance with physical activity guidelines: prevalence in a population of children and youth. *Ann Epidemiol.* 2002;12:303–308

10. Goodman E, Whitaker RC. A prospective study of the role of depression in the development and persistence of adolescent obesity. *Pediatrics.* 2002;110:497–504

11. Patrick K, Norman GJ, Calfas KJ, et al. Diet, physical activity, and sedentary behaviors as risk factors for overweight in adolescence. *Arch Pediatr Adolesc Med.* 2004;158:385–390

12. Norman AC, Drinkard B, McDuffie JR, Ghorbani S, Yanoff LB, Yanovski JA. Influence of excess adiposity on exercise fitness and performance in overweight children and adolescents. *Pediatrics.* 2005;115:e690–e696

13. Stockman NK, Schenkel TC, Brown JN, Duncan AM. Comparison of energy and nutrient intakes among meals and snacks of adolescent males. *Prev Med.* 2005;41:203–210

14. Henricson C, Roker D. Support for the parents of adolescents: a review. *J Adolesc.* 2000;23:763–783

15. Steinberg L, Morris AS. Adolescent development. *Annu Rev Psychol.* 2001;52:83–110

Late Adolescent and Young Adult

11.1 Background

The rising prevalence of obesity and morbid obesity in adolescence means that more adolescents will be experiencing obesity-related comorbid conditions such as type 2 diabetes, nonalcoholic steatohepatitis, dyslipidemia, hypertension, and pulmonary disease than ever before. Almost 80% of adolescents with obesity will go on to become adults with obesity,[1] and in adulthood, obesity also increases the risks of cancer of the breast, colon, prostate, endometrium, kidney, and gallbladder[2] and contributes to significant functional disability because of osteoarthritis. All these will necessitate screening at increasingly earlier ages.

Adults with morbid obesity have a 50% to 100% increased risk of premature death compared with adults of normal weight, and even modest weight increases of 10 to 20 lb (4.5–9.1 kg) can increase mortality.[3] In addition to nutrition and physical activity health behaviors, inadequate or excess sleep has been associated with hyperglycemia in adolescents with obesity.[4] A study from Norway of 14- to 19-year-olds who were followed 31.5 years found they had a 30% higher mortality if their body mass index (BMI) was between 85% and 95% and an 80% (for males) to 100% (for females) higher mortality if their BMI was greater than 95% for age in adolescence.[5] Psychological morbidity is also a significant factor in the life of adolescents with obesity. In a study of 7th to 12th graders, adolescents who were depressed had a higher rate of obesity at follow-up, whereas baseline obesity did not predict depression, indicating that obesity can be the outcome of psychological morbidity.[6] The first year of college is associated with excess weight gain and attention to maintaining a healthy lifestyle should be part of anticipatory guidance for teens.[7]

The developmental tasks of adolescence need to be taken into account in the prevention and treatment of obesity, bearing in mind that family involvement is still crucial to provide support for the teen. Evolution of a healthy self-image is one of the important steps toward adulthood, and self-esteem is found to be lower in obese adolescents than peers of normal weight.[8] Adolescents who experience the negative effects of weight-based teasing may cope using avoidance, increased food consumption, and binge eating. There was a dose response on skipping school or decrease in grades for each teasing experience.[9]

The effects of adolescent obesity on body image may persist into adulthood; women who were obese as adolescents have persistent severe disturbances in body image, in contrast to women who become obese as adults.[10]

Another late adolescence task is developing a plan for social and economic stability. Obesity in female adolescents is linked to lower education levels, lower household incomes, and higher poverty rates in adulthood.[11] Lower college acceptance and less likelihood of marriage were also found among women with obesity.[2,12]

11.2 Prevention: Conversations With Teens (BALANCE)

Prevention touch points for teens include **belief, assessment, lifestyle, activity, nutrition, child/adolescent,** and **environment** (BALANCE).

Belief

- Obesity prevention continues to be important in this age group because the risk for obesity continues into adulthood. Obesity rates continue to rise in adulthood—in a survey of adults older than 20 years of age during 1999–2000, 65% were overweight or obese and a corresponding 27% of high school students were overweight or obese.[13]
- Teens may need to be reminded that excess weight gain can still occur, and continued attention on nutrition and activity is important.
- It may also be helpful to discuss obesity prevention in the overall context of health prevention issues; family history can be a useful entry point into this discussion for the young adult.

Assessment

- Self-monitoring may be a valuable technique to manage weight in this age group.
- Female college freshman who received feedback on their weight change gained little or no weight over a semester, compared with a control group that gained an average of 6.6 lb (3.0 kg).[14]

Lifestyle

- Irregular schedules and decreased sleep may contribute to weight gain.[15] It is worth going over the importance of scheduling activity, meals, and sleep, as well as the relationship of structure to maintaining healthy behaviors.
- Time management and priority setting are important skills when asking a teen to consider attending to regular meals and exercise.
- Families can provide support by providing a regular dinnertime, healthy available snacks, and opportunities for exercise, such as YMCA memberships. The adolescent can be encouraged to set aside time to take advantage of these opportunities.

Activity

- The older teen and young adult may be moving out of competitive activities and looking for options to maintain physical activity in the course of day-to-day activities.
- Optimizing opportunities, such as walking to school or work, looking for a part-time job that involves physical activity, and engaging in social activities that involve physical activity, can all be helpful.
- Learning a lifetime sport such as tennis, golf, or biking should be encouraged.

Nutrition

- Frequency of fast food consumption is associated with greater weight gain and greater increase in insulin resistance.[16] It is important to help adolescents find simple, nutritious alternatives to fast food.
- Unregulated eating often increases snacking, consuming fast or convenience food, and skipping meals.
- Eating patterns may veer into bingeing, bulimia, grazing, fad diets, or restrictive eating or anorexia. The following questions[17] can help to start a conversation about binge eating behavior. Does the adolescent
  1. Eat much more quickly than usual during binge episodes?
  2. Eat until uncomfortably full?
  3. Eat large amounts of food even when not really hungry?
  4. Eat alone because of embarrassment about the amount of food eaten?
  5. Feel disgusted, depressed, or guilty after overeating?
- Patterns of emotional eating may also occur. Attention to a diet history that takes into account dietary behaviors and feelings is important.
- If an eating disorder is suspected, consider the American Academy of Pediatrics clinical report, "Identification and Management of Eating Disorders in Children and Adolescents"[18] (see page 185).

Child/Adolescent

Attention to mental health is important as teens prepare for the next phase of development. Depression in adolescence is associated with an additional increased risk of obesity in young adulthood.[19]

High-risk health behaviors may be more common in this age group and include risk for obesity. Late adolescents and young adults (18–24 years of age) have a higher prevalence of smoking, greater increases in smoking, larger increase in obesity, and a higher level of sedentary behavior compared with adults (25–74 years of age).[20]

Environment

- It is helpful to get a picture of the adolescent's day, including place and time of eating, structured and unstructured activity, screen time, homework, and job and home responsibilities.
- Working with late adolescents and young adults on strategies to buffer an obesity-promoting environment is important—independent living or entrance to college can be opportunities for this interaction.

11.3 Intervention

When an adolescent has a BMI greater than 85% but less than 95% or is crossing growth percentiles in an upward direction, it is time for a more in-depth look at eating and activity, especially related to unregulated eating, an increase in sedentary time, and poor food choices—all of which can contribute to the risk of becoming an adult with obesity. In addition to reemphasizing concepts covered previously, teens and families may need to pay more attention to their ability to provide and influence nutrition and activity by focusing on *energy balance, structure,* and *modeling healthy behavior* (discussed next).

Energy Balance

Change in lifestyle and increased pressures of college, work, and social life may cause shifts in energy balance that are not immediately apparent to the teen. Self-assessment is important; diet and activity records can be a start to focus attention on daily choices. Connections between eating and study habits, workplace environments, and social eating are all important to tease out to allow the teen to begin making conscious choices about nutrition and activity.

Structure

Older adolescents and young adults are becoming increasingly independent of family meal structure, because they have irregular work hours and are often juggling the demands of school, work, and social lives. Energy balance may have as much to do with time management as unhealthy eating choices and sedentary behavior. Teens may see increased freedom at college as the absence of structure and need help seeing that scheduling meals, activity, and sleep may help correct weight gain. Teens may seek help from programs and dietary supplements for weight loss. They will benefit from a careful discussion of these options aimed at assessing efficacy and health benefits and harms.

Modeling Healthy Behavior

It is important to ask a teen what is being used as a model for decision making about eating and activity. This can be a thought-provoking question that can stimulate discussion about healthy behaviors. It is important to continue discussing health risks and family history with a teen who is already overweight by exploring models of health behavior he or she was exposed to as a child as a basis for taking care of his or her own health.

11.4 Treatment

It is time to initiate a focused treatment strategy when a teen's BMI is greater than 95% and you are dealing with excess adiposity. It is important to review the issues discussed in the previous 2 sections because these are the building blocks of good nutrition and activity habits. However, you will also have to focus on the barriers to change that may have prevented parents, families, and teens from implementing these strategies.

A useful way to begin is to obtain a family history focused on obesity-related comorbidities, which can serve to emphasize the health risks involved and the necessity of taking action early once obesity is identified.

11.5 Family History

Family history should be updated at this time, with attention to obesity-related comorbidities, the family weight trajectory, eating behaviors, and mental health diagnosis (Table 11.1).

Table 11.1. Family History, Late Adolescent and Young Adult

Complete or update this family history targeted toward obesity and related comorbidities.

	Mother	Father	Maternal Grandmother	Maternal Grandfather	Paternal Grandmother	Paternal Grandfather	Sibling 1	Sibling 2
Obesity	☐	☐	☐	☐	☐	☐	☐	☐
Cardiovascular disease	☐	☐	☐	☐	☐	☐	☐	☐
High blood pressure	☐	☐	☐	☐	☐	☐	☐	☐
Stroke	☐	☐	☐	☐	☐	☐	☐	☐
High cholesterol	☐	☐	☐	☐	☐	☐	☐	☐
High triglyceride level	☐	☐	☐	☐	☐	☐	☐	☐
Type 1 or 2 diabetes	☐	☐	☐	☐	☐	☐	☐	☐
Liver disease	☐	☐	☐	☐	☐	☐	☐	☐
Bariatric surgery	☐	☐	☐	☐	☐	☐	☐	☐
Polycystic ovarian disease	☐	☐	☐	☐	☐	☐	☐	☐
Binge eating disorder	☐	☐	☐	☐	☐	☐	☐	☐
	☐	☐	☐	☐	☐	☐	☐	☐
	☐	☐	☐	☐	☐	☐	☐	☐

11.6 Review of Systems

The review of systems can also serve as a point of departure to discuss obesity-related comorbidities, pointing out particular risk factors as they relate to increasing BMI.

- Skin: Acanthosis nigricans, striae, acne, hirsutism
- Head, eyes, ears, nose, and throat (HEENT): Headache, snoring, sleep disturbance, daytime napping, attention problems, poor school functioning, irritability, visual disturbance
- Lungs: Asthma, shortness of breath during exercise, cough at end of exercise, decreased exercise tolerance, smoking
- Cardiac: Hypertension, hyperlipidemia, chest pain, dizziness or shortness of breath during exercise
- Abdomen: Gastroesophageal reflux, stomach pain before or after eating, chronic diarrhea or constipation, morning anorexia, right upper quadrant discomfort or pain
- Musculoskeletal: Limping, hip pain or decreased motion, knee pain, bowing, ankle pain
- Genitourinary: Enuresis, delayed pubertal development, irregular or absent menses
- Psychological: Symptoms of depression, anxiety, low self-esteem, self-injury or suicidal ideation, sleep disturbance

11.7 Physical Examination

- Height
- Weight
- BMI + previous BMI measurements
- Blood pressure
- General: Height deceleration or poor linear growth, centripetal or visceral fat distribution
- Skin: Acanthosis nigricans (neck, axilla, groin), acne, cervical fat pad, striae, hirsutism
- HEENT: Funduscopic examination for papilledema, tonsillar hypertrophy, thyroid enlargement
- Cardiopulmonary: Wheezing, poor ventilation, heart murmur
- Abdominal: Hepatomegaly
- Musculoskeletal: Range of motion, genu varum, limp, hip or knee pain, ankle pain
- Genitourinary: Tanner stage

11.8 Family Constellation and Social History

Information about where the family and adolescent are in terms of decision making and independence can be helpful in working with the adolescent to individualize lifestyle change.

- Who is living at home with the adolescent?
- Who is responsible for purchasing and preparing meals?
- Does the family eat together?
- How much of a priority is improving nutrition and physical activity to the adolescent?

11.9 Questions for the Family

Family dynamics and communication are important when adolescents are trying to make changes in lifestyle. Questions from Table 11.2 may help you focus on family factors that can facilitate or hamper change.

11.10 Teen Touch Points

Teen touch points focus on helping teens initiate and maintain change by helping them believe change can occur, identify the change needed, value the outcome of the change, know how to change, and have the energy to change and sustain the change.

- ***Believe that change can occur.***
  - Building on success is crucial. Finding ways that succeeded in the past and translating skills and behaviors to weight loss can help the young person believe that change is possible.
  - Engaging a support network is also important because teens often think they have to do this alone. Parents, extended family, and friends can all be helpful in encouraging the teen.
  - Specifically asking, "How can your mother, father, or other family member best help you?" often opens the door for dialogue and allows the teen to have a role in organizing his or her own support system.

Table 11.2. Questions for the Family, Late Adolescent and Young Adult	Never	Seldom	Sometimes	Often	Always
Parents and adolescent agree on nutritional issues.	☐	☐	☐	☐	☐
Parents understand the principles of adolescent development.	☐	☐	☐	☐	☐
Parents are interacting with the young adult to guide and support responsible decision making.	☐	☐	☐	☐	☐

- *Identify the change.*
    - The concept of incremental change may still be difficult for the teen to grasp in an environment that gives the message of all or nothing. You may need to work with the young person to get the change down to a doable level.
    - Providing background information about nutrition and activity is important. Allow the teen decide where to start the change process. Often the teen has already thought about what he or she might do to improve nutrition and activity—this is a good place to start.
- *Value the outcome.*
    - It is important to help identify what values underpin decision making in this age group.
    - A teen may be more interested and initially committed to stabilizing weight, reducing cholesterol, or feeling more in control of eating than weight loss.
    - It is important to start "where the patient is" when beginning the treatment process.
- *Know how to change.* Setting a goal is important, as is developing a strategy for change. Self-knowledge is a key ingredient for establishing a plan. By this age most young adults know how they operate in the world (planners, procrastinators, emotional decision makers, analytical thinkers, independents, and/or influenced by friends). Using this self-knowledge can help you and the teen individualize a pathway of activity and nutrition change.
- *Have the energy to change and sustain.* Joining a group that is engaged in activity, volunteering, or pursuing a special interest can provide emotional support for the late adolescent and build positive relationships and skills. Adult weight management groups may be appropriate for some older teens as well. The ability to recognize stress and use stress management techniques is important, and skill building in this area can be taught.

11.11 Developmental Touch Point

At this stage of development adolescents are working on independence and a positive identity that allows for goal achievement. Sexual identity is established, and close personal friendships and relationships are fostered. Vocational decisions are being considered, and individual capabilities are being self-assessed.

11.12 Nutrition and Activity Questions and Approaches

Parents or the young adult can answer the nutrition and activity questions in Table 11.3, which can provide a focal point for targeted intervention (Table 11.4) in a brief encounter. Questions answered "Often" or "Always" can be targeted first for change.

11.13 A Case in Point: BL

BL is a 17-year-old white girl who comes with her mother to your office because her mother is concerned about her weight. BL has been overweight since the beginning of 1st grade; her current weight is 236 lb (107.0 kg), and her height is 5′6″ (167.6 cm). You calculate her BMI to be 38.1 (>95%).

When you ask BL if she is concerned about her weight, she responds with a fairly emphatic, "No."

BL is a good student, is a junior in high school, and is planning on majoring in English in college. She is not engaged in any extracurricular activities, likes to read, and was involved in several school plays.

You take a family history and find that the mother's cholesterol was 245 mg/dL before she started taking medication. BL's father has treated hypertension, and the paternal grandfather had a myocardial infarction and bypass surgery.

BL's review of systems, except for her weight, is essentially negative. Upon physical examination, you find her blood pressure is elevated at 124/82 mm Hg and she has a minor degree of abdominal striae; otherwise, it is a negative physical examination.

You asked BL to fill out the questions in Table 11.3 and she answered "Often" or "Always" to having an unhealthy snack and lunch at school (question 17), having a limited intake of vegetables (question 13), skipping breakfast (question 16), and having a preference for quiet activities (question 3).

When you ask how easy it would be for her to change these behaviors, she fills out "Impossible" or "Could Try" for all of them, saying that she really is not concerned about her weight and does not think she needs to change anything.

The mother believes that BL's weight is keeping her from doing the things she should be doing at her age, such as dating and being more involved in extracurricular and social activities. The mother is also worried about what it will be like at college for BL unless she learns to make better food choices.

Table 11.3. Nutrition and Activity Questions, Late Adolescent and Young Adult

These questions can be answered by the young adult (or parent) and provide a focal point for targeted intervention in a brief encounter. First have the young adult (or parent) answer these questions about the presence or absence of behaviors that promote weight gain; then refer to Table 11.4.

Please answer the following for the statements below: Does your adolescent…?

	Never	Seldom	Sometimes	Often	Always
1. Not have time to participate in physical activity every day.	☐	☐	☐	☐	☐
2. Not have a favorite way to be active (ie, sports team, riding bikes, etc).	☐	☐	☐	☐	☐
3. Prefer quiet activities.	☐	☐	☐	☐	☐
4. Seem unmotivated to get active.	☐	☐	☐	☐	☐
5. Lack interest in activities with friends or extracurricular activities.	☐	☐	☐	☐	☐
6. Stay indoors after school.	☐	☐	☐	☐	☐
7. Sleep less than 8 or more than 11 hours a night.	☐	☐	☐	☐	☐
8. Watch television or play with computer/video games in his or her bedroom.	☐	☐	☐	☐	☐
9. Spend more than 2 hours watching television, playing video games, or using a computer each day.	☐	☐	☐	☐	☐
10. Eat in front of the television or computer.	☐	☐	☐	☐	☐
11. Eat late at night or right before bed.	☐	☐	☐	☐	☐
12. Eat when bored.	☐	☐	☐	☐	☐
13. Have a limited intake of vegetables.	☐	☐	☐	☐	☐
14. Have a limited intake of fruits.	☐	☐	☐	☐	☐
15. Have a limited intake of dairy foods (yogurt, cheese, milk).	☐	☐	☐	☐	☐
16. Skip breakfast.	☐	☐	☐	☐	☐
17. Have unhealthy snack and lunch at school.	☐	☐	☐	☐	☐
18. Frequent the school vending machines for snacks and drinks.	☐	☐	☐	☐	☐
19. Eat more than 1 snack between meals a day.	☐	☐	☐	☐	☐
20. Graze between meals.	☐	☐	☐	☐	☐
21. Choose fruit or vegetables when making snacks.	☐	☐	☐	☐	☐
22. Overeat after school.	☐	☐	☐	☐	☐
23. Drink juice or sugared beverages between meals.	☐	☐	☐	☐	☐
24. Eat meals alone.	☐	☐	☐	☐	☐
25. Feel bad about himself or herself.	☐	☐	☐	☐	☐
26. Eat at fast-food restaurants.	☐	☐	☐	☐	☐
27. Choose healthy foods when eating out at restaurants or with friends.	☐	☐	☐	☐	☐
28. Seem depressed.	☐	☐	☐	☐	☐

Questions answered "Often" or "Always" in Table 11.3 can be targeted first for change. Using these specific questions, ask the parent, "How willing are you to…?"

Please answer the following for the statements below: How willing are you to…?

	Impossible	Could Try	Could Do Sometimes	Could Do Often	Easy
1. Schedule time for your teen to be active every day.	☐	☐	☐	☐	☐
2. Find extracurricular activities your teen will enjoy and add activity to his or her lifestyle.	☐	☐	☐	☐	☐
3. Plan an activity you can do with your teen.	☐	☐	☐	☐	☐
4. Have your teen partner with a family member/friend in a physical activity.	☐	☐	☐	☐	☐
5. Encourage a peer group activity to be a part of after-school time.	☐	☐	☐	☐	☐
6. Develop a plan to increase sleep for your teen.	☐	☐	☐	☐	☐
7. Move televisions, video games, and computers out of your teen's bedroom.	☐	☐	☐	☐	☐
8. Reduce time spent watching television, playing video games, or using the computer.	☐	☐	☐	☐	☐
9. Encourage activities other than screen time, such as playing board games, reading, and doing chores.	☐	☐	☐	☐	☐
10. Turn off the television during meals and snacks.	☐	☐	☐	☐	☐
11. Help your teen find activities to do instead of munching.	☐	☐	☐	☐	☐
12. Offer vegetables at meals and as snacks.	☐	☐	☐	☐	☐
13. Offer fruits at meals and as snacks.	☐	☐	☐	☐	☐
14. Offer dairy products at meals and as snacks.	☐	☐	☐	☐	☐
15. Schedule time for breakfast each day.	☐	☐	☐	☐	☐
16. Help your teen prepare healthier school snacks ahead of time.	☐	☐	☐	☐	☐
17. Pack a school lunch and snack; limit extra money for vending machines.	☐	☐	☐	☐	☐
18. Schedule regular meals.	☐	☐	☐	☐	☐
19. Keep only healthy snacks in the house.	☐	☐	☐	☐	☐
20. Change from juice or soda to water between meals.	☐	☐	☐	☐	☐
21. Eat meals together.	☐	☐	☐	☐	☐
22. Limit how often you buy/serve fast food.	☐	☐	☐	☐	☐
23. Learn how to choose healthier options when dining out.	☐	☐	☐	☐	☐
24. Have a pediatrician, counselor, or therapist evaluate for depression.	☐	☐	☐	☐	☐

You acknowledge BL's and the mother's feelings. You point out that obesity-related comorbidities are in the family history and that BL's blood pressure is elevated. You express your concerns about BL's current and future health and ask her to get laboratory studies to further evaluate her health status. She and her mother agree, and you schedule an appointment for them to come back in 3 to 4 weeks and review the laboratory work.

Second Visit

BL returns and her weight is unchanged. You received BL's laboratory studies, which are all normal except for elevated total cholesterol of 276 mg/dL and a low high-density lipoprotein (HDL) of 34 mg/dL.

You begin the visit by reviewing the laboratory data and elevated cholesterol, as well as the positive family history for hypercholesterolemia and heart disease. BL is somewhat upset by having a high cholesterol and asks what she can do about it. Her mother reiterates her concern about BL's weight and eating habits. You review the positive family history for hypercholesterolemia and heart disease.

You go back to BL's original questionnaire and point out that school lunches and snacks are generally higher in fats and calories, both of which can contribute to elevations in cholesterol, and mention that vegetables are a natural source of fiber that can help lower cholesterol. You ask BL if she could pack a lunch or make a healthier choice at school, and she says she thinks she can. You ask BL if she can think of a way she can start eating more vegetables; she says she could eat salad. You ask the mother to provide salad ingredients instead of snack food for BL's after-school snack to which she agrees.

You give BL a diet and activity record to complete and some background information on recommended food groups and portion sizes. You ask BL to schedule a return visit in 1 month.

Third Visit

BL comes back with her diet and activity records. Her weight is 234 lb (106.1 kg), her height is 5´6˝ (167.6 cm), and her blood pressure is 120/79 mm Hg. Her review of systems and physical examination are unremarkable. She packs a lunch most of the time and is not having any problems with this change. She started eating a salad after school but is drifting to the snack food her brother eats. The mother is impatient with BL, who says she nags at her a lot.

You review BL's choices and reinforce the positive changes she made. You note her lower weight and blood pressure and encourage her to continue. You reassure the mother that BL is making progress and to try to stay positive. You order a repeat cholesterol test to be done right before her next visit in 4 to 5 weeks.

Fourth Visit

BL returns with her laboratory work. Her cholesterol is 252 mg/dL, and her HDL is 35 mg/dL. Her weight is 232 lb (105.2 kg), and her blood pressure is 120/80 mm Hg. BL's diet records show that she is packing her lunch and is able to eat salad most days after school. She is also involved in the Spanish club at school. You reinforce BL's positive changes, but her mother notes that she should be doing more, taking more responsibility, and that her weight is not changing enough. You encourage the mother, pointing out that this is the first time BL lost weight since she was in 1st grade.

You ask BL if she is ready to make more changes, to which she says she is because she would like to lower her cholesterol. She shares that she is worried about the family history of heart attacks. You review her initial questions and ask if she could begin eating a nonsugared cereal for breakfast. You also go over some ways she could increase her activities of daily living, such as walking around the block before coming in from the bus stop after school, taking on dog-walking chores, and thinking about increasing her walking when she is out with friends. She thinks she will try these ideas, and you ask her to schedule an appointment in 4 to 5 weeks.

Fifth Visit

Having just turned 18, BL comes by herself to this visit. She brings diet records and notes that her mother is still nagging her all the time about her weight and eating habits. BL's weight is 231 lb (104.8 kg), and her blood pressure is 120/82 mm Hg. Her review of systems and physical examination are normal. You note that she is eating breakfast and walking off and on. You spend some time talking to BL about how she is handling her mother's nagging. She said it bothers her, and she often gets stubborn and eats what she knows she should not. You ask about her goals, and she says she is used to her weight, so it does not bother her that much. However, having normal cholesterol is important to her. You ask if she can make the changes you talked about "for her" and not her mother. You schedule her next visit in 6 weeks with repeat laboratory studies.

Sixth Visit

BL comes back with her laboratory values, which show a cholesterol level of 226 mg/dL and HDL cholesterol of 38 mg/dL, with a blood pressure reading of 118/76 mm Hg. Her weight is 225 lb (102.1 kg). She got a summer job at the local mall and is walking with friends during her breaks. She eats breakfast and packs a lunch and notes that she is making healthy choices when going out with friends. She is pleased with the results of her laboratory work and asks you to write down the results so that she can show her mother. She is looking forward to her senior year. You schedule her next visit for 6 to 8 weeks.

References

1. Whitaker RC, Wright JA, Pepe MS, Seidel KD, Dietz WH. Predicting obesity in young adulthood from childhood and parental obesity. *N Engl J Med.* 1997;337:869–873

2. Gortmaker SL, Must A, Perrin JM, Sobol AM, Dietz WH. Social and economic consequences of overweight in adolescence and young adulthood. *N Engl J Med.* 1993;329:1008–1012

3. Warman JL. The application of laparoscopic bariatric surgery for treatment of severe obesity in adolescents using a multidisciplinary adolescent bariatric program. *Crit Care Nurs Q.* 2005;28:276–287

4. Koren D, Levitt Katz LE, Brar PC, Gallagher PR, Berkowitz RI, Brooks LJ. Sleep architecture and glucose and insulin homeostasis in obese adolescents. *Diabetes Care.* 2011;34(11):2442–2447. Epub 2011 Sep 20

5. Engeland A, Bjorge T, Sogaard AJ, Tverdal A. Body mass index in adolescence in relation to total mortality: 32-year follow-up of 227,000 Norwegian boys and girls. *Am J Epidemiol.* 2003;157:517–523

6. Goodman E, Whitaker RC. A prospective study of the role of depression in the development and persistence of adolescent obesity. *Pediatrics.* 2002;110:497–504

7. Gow RW, Trace SE, Mazzeo SE. Preventing weight gain in first year college students: an online intervention to prevent the "freshman fifteen." *Eat Behav.* 2010;11(1):33–39

8. Strauss CC, Smith K, Frame C, Forehand R. Personal and interpersonal characteristics associated with childhood obesity. *J Pediatr Psychol.* 1985;10:337–343

9. Puhl RM, Luedicke J. Weight-based victimization among adolescents in the school setting: emotional reactions and coping behaviors. *J Youth Adolesc.* Epub 2011 Sep 15

10. Stunkard A, Mendelson M. Obesity and body image. 1. Characteristics of disturbances in the body image of some obese persons. *Am J Psychiatry.* 1967;123:1296–1300

11. Sargent JD, Blanchflower DG. Obesity and stature in adolescence and earnings in young adulthood. Analysis of a British birth cohort. *Arch Pediatr Adolesc Med.* 1994;148:681–687

12. Dietz WH. Childhood weight affects adult morbidity and mortality. *J Nutr.* 1998;128(2 suppl):411S–414S

13. Centers for Disease Control and Prevention. Overweight among students in grades K-12—Arkansas, 2003-04 and 2004-05 school years. *MMWR Morb Mortal Wkly Rep.* 2006;55:5–8

14. Levitsky DA, Garay J, Nausbaum M, Neighbors L, Dellavalle DM. Monitoring weight daily blocks the freshman weight gain: a model for combating the epidemic of obesity. *Int J Obes (Lond).* 2006;30:1003–1010

15. Gangwisch JE, Malaspina D, Boden-Albala B, Heymsfield SB. Inadequate sleep as a risk factor for obesity: analyses of the NHANES I. *Sleep.* 2005;28:1289–1296

16. Pereira MA, Kartashov AI, Ebbeling CB, et al. Fast-food habits, weight gain, and insulin resistance (the CARDIA study): 15-year prospective analysis. *Lancet.* 2005;365:36–42

17. WIN Weight-Control Information Network (NIDDK). Binge eating disorder. win.niddk.nih.gov/publications/binge.htm. Accessed June 21, 2006

18. Rosen DS, American Academy of Pediatrics Committee on Adolescence. Identification and management of eating disorders in children and adolescents. *Pediatrics.* 2010;126:1240–1253

19. Franko DL, Striegel-Moore RH, Thompson D, Schreiber GB, Daniels SR. Does adolescent depression predict obesity in black and white young adult women? *Psychol Med.* 2005;35:1505–1513

20. Winkleby MA, Cubbin C. Changing patterns in health behaviors and risk factors related to chronic diseases, 1990-2000. *Am J Health Promot.* 2004;19:19–27

12 Obesity Health Strategies for Practices: Identification, Prevention, Intervention, and Treatment

12.1 Practice Interventions

Every pediatrician will need to address obesity in his or her practice. Pediatric subspecialists are currently engaged in treating the comorbidities of obesity previously seen only in adults: type 2 diabetes, nonalcoholic steatohepatitis, hypertension and hyperlipidemia, sleep apnea, and polycystic ovarian disease. Hospitalists are caring for seriously ill obese patients and need to prepare to treat obesity-related disease in an inpatient setting. Primary care pediatricians will need to be able to increase their practice capacity to identify, prevent, intervene, and treat the child and family with obesity.

12.2 Identification of Weight Status

Risk Factors

No physician should miss the opportunity to identify the obesity risk status of a child or an adolescent. Risk for obesity can be increased by parental obesity,[1] a history of maternal diabetes,[2] maternal smoking,[3] intrauterine growth retardation,[4] and obesity-associated genetic syndromes.[5] Questions about these factors should be routinely incorporated into every child's medical history.

Body Mass Index

Calculating and categorizing a patient's body mass index (BMI) is the first step in evaluating health risk; every child should have his or her BMI and BMI percentile routinely measured and plotted on the BMI curve.[6] Practice patterns should be addressed to incorporate this in the staff's routine. Sharing growth and BMI charts with parents and families is a first step toward bringing up the issue of healthy growth and opening the door for discussion about family patterns of nutrition, activity, and sedentary behavior.

12.3 Prevention

The extent and severity of the obesity epidemic dictates that practice strategies need to be put in place to incorporate obesity prevention into the office routine. Pediatricians and other health care professionals can provide parents and patients with information about the etiology of obesity, developmentally appropriate nutrition and activity balance, and family-based lifestyle change. Adolescents perceive their providers as valuable sources of information about weight.[7] Research on primary care prevention of obesity is still evolving, but some basic recommendations can be made.

Promote Breastfeeding

Breastfeeding should be encouraged and supported for all newborns.[8] Pediatricians can

- Advocate for breastfeeding-friendly hospitals.
- Provide lactation support for all mothers, especially mothers who are obese, to encourage initiation and maintenance.
- Encourage mothers and families who formula-feed to recognize satiety cues.

Encourage Healthy Eating

Families should be provided with guidelines that explain age-appropriate food group composition, servings, and portions sizes.

- Fruit and vegetable consumption should be increased to meet dietary requirements (5 servings a day).[6]
- Parents and families should be encouraged to model healthy eating.
- Parents should choose what is available to eat at meals and snacks but allow children to choose whether to eat and how much.[6]

Limit Juice and Sugar-Sweetened Beverages

The American Academy of Pediatrics (AAP) recommends that juice intake be limited, with the following specific suggestions[9]:

- Juice should not be introduced into an infant's diet before 6 months of age.
- Infants should not be given juice from bottles, and when given in cups, it should not be made available so that infants consume juice throughout the day. Infants should not be given juice at bedtime.

- Juice intake should be limited to 4 to 6 oz a day for children 1 to 6 years of age. Juice intake should be limited to 8 to 12 oz or 2 servings per day for children 7 to 18 years of age.
- Children should be encouraged to eat whole fruits to meet their recommended daily fruit intake.
- The consumption of sugar-sweetened beverages should be reduced[10] or eliminated.

Reduce Screen Time

Studies in school interventions show that reducing screen time (eg, television, computer) can prevent obesity.[11,12] The AAP recommends[13]

- Limiting children's total time with entertainment media to no more than 1 to 2 hours of quality programming per day
- Removing television sets from children's bedrooms
- Discouraging television viewing for children younger than 2 years of age and encouraging more interactive activities that will promote proper brain development, such as talking, playing, singing, and reading together
- Encouraging alternative entertainment for children, including reading, athletics, hobbies, and creative play

Encourage Physical Activity

Physical activity is part of healthy development in children and lays the groundwork for lifelong habits that will support activity in adulthood. The AAP recommends encouraging physical activity as part of an obesity prevention strategy.[14]

- Determine physical activity levels of the child and family members at regular health care visits.
- Encourage children and adolescents to be physically active for at least 60 minutes per day, which may be accumulated in smaller increments.
- Events should be of moderate intensity and include a wide variety of activities as part of sports, recreation, transportation, chores, work, planned exercise, and school-based physical education classes. These activities should be primarily unstructured and fun if they are to achieve best compliance.
- Identify any barriers the child, youth, or parent might have against increasing physical activity, which could include lack of time, competing interests, perceived lack of motor skills, and fear of injury of the child.
- Parents might be additionally concerned about financial and safety issues. Efforts must be made to work with the family to educate them on the importance of lifelong physical activity and to identify potential strategies to overcome some of their barriers.
- Advise parents to support their child or youth in developmentally and age-appropriate sports and recreational activities. The child's favorite types of physical activity should be a priority; these might best occur in the school setting during extracurricular activities in which parents or grandparents can take part as leaders and coaches.
- Recommend that parents become good role models by increasing their own level of physical activity. Parents should also encourage physical activities that family members of all ages and abilities can do together.
- Parents should encourage children to play outside as much as possible. Safety should be promoted with the use of appropriate protective equipment (eg, bicycle helmets, life jackets).
- These obesity prevention messages should permeate the practice and be delivered at every opportunity. An easy way to frame obesity prevention messages is by using a framework such as 5-2-1-0 (Figure 12.1), which can help guide setting goals.

R̸ for Healthy Active Living

Name _____ Date _____

Ideas for Living a Healthy Active Life

5 Eat at least 5 fruits and vegetables every day.

2 Limit screen time (for example, TV, video games, computer) to 2 hours or less per day.

1 Get 1 hour or more of physical activity every day.

0 Drink fewer sugar-sweetened drinks. Try water and low-fat milk instead.

My Goals (choose one you would like to work on first)

☐ Eat _____ fruits and vegetables each day.
☐ Reduce screen time to _____ minutes per day.

☐ Get _____ minutes of physical activity each day.
☐ Reduce number of sugared drinks to _____ per day.

_____
Patient or Parent/Guardian signature

_____
Doctor signature

From Your Doctor

American Academy of Pediatrics
DEDICATED TO THE HEALTH OF ALL CHILDREN™

Healthy Active Living
An initiative of the American Academy of Pediatrics

Figure 12.1. Rx for Healthy Active Living

12.4 Intervention

When a child or teen has a BMI greater than 85% but less than 95% or is crossing growth percentiles in an upward direction, these prevention messages should be intensified. At this point, recommended nutrition and activity lifestyle changes should be coupled with strategies to help parents and families implement them. Several strategies are recommended to help parents and families regain control of excess weight gain; these include controlling the nutrition and activity environments, setting goals, monitoring behavior, rewarding success, problem solving, and using parenting skills.[15]

A family history of obesity-related comorbidities should be obtained, a complete physical examination performed, and a lipid profile and liver enzymes measured, with other laboratory studies as clinically determined.[15]

Managing the Nutrition and Activity Environments

Micromanaging eating and activity behaviors can be exhausting for families. Family-based environmental change can set new norms for eating and activity that do not need to be renegotiated every time. Examples of managing the environment include:

- Eliminating sugar-sweetened beverages from the home
- Increasing the number of meals prepared at home
- Serving food restaurant style—placing appropriate portions on the plate—rather than family style, where dishes on served on the table
- Reducing screen time to 2 hours a day for children and family members older than 2 years of age
- Not eating in front of the television
- Removing the television from the bedroom
- Planning after-school time to include activities and outdoor time

Setting Goals

Help the family set incremental, achievable goals for behavior change in a setting that allows discussion between family members and the pediatrician.

- Goals can be environmental and involve parental behavior.
- Goals can be individual, such as a child committing to spending time outdoors every day or joining one after-school activity.
- Goals can be relational, such as the parents and the child agreeing to partner with each other on a daily walk or parents increasing their praise of the child for following the television schedule.

Monitoring Behavior

Monitoring behavior helps families stay on course with change. Monitoring should occur in a setting where behavior can be discussed in a nonjudgmental way; this will identify setbacks and allow needed changes to occur. Examples of monitoring could include keeping track of

- Sugar-sweetened beverages consumed each day
- Activities (using an activity log)
- Screen time
- Outdoor time
- Parents' success in achieving environmental change

Rewarding Success

Managing weight is hard work; parents and families can become focused on what is not being done and forget to reward their successes. Reminding parents to praise and give attention to the positive can help fuel the next steps toward change. For example,

- Rewards should be for short-term gains (ie, something done that day).
- Parents should let the child know what behaviors will be rewarded and how, and parents need to be consistent.
- Parents should reward with time, attention, and activity.

Problem Solving

Skills families need most are the ones that enable them to evaluate progress, identify problems, identify solutions, and try new behaviors. This is similar to the Deming cycle of plan, do, study, act, which is used in quality improvement. Examples of issues that require problem solving are

- After-school hunger
- Emotional eating
- Resistance to change
- Parties
- Eating out
- Eating with friends

Using Parenting Skills

Initiating and maintaining lifestyle change requires parenting skills. Firm, consistent parenting that supports the child's autonomy and self-sufficiency while setting appropriate boundaries is likely to be the most effective parenting strategy. Parents willing to partner with their child, communicate expectations, and reward progress allow weight management to occur in a positive setting. Examples of helpful parenting skills include:

- Setting reasonable boundaries and allowing children to choose within those boundaries

- Setting limits and saying no in a reasonable, consistent way
- Modeling the expected behaviors
- Communicating expectations clearly in a developmentally appropriate manner

Strategies for accomplishing this work in a practice setting need to be developed. Additional visits, group visits, and use of nursing personnel, nutritionists, and psychologists can all be considered.

12.5 Treatment

A BMI greater than 95% for age and gender is a strong indicator of obesity in a child and has a high correlation with increased adiposity.[16] At this point, 3 things must occur: screening for obesity-related comorbidities, treatment of obesity, and treatment of any identified comorbidities.

Screening for Obesity-Related Comorbidities

When obesity is identified, appropriate history, review of systems, physical examination, and laboratory testing need to be part of the practice routine. Remember that the presence of 1 comorbid condition does not rule out additional comorbidities and signs and symptoms of many may be present at the same time (Table 12.1). Laboratory studies include a lipid profile, liver enzymes, fasting glucose, and any other studies that are clinically indicated.[15]

In addition to comorbidities, obesity-related emergencies can also occur (see Chapter 1 for additional information).

Treatment of Obesity

The preventive and intervention approaches previously discussed should be intensified in treating the obese child and family. Specific randomized controlled trials for obesity treatment were evaluated by the Cochrane Review[17] and the US Preventative Health Services Task Force (USPHSTF).[18] The USPHSTF report notes that successful programs were moderate- to high-intensity with more than 25 hours of contact with the child and/or the family over a 6-month period. Improved weight status is defined as an absolute and/or relative decrease in BMI 12 months after the beginning of the intervention. Evidence was limited on the long-term sustainability of BMI changes achieved through behavioral interventions and on the trajectory of weight gain in children and adolescents. The programs reviewed in the USPHSTF report included:

- Interventions with the main focus on changes in physical activity and sedentary behavior
- Interventions in which the main focus is behavioral therapy compared with usual care or no treatment
- Interventions comparing behavior therapy at varying degrees of family involvement
- Interventions comparing cognitive-behavioral therapy with relaxation
- Interventions comparing behavioral therapy with mastery criteria and contingent reinforcement
- Interventions comparing problem solving with usual care or behavioral therapy

Table 12.1. Screening and Treatment for Obesity-Related Comorbidities

Type 2 Diabetes	
History	Maternal diabetes during pregnancy, small for gestational age, intrauterine growth retardation, family history of diabetes
Review of systems	Polyuria; polydipsia; nocturia; recurrent vaginal, bladder, or other infections; recent weight loss
Physical examination	Acanthosis nigricans
Laboratory	Elevated fasting glucose, glycosuria, positive glucose tolerance test, hyperinsulinemia
Treatment	Referral to a pediatric endocrinologist for treatment with metformin or insulin and lifestyle change
Nonalcoholic Steatohepatitis	
History	No specific history; some cases have other family members affected
Review of systems	Possible nausea and right upper quadrant discomfort
Physical examination	Hepatomegaly
Laboratory/imaging	Elevated serum aminotransferase levels, echogenicity of liver on ultrasound
Treatment	Referral to a pediatric gastroenterologist for evaluation and definitive diagnosis, weight loss

Hypertension

History	Family history of hypertension or other obesity-related comorbidity
Review of systems	Usually asymptomatic
Physical examination	Elevated systolic and/or diastolic blood pressure
Laboratory/imaging	Evaluation for other causes of hypertension as indicated
Treatment	Referral to a pediatric hypertension specialist, dietary treatment, pharmacologic treatment

Dyslipidemia

History	Family history of lipid disorders, cardiovascular disease
Review of systems	Asymptomatic; other obesity comorbidities, particularly signs of metabolic syndrome
Physical examination	No specific signs; acanthosis nigricans may indicate metabolic syndrome
Laboratory/imaging	Lipid panel
Treatment	Referral to a lipid specialist, dietary management

Sleep Apnea

History	Family history of sleep apnea
Review of systems	Snoring, snoring with apnea, daytime tiredness, napping, poor concentration in school, enuresis
Physical examination	Large tonsils or adenoids
Laboratory/imaging	Nighttime polysomnography
Treatment	Referral to a pediatric pulmonologist, weight loss

Slipped Capital Femoral Epiphysis

History	Knee or hip pain
Review of systems	Knee or hip pain, limp
Physical examination	Limp, pain in knee or hip
Laboratory/imaging	Hip and knee films
Treatment	Immediate referral to pediatric orthopedist

Blount Disease

History	Bowing
Review of systems	Bowing (tibia vera), knee pain, limp
Physical examination	Bowing, knee pain, limp
Laboratory/imaging	Knee films
Treatment	Referral to pediatric orthopedist

Depression

History	Family history of depression, history of abuse, psychological trauma, teasing, low self-esteem
Review of systems	Loss of interest, anger, irritability, sadness, suicidal ideation
Physical examination	No signs; may have sad, irritable appearance with lack of self-care
Laboratory/imaging	None
Treatment	Mental health referral for counseling or pharmacologic treatment

Interventions With the Main Focus on Changes in Physical Activity and Sedentary Behavior.

Increasing exercise is a therapeutic strategy in treating obesity; however, few randomized, controlled trials have been performed.[17] In a study reviewed by the Cochrane report, girls who were obese had exercise added to a family-based dietary weight control program.[19] Both groups lost weight, but the exercise group had significantly larger decreases in overweight percentages at 6 months; however, this difference did not persist at 12 months. Children in the exercise group had supervised exercise 3 times a week that changed to walking 3 miles with a parent 3 times a week in the maintenance phase.[19] In another reviewed study, exercise increased fat-free mass in a group of adolescents when added to an intervention providing dietary advice.[20]

Exercise is reported to confer a metabolic benefit in children with obesity, with reductions of adiponectin after a 3-month exercise intervention that also lowered fat mass, insulin resistance, and hyperinsulinemia without significantly altering weight.[21]

Lifestyle activities are defined as "interventions [that] allow a person to individualize his/her physical activity programs to include a wide variety of activities that are at least of moderate intensity and to accumulate bouts of these activities in a manner befitting his/her life circumstances."[22] In a randomized, controlled study evaluated by the Cochrane review,[17] lifestyle exercise was compared with aerobic exercise and low-intensity calisthenics as an intervention for obesity in 5- to 8-year-old children. All groups were trained in behavioral therapy–type strategies, and all children lost weight during the active treatment period. Lifestyle exercise was found to result in significantly lower overweight percentage than in children in the aerobic and callisthenic groups.[23]

Decreasing sedentary behavior is also one of the strategies applied to treating obesity in children and is shown to result in a decreased overweight percentage.[24] Exercise was compared with decreasing sedentary behavior in a study of 8- to 12-year-old children with obesity. Parents decreased sedentary behavior by limiting television watching cues (eg, turning television to face the wall) and providing physical activity equipment. Children self-monitored their physical activity. At the end of 1 year, children in the group that decreased sedentary behavior had greater decreases in overweight percentage and body fat percentage versus the exercise and combined groups. The children whose sedentary activity was decreased also had lower caloric intake and a likely increase for high-intensity exercise than those children in the exercise group. All children had increased fitness at the end of the study.

Another study of 8- to 12-year-olds with obesity compared increased physical activity with decreased sedentary behavior.[25] There were no differences between groups, but both groups showed decreases in overweight percentage as a result of the intervention. These studies suggest that increasing exercise, including lifestyle exercise, and implementing strategies to reduce sedentary time are valuable and necessary additions to obesity treatment plans.

Interventions in Which the Main Focus Is Behavioral Therapy Compared With Usual Care or No Treatment.

Obesity treatment plans in children rely on family-based lifestyle change and need to include a behavioral component. Several randomized, controlled trials[17] reported a positive effect when behavioral therapy is added to the intervention. In a study of 5- to 8-year-old girls with obesity, behavioral treatment (ie, training in self-monitoring, praise, modeling, contracting) was compared with an educational intervention.[23] At 12 months there were significant differences in the overweight percentage in the behavioral group compared with that of the educational intervention group.

In another study, a behavioral intervention for 6- to 13-year-olds with obesity was compared to a waiting list control group with no intervention.[26] Both behavioral groups had significantly greater decreases in overweight percentage than the control group, but they were not different from each other.

An evaluation of the Shapedown program for adolescents showed that a 15-month intervention significantly improved relative weight, weight-related behavior, and depression at 1 year compared with a control group.[27]

In a different study, a comparison was made between children with obesity in a control group who had medical checkups, dietitian advice, and negotiated changes in dietary behavior and a group who had the addition of family therapy to the conventional treatment. Children in the family therapy group had a smaller increase in BMI and reduced skinfold thickness over 18 months compared with the conventional group.[28] There was no difference between the conventional therapy group and control group.

Interventions Comparing Behavior Therapy at Varying Degrees of Family Involvement.

Parent involvement is important. When parent behavioral training was added to a multicomponent behavioral weight management program involving obese 8- to 12-year-olds and their parents, there was a greater decrease in overweight percentage than in a group without the parent training.[29]

Parents are more effective as the exclusive agents of changes than when children are responsible for their own weight loss, with greater weight reduction in the parent-only intervention group.[30–32]

When child self-regulation was emphasized in a parent-child multicomponent behavioral weight management program, there was a trend toward decreased gain in overweight percentage over a 3-year period in the child self-regulation group.[33]

No difference was found in a study of African American girls, 14 years of age, in a weight management program between treating the child alone, mother and child in the same session, or mother and child in different sessions.[34]

Interventions Comparing Cognitive-Behavioral Therapy With Relaxation.

The addition of cognitive-behavioral therapy did not seem to make a difference in outcome when added to standard behavioral therapy weight management programs in the studies included in the Cochrane review.[17] In children 7 to 13 years of age with obesity, at 6 months both groups had significant reduction in overweight percentage but were not different from each other.[35]

A second study included a 6-week patient rehabilitation program for children and adolescents. Both groups, the standard behavioral group and a group with added cognitive-behavioral therapy, had significant weight loss at 6 weeks and 1 year but were not different from each other.[36]

Interventions Comparing Behavioral Therapy With Mastery Criteria and Contingent Reinforcement.

Adding mastery of parenting skills to standard behavior change strategies was compared with the standard therapy over 26 weekly and 6 monthly meetings in a group of children with obesity. Weight loss was better at 1 year in the parenting skills group, but there was no difference between groups at 2 years.[37]

Interventions Comparing Problem Solving With Usual Care or Behavioral Therapy.

Family involvement is important in any obesity treatment plan.[6] Specific strategies for including problem-solving skills in obesity intervention were reviewed.[17] In a study to investigate the effect of including problem-solving training in a weight loss group,[38] parents were trained in problem-solving exercises related to weight control. They received training in self-monitoring, stimulus control strategies, family support, cognitive restructuring, peer relations, and maintenance

strategies; in addition, the control group received diet and exercise information. A third group received only instructional materials. Six months after the 8-week intervention, the problem-solving and behavioral groups had significantly decreased their overweight percentage compared with the instruction-only group. Children in the problem-solving group had significantly greater decreases in overweight percentage than children in the behavioral group.[38] Results of another study showed no difference between groups in a family-based behavioral program and either child or child-parent teaching of problem solving.[39]

As a result of this review, the Cochrane reviewers stated that practitioners need to consider issues that affect sustainability and environmental change while addressing behavior change in a complex set of circumstances in which families currently find themselves. Family involvement and support of families is crucial.[17]

References

1. Whitaker RC, Wright JA, Pepe MS, Seidel KD, Dietz WH. Predicting obesity in young adulthood from childhood and parental obesity. *N Engl J Med.* 1997;337:869–873

2. Pettitt DJ, Aleck KA, Baird HR, Carraher MJ, Bennett PH, Knowler WC. Congenital susceptibility to NIDDM. Role of intrauterine environment. *Diabetes.* 1988;37:622–628

3. Raum E, Küpper-Nybelen J, Lamerz A, Hebebrand J, Herpertz-Dahlmann B, Brenner H. Tobacco smoke exposure before, during, and after pregnancy and risk of overweight at age 6. *Obesity (Silver Spring).* Epub 2011 May 26

4. Gluckman PD, Hanson MA. The consequences of being born small—an adaptive perspective. *Horm Res.* 2006;65(suppl 3):5–14

5. Hassink S. Problems in childhood obesity. In: Bray GA, ed. *Office Management of Childhood Obesity.* Philadelphia, PA: Saunders; 2004:73–90

6. Dietz WH, Robinson TN. Clinical practice. Overweight children and adolescents. *N Engl J Med.* 2005;352:2100–2109

7. Marks A, Malizio J, Hoch J, Brody R, Fisher M. Assessment of health needs and willingness to utilize health care resources of adolescents in a suburban population. *J Pediatr.* 1983;102:456–460

8. Arenz S, Ruckerl R, Koletzko B, von Kries R. Breast-feeding and childhood obesity—a systematic review. *Int J Obes Relat Metab Disord.* 2004;28:1247–1256

9. American Academy of Pediatrics Committee on Nutrition. The use and misuse of fruit juice in pediatrics. *Pediatrics.* 2001;107:1210–1213

10. Ludwig DS, Peterson KE, Gortmaker SL. Relation between consumption of sugar-sweetened drinks and childhood obesity: a prospective, observational analysis. *Lancet.* 2001;357:505–508

11. Robinson TN. Reducing children's television viewing to prevent obesity: a randomized controlled trial. *JAMA.* 1999;282:1561–1567

12. Gortmaker SL, Peterson K, Wiecha J, et al. Reducing obesity via a school-based interdisciplinary intervention among youth: Planet Health. *Arch Pediatr Adolesc Med.* 1999;153:409–418

13. American Academy of Pediatrics Committee on Public Education. Children, adolescents, and television. *Pediatrics.* 2001;107:423–426

14. American Academy of Pediatrics Council on Sports Medicine and Fitness and Council on School Health. Active healthy living: prevention of childhood obesity through increased physical activity. *Pediatrics.* 2006;117:1834–1842

15. Barlow SE. Expert committee recommendations regarding the prevention, assessment, and treatment of child and adolescent overweight and obesity: summary report. *Pediatrics.* 2007;120(suppl 4):S164–192

16. Freedman DS, Wang J, Maynard LM, et al. Relation of BMI to fat and fat-free mass among children and adolescents. *Int J Obes (Lond).* 2005;29:1–8

17. Summerbell CD, Ashton V, Campbell KJ, Edmunds L, Kelly S, Waters E. Interventions for treating obesity in children. *Cochrane Database Syst Rev.* 2003;3:CD001872

18. US Preventive Services Task Force, Barton M. Screening for obesity in children and adolescents: US Preventive Services Task Force recommendation statement. *Pediatrics.* 2010;125(2):361–367

19. Epstein LH, Wing RR, Penner BC, Kress MJ. Effect of diet and controlled exercise on weight loss in obese children. *J Pediatr.* 1985;107:358–361

20. Schwingshandl J, Sudi K, Eibl B, Wallner S, Borkenstein M. Effect of an individualised training programme during weight reduction on body composition: a randomised trial. *Arch Dis Child.* 1999;81:426–428

21. Balagopal P, George D, Yarandi H, Funanage V, Bayne E. Reversal of obesity-related hypoadiponectinemia by lifestyle intervention: a controlled, randomized study in obese adolescents. *J Clin Endocrinol Metab.* 2005;90:6192–6197

22. Dunn AL, Andersen RE, Jakicic JM. Lifestyle physical activity interventions. History, short- and long-term effects, and recommendations. *Am J Prev Med.* 1998;15:398–412

23. Epstein LH, Wing RR, Woodall K, Penner BC, Kress MJ, Koeske R. Effects of family-based behavioral treatment on obese 5- to 8-year-old children. *Behav Ther.* 1985;16:205–212

24. Epstein LH, Valoski AM, Vara LS, et al. Effects of decreasing sedentary behavior and increasing activity on weight change in obese children. *Health Psychol.* 1995;14:109–115

25. Epstein LH, Paluch RA, Gordy CC, Dorn J. Decreasing sedentary behaviors in treating pediatric obesity. *Arch Pediatr Adolesc Med.* 2000;154:220–226

26. Senediak C, Spence SH. Rapid versus gradual scheduling of therapeutic contact in a family based behavioural weight control programme for children. *Behav Psychother.* 1985;13:265–287

27. Mellin LM, Slinkard LA, Irwin CE. Adolescent obesity intervention: validation of the SHAPEDOWN program. *J Am Diet Assoc.* 1987;87:333–338

28. Flodmark CE, Ohlsson T, Ryden O, Sveger T. Prevention of progression to severe obesity in a group of obese schoolchildren treated with family therapy. *Pediatrics.* 1993;91:880–884

29. Israel AC, Stolmaker L, Andrian CA. The effects of training parents in general child management skills on a behavioral weight loss program for children. *Behav Ther.* 1985;16:169–180

30. Golan M, Fainaru M, Weizman A. Role of behaviour modification in the treatment of childhood obesity with the parents as the exclusive agents of change. *Int J Obes Relat Metab Disord.* 1998;22:1217–1224

31. Golan M, Weizman A, Apter A, Fainaru M. Parents as the exclusive agents of change in the treatment of childhood obesity. *Am J Clin Nutr.* 1998;67:1130–1135

32. Golan M, Weizman A, Fainaru M. Impact of treatment for childhood obesity on parental risk factors for cardiovascular disease. *Prev Med.* 1999;29:519–526

33. Israel AC, Guile CA, Baker JE, Silverman WK. An evaluation of enhanced self-regulation training in the treatment of childhood obesity. *J Pediatr Psychol.* 1994;19:737–749

34. Wadden TA, Stunkard AJ, Rich L, Rubin CJ, Sweidel G, McKinney S. Obesity in black adolescent girls: a controlled clinical trial of treatment by diet, behavior modification, and parental support. *Pediatrics.* 1990;85:345–352

35. Duffy G, Spence SH. The effectiveness of cognitive self-management as an adjunct to a behavioural intervention for childhood obesity: a research note. *J Child Psychol Psychiatry.* 1993;34:1043–1050

36. Warschburger P, Fromme C, Petermann F, Wojtalla N, Oepen J. Conceptualization and evaluation of a cognitive-behavioural training programme for children and adolescents with obesity. *Int J Obes Relat Disord.* 2001;25(suppl 1):S93–S95

37. Epstein LH, McKenzie SJ, Valoski A, Klein KR, Wing RR. Effects of mastery criteria and contingent reinforcement for family-based child weight control. *Addict Behav.* 1994;19:135–145

38. Graves T, Meyers AW, Clark L. An evaluation of parental problem-solving training in the behavioral treatment of childhood obesity. *J Consult Clin Psychol.* 1988;56:246–250

39. Epstein LH, Paluch RA, Gordy CC, Saelens BE, Ernst MM. Problem solving in the treatment of childhood obesity. *J Consult Clin Psychol.* 2000;68:717–721

13

School and Community Efforts

13.1 The Overweight or Obese Child and the School Setting

Schools provide a daily nutrition and activity environment for more than 95% of US children.[1] A variety of obesity prevention and treatment strategies, including improving nutrition education, increasing physical activity, reducing television viewing, and decreasing availability of high-calorie drinks and snacks, have been tried in schools. Somewhat similar to the family setting, issues of access, knowledge, attitudes, beliefs, and behavior play a role in shaping these environments for children. To engage in obesity prevention and treatment, it is important that the pediatrician understand the role that school plays in the daily lives of children and their families.

13.2 The Individual Patient

Each child with obesity will have a unique interaction with the school environment. It is important to understand the particular school-based nutrition and activity factors that affect energy balance in each individual situation.

Access to Food

School breakfast and lunch programs are important to many children. It is critical that families and pediatricians know what is served, in what portions, and what discretion children have over choices and amounts of foods. School menus can be very helpful, but it is always important to ask the child or adolescent what is actually eaten and what food is left from the school meal. Trading food and buying extra snacks are not unusual behaviors and should be asked about. Some schools use credit cards funded by the parents monthly for food purchases; asking about how fast this money is spent can also give an idea of extra food consumption. Meal skipping can occur and disrupt eating patterns. Some children simply do not like what is offered and will wait until they get home to eat or will feel self-conscious about eating in front of others; others will feel rushed by long lines and little time, grab a snack, and skip a regular meal. It is important to understand these meal patterns so that you can help families

find solutions. Packing a lunch can help provide needed nutritional changes. Families may need suggestions for selecting healthy options for a packed lunch. Pediatricians should also be advocates for providing the healthiest possible breakfast and lunch options.

Snacking can occur as a planned part of the school day. Many schools provide morning snacks for younger children. Snacks and sweetened beverages can also be provided as special treats and rewards, such as for birthday parties or class achievements. Snacking is a routine part of after-school programs, and snacks can often be purchased from school stores or vending machines. Families can pack a snack to substitute for the one at school, lobby with schools to remove vending machines or provide healthier alternatives, or limit the amount of money the child has to purchase these items. Sports programs are an integral part of school activities, but there may be occasions where high-energy dense snacks and drinks are consumed. Parents and coaches should use these events as opportunities to provide healthy snacks and plenty of water as a way to model healthy eating.

Access to Physical Activity

Physical education classes may take place every day or not at all. It is important to ask about the frequency of physical education, as well as time spent in actual activity and skill development. These classes, in addition to regular curriculum, should provide an opportunity for honing age-appropriate skills and developing interest in noncompetitive activities that could provide lifelong activity. Children like activity to be fun, geared to their skill level, and inclusive. Pediatricians should make every effort to keep children with obesity involved in physical education. Adaptive gym and alternatives, such as participating in a walking club or walking during class, can be used as ways to encourage children who are obese to stay active.

Extracurricular sports can play a large role in providing daily physical activity for children. However, these competitive sports may quickly move out of reach for a child with obesity. Pediatricians should encourage schools to maintain intramural sports and provide as many lifestyle activities after school as possible. Sometimes reengaging the child or adolescent needs to start with participating in *any* planned after-school activity, club, or group to break the cycle of watching television, using a computer, and being sedentary. Families may need to be encouraged to find extracurricular options available at school that go beyond competitive sports.

Educational Opportunities

Opportunities for increasing students' knowledge of good nutrition, importance of activity, media savvy, and importance of television reduction have been studied in schools. Changing knowledge and beliefs of children may be a powerful tool that school programs can provide to combat obesity. Curriculum changes, extracurricular classes, and support groups are all mechanisms used to accomplish these goals. Pediatricians can play a role as invited classroom speakers, in training faculty, and meeting with parents to get the message out about obesity prevention and treatment. Pediatricians can also be available as resources for school boards and school wellness committees and encourage needed policy changes, such as reducing soda and juice availability. Many schools are beginning to report body mass index (BMI) percentiles; pediatricians have a clear role in helping school nurses and the families who receive this information interpret and act on it.

13.3 Advocacy in the School

Pediatricians are often in a position to advocate for change in schools and provide support and expertise to school personnel. Schools face many challenges in providing healthy meals and snacks. Competitive foods (foods of minimal nutritional value that are sold in competition with school meals in snack bars, school stores, and vending machines) tempt students. Offering these foods also sends a mixed message to students and may devalue lessons given in class about good nutrition. Food service personnel may have limited training, space, and time, as well as inadequate facilities in which to prepare food.[2]

Pediatricians can encourage some additional community efforts in their neighborhoods and neighborhood schools. They can promote safe walking and biking to school by asking questions such as, "Does the school have places to lock a bicycle?" "Where would kids safely keep their helmets if they biked to school?" or "Is there a safe walking route to school?" Similarly, pediatrician support for "the walking school bus," a system whereby parents act as school guards and make sure there are safe routes to school, can be invaluable.

Pediatricians can also support "mixed use" polices, where schools open their schoolyards on weekends and evenings for free play. Many jurisdictions have had legal barriers to doing this (eg, school district liability, in case of injury, etc). Yet, there are groups that are working on these and have successfully overcome these barriers, making physical activity far more accessible to children. Encouraging community gardens and school gardens are great ways for schools to make "trying new vegetables" a part of their health curriculum.

In the following sections, some specific school and early childhood programs will be reviewed to provide background for the kinds of changes and implementation strategies that are used. In a review of obesity prevention program studies, the Cochrane review published an analysis of obesity prevention trials lasting at least 12 weeks.[3] These studies were all randomized, controlled trials, performed in the school setting.

13.4 Early Childhood Settings[3]

Special Supplemental Nutrition Program for Women, Infants, and Children

The Special Supplemental Nutrition Program for Women, Infants, and Children (WIC) would seem a logical place to start for obesity prevention. To date, most studies in this population are feasibility studies. In one study, Bright Futures guidelines were incorporated into the content of every 2-month educational group and twice-yearly sessions with a nutritionist. Six key messages were used:

1. Increase physical activity.
2. Monitor mealtime behavior.
3. Limit household television viewing.
4. Drink water instead of sweetened beverages.
5. Consume 5 fruits or vegetables daily.
6. Increase family activities to promote fitness.

Parents were encouraged to serve as role models. Compared with a control group, participants reported increased frequency of active play with the child and of offering the child water instead of sweetened beverages.[4]

Preschool[3]

In the preschool group (2.6–5.5 years of age), a study in a child care setting involved seven 1-hour sessions on reducing television viewing by encouraging reading with informational packets sent home to parents. Children were watching 11.9 hours (intervention group) and 14.0 hours (control group) per week of television and videos before the intervention. Although BMI did not change, children reduced their television viewing by 3.1 hours per week, whereas the control group increased their viewing by 1.6 hours per week.[5]

Home Visits

A trial of home visitation with a group of preschool-aged boys (14–30 months of age) focused on parenting skills to develop appropriate diet and activity behavior in a Native American population compared with a parenting skills intervention alone. At the end of 12 weeks, energy intake was increasing for those in the control group and decreasing for the intervention group, although there were no differences in BMI. Mothers in the intervention group were also engaging in less restrictive feeding.[6]

13.5 School Settings[3]

Sweetened Beverage Reduction

In a study in the UK, 644 schoolchildren, 7 to 11 years of age, received three 1-hour sessions (1 per term) focused on reducing carbonated beverage consumption. Self-reported soft drink consumption decreased approximately 58 mL per day, but there was no significant difference in BMI z scores between groups.[7]

Increased Physical Activity[3]

In a trial of 292 kindergarten children in Thailand (mean age of 4.5 years), 35 minutes of aerobic exercise (15-minute walk before school and 20-minute aerobic dance after the afternoon nap) was added 3 times a week for 29.6 weeks to the usual physical education. Thirteen months after the intervention there was a suggestion of a greater decrease in BMI of the control group versus the intervention group, but no statistically significant difference was found between groups in BMI or triceps skinfold.[8]

In a US trial called project SPARK, 549 children (mean age of 9.25 years) were provided with high levels of physical activity in three 30-minute sessions a week. There was a trend toward lower triceps and calve skinfolds in the control group, but there were no significant differences between the groups at 2 years of age.[9]

Improved Nutrition and Increased Physical Activity[3]

The APPLES study[10] included 634 children, 7 to 11 years of age, in 10 schools. This was a 1-year study targeting parents, teachers, and food service staff. Schools individualized plans to include modification of meals, physical education and recess, and classroom education. The intervention team included a dietitian, pediatrician, health promotion specialist, psychologist, obesity physician, and nutritional epidemiologist. There was no difference in BMI at 1 year, but children who had the intervention had higher vegetable consumption than those in the control group.

A school study from England[11] of children 5 to 7 years of age tracked the independent effects of nutrition intervention alone, physical activity alone, a combined intervention, and a control group. The intervention took place at lunchtime clubs and was delivered by the intervention team, which included parents. Reinforcing health messages, food tasting, and noncompetitive activities were targeted. After 20 weeks there was no change in overweight or obesity. Physical activity did increase on the playground and fruit and vegetable consumption increased, but there was no decrease in snack food.

A 24-week obesity prevention program in the United States[12] included 201 girls, 9 to 12 years of age, with a BMI greater than 75%. This intervention included social support and nutrition education 4 times a week for 16 weeks. Once a week, community instructors led groups in dance, self-defense, and swimming. Nutrition advice was to avoid dieting, increase fruit and vegetable consumption, and decrease sugar intake. After the intervention, the girls met weekly for 2 months for lunch and discussion. At the end of the study there was no difference in BMI between the control and intervention groups, but those in the intervention group did progress toward physical activity on the stages of change model.

Six hundred six children, 9 to 10 years of age,[13] were randomly assigned to play, play and physical education, physical education only, and a control group. The intervention promoted more walking, and teachers taught play activities and encouraged self-directed activities with the goal of 30 minutes of activity outside school a day. At 12 weeks there was no difference in BMI among groups, but those in the intervention group had an increase in physical activity, especially among girls.

Television Viewing Reduction[3]

In a study to reduce television viewing, children 8 to 10 years of age[14] were exposed to 18 lessons of 30 to 50 minutes incorporated into the curriculum. Self-monitoring, self-reporting of television and video use, and adoption of a 7-hour-a-week budget were encouraged. After 6 months, the intervention group showed a significant decrease in television viewing and meals eaten in front of the television, as well as in all measures of body fatness, BMI, waist circumference, and waist-to-hip ratio.

Improved Nutrition, Increased Physical Activity, and Decreased Television Viewing[3]

Planet Health[15] is a school obesity prevention intervention that included 1,295 children 11 to 12 years of age. The intervention was designed to be delivered by teachers in multiple subject areas—language arts, math, science, social studies, and physical education—and included information on promoting physical activity, modifying dietary intake, and providing a strong emphasis on reducing television viewing. After 18 months, the percentage of girls with obesity in the intervention schools was reduced compared with controls. There was no significant difference in outcome for the boys. There was also greater remission of obesity in girls in the intervention group than those in the control group. Television viewing hours were reduced among boys and girls, and girls increased their fruit and vegetable consumption. Television reduction predicted obesity change in the girls but not in boys. Analysis of the cost benefit was performed and worked out to $4,305 per quality-of-life year saved, with a net savings of $7,313 to society.[16]

Teachers found Planet Health to be feasible and acceptable. Difficulties in implementation mentioned were lack of time for planning, lack of curriculum reinforcement in school meal programs, presence of vending machines in schools, and lack of reinforcement in the children's homes.[17]

A study of 410 German children, 5 to 7 years of age, incorporated nutrition education and activity breaks into the school curriculum. Emphasis was on increased fruit and vegetable consumption, reduced high-fat food consumption, 1 hour of activity a day, and decreased television viewing to less than 1 hour a day. At 1 year there was no change in BMI, but triceps skinfold measurements decreased in the intervention group. There was no difference in overweight percentage in either group.[18]

13.6 Comprehensive School Health Program Changes

A review of schools following Centers for Disease Control and Prevention (CDC) guidelines for healthy eating programs, which include recommendations for school policies, curriculum change, instructions to students, integration of school food services and nutrition education, staff training, family and community involvement, and program evaluation,[19] was conducted to determine the effective of these

recommendations. Students from schools following these guidelines had lower rates of overweight and obesity, higher consumption of fruits and vegetables, less caloric intake from fat, higher dietary quality, more participation in physical activities, and less participation in sedentary activities compared with students who were provided only with healthier menu alternatives or no nutritional plan.[20]

In summary, the Cochrane reviewers[3] believed that sustainability and environmental change combined with behavior change and family support are important factors in determining a positive outcome for these interventions. In a recent review of obesity interventions, the CDC stated, "When planning future interventions aimed at weight-control outcomes, considering interventions that produced modest but positive changes in weight-related measures might be useful. These interventions are 1) including nutrition and physical activity components in combination, 2) allotting additional time to physical activity during the school day, 3) including non-competitive sports (eg, dance), and 4) reducing sedentary activities, especially television viewing."[21]

Programs that are successful in a research setting need to be translated into the wider school environment. Factors thought to be important in terms of initiating and maintaining a school-based obesity program include[22]

- Relative advantage—Innovation is better that the status quo.
- Compatibility—Innovation is consistent with current values of the school.
- Low complexity—The innovation is not difficult to understand and use.
- Observability—The results are noticeable to others.
- "Trialability"—The innovation can be tried out on a partial or temporary basis.

13.7 Advocacy for Healthier Communities

Pediatricians can be powerful voices for improving community access to healthy foods and physical activity. As child health experts, pediatricians have knowledge and experience that can inform community health change. Participating in local community coalitions, testifying at community councils and state legislatures, and speaking at meetings of community organizations are a few ways to take the message of the importance of healthy lifestyle change beyond the clinic walls. Taking advantage of media opportunities to write or speak about childhood obesity and healthy lifestyles is another way to extend your voice. The AAP offers resources for pediatricians at www.aap.org/obesity.

References

1. Resnicow K. School-based obesity prevention. Population versus high-risk interventions. *Ann NY Acad Sci.* 1993;699:154–166

2. Gross SM, Cinelli B. Coordinated school health program and dietetics professionals: partners in promoting healthful eating. *J Am Diet Assoc.* 2004;104:793–798

3. Summerbell CD, Waters E, Edmunds LD, Kelly S, Brown T, Campbell KJ. Interventions for preventing obesity in children. *Cochrane Database Syst Rev.* 2005;3:CD001871

4. McGarvy E, Keller A, Forrester M, Williams E, Seward D, Suttle DE. Feasibility and benefits of a parent-focused preschool child obesity intervention. *Am J Public Health.* 2004;94:1490–1495

5. Dennison BA, Russo TJ, Burdick PA, Jenkins PL. An intervention to reduce television viewing by preschool children. *Arch Pediatr Adolesc Med.* 2004;158:170–176

6. Harvey-Berino J, Rourke J. Obesity prevention in preschool Native-American children: a pilot study using home visiting. *Obes Res.* 2003;11:606–611

7. James J, Thomas P, Cavan D, Kerr D. Preventing childhood obesity by reducing consumption of carbonated drinks: cluster randomized controlled trial. *BMJ.* 2004;328:1237

8. Mo-suwan L, Pongprapai S, Junjana C, Peutpaiboon A. Effects of a controlled trial of a school-based exercise program on the obesity indexes of preschool children. *Am J Clin Nutr.* 1998;68:1006–1111

9. Sallis JF, McKenzie TL, Alcaraz JE, Kolody B, Hovell MF, Nader PR. Project SPARK. Effects of physical education on adiposity in children. *Ann NY Acad Sci.* 1993;699:127–136

10. Sahota P, Rudolf MC, Dixey R, Hill AJ, Barth JH, Cade J. Randomised controlled trial of primary school based intervention to reduce risk factors for obesity. *BMJ.* 2001;323:1029–1032

11. Warren JM, Henry CJ, Lightowler HJ, Bradshaw SM, Perwaiz S. Evaluation of a pilot school programme aimed at the prevention of obesity in children. *Health Promot Int.* 2003;18:287–296

12. Neumark-Sztainer D, Story M, Hannan PJ, Rex J. New Moves: a school-based obesity prevention program for adolescent girls. *Prev Med.* 2003;37:41–51

13. Pangrazi RP, Beighle A, Vehige T, Vack C. Impact of Promoting Lifestyle Activity for Youth (PLAY) on children's physical activity. *J Sch Health.* 2003;73:317–321

14. Robinson TN. Reducing children's television viewing to prevent obesity: a randomized controlled trial. *JAMA.* 1999;282:1561–1567

15. Gortmaker SL, Peterson K, Wiecha J, et al. Reducing obesity via a school-based interdisciplinary intervention among youth: Planet Health. *Arch Pediatr Adolesc Med.* 1999;153:409–418

16. Wang LY, Yang Q, Lowry R, Wechsler H. Economic analysis of a school-based obesity prevention program. *Obes Res.* 2003;11:1313–1324

17. Wiecha JL, El Ayadi AM, Fuemmeler BF, et al. Diffusion of an integrated health education program in an urban school system: Planet Health. *J Pediatr Psychol.* 2004;29:467–474

18. Muller MJ, Asbeck I, Mast M, Lagnase L, Grund A. Prevention of obesity—more than an intention. Concept and first results of the Kiel Obesity Prevention Study (KOPS). *Int J Obes Relat Metab Disord.* 2001;25(suppl 1):S66–S74

19. Centers for Disease Control and Prevention. Guidelines for school health programs to promote lifelong healthy eating. *MMWR Recomm Rep.* 1996;45(RR-9):1–41

20. Veugelers PJ, Fitzgerald AL. Effectiveness of school programs in preventing childhood obesity: a multilevel comparison. *Am J Public Health.* 2005;95:432–435

21. Katz DL, O'Connell M, Yeh MC, et al. Public health strategies for preventing and controlling overweight and obesity in school and worksite settings: a report on recommendations of the Task Force on Community Preventive Services. *MMWR Recomm Rep.* 2005;54(RR-10):1–12

22. Rogers EM. Diffusion of preventive innovations. *Addict Behav.* 2002; 27:989–999

A.1

BALANCE for a Healthy Life:
Patient Handouts for Your Practice

Index

AVOIDING FOOD TRAPS

Food traps are situations and places that make it difficult to eat right. We all have them. The following tips may help you avoid some of the most common traps.

Food Trap #1: Vacations, Holidays, and Other Family Gatherings

Vacations

When on a trip, don't take a vacation from healthy eating and exercise.

What you can do

- ☐ Plan your meals. Will all your meals be from restaurants? If so, can you split entrees and desserts to keep portions from getting too large? Can you avoid fast food? Can you bring along your own healthy snacks?
- ☐ Stay active. Schedule time for physical activities such as taking a walk or swimming in the hotel pool.

Holidays

It's easy to overeat during holidays. But you don't need to fear or avoid them.

What you can do

- ☐ Approach the holidays with extra care. Don't lose sight of what you and your child are eating. Plan to have healthy foods and snacks on hand. Bring a fruit or veggie tray with you when you go to friends and family.
- ☐ Celebrate for the day, not an entire month! Be sure to return to healthy eating the next day.

Other Family Gatherings

In some cultures, when extended families get together, it can turn into a food feast, from morning to night.

What you can do

- ☐ Eat smaller portions. Avoid overeating whenever you get together with family. Try taking small portions instead.
- ☐ Get family support. Grandparents, aunts, and uncles can have an enormous effect on your child's health. Let them know that you'd like their help in keeping your child on the road to good health.

Food trap #2: Snack Time

The biggest time for snacking is after school. Kids come home wound up, stressed out, or simply bored, so they reach for food.

What you can do

- ☐ **Offer healthy snacks** such as raw vegetables, fruit, light microwave popcorn, vegetable soup, sugar-free gelatin, or fruit snacks.
- ☐ **You pick the snack.** When children are allowed to pick their own snacks, they often make unhealthy choices. Talk to your child about why healthy snacks are important. Come up with a list of snacks that you can both agree on and have them on hand.
- ☐ **Keep your child entertained.** Help your child come up with other things to do instead of eating, such as playing outside, dancing, painting a picture, flying a kite, or taking a walk with you.
- ☐ **Make sure your child eats 3 well-balanced meals a day.** This will help cut down on the number of times he or she needs a snack.

Food trap #3: Running Out of Time

Finding time every day to be physically active can be very difficult. However, if you plan ahead, there are ways to fit it in.

What you can do

- ☐ **Make a plan.** Sit down with your child and plan in advance for those days when it seems impossible to find even 15 minutes for physical activity.
- ☐ **Have a plan B** ready that your child can do after dark, such as exercising to a workout video.
- ☐ **Make easy dinners.** If you run out of time to make dinner, don't run to the nearest fast-food restaurant. Remember, dinners don't have to be elaborate. They can be as simple as a sandwich, bowl of soup, piece of fruit, and glass of milk.

Remember

Your job is to provide good nutrition to your child and family and encourage regular physical activity. Stay positive and focus on how well your child is doing in all areas of life. It can help keep nutrition and activity change moving along.

Belief, **A**ssessment, **L**ifestyle, **A**ctivity, **N**utrition, **C**hild, **E**nvironment

Adapted from American Academy of Pediatrics. *A Parent's Guide to Childhood Obesity: A Road Map to Health.* Hassink SG, ed. Elk Grove Village, IL: American Academy of Pediatrics; 2006
The information contained in this publication should not be used as a substitute for the medical care and advice of your pediatrician. There may be variations in treatment that your pediatrician may recommend based on individual facts and circumstances.

EVERYONE GET FIT

A generation ago, most kids came home from school, had a snack, and then went outside until they were called in for dinner. Most children, it seemed, were active without being told to do so. Today we are seeing an epidemic of obesity, and the lack of interest in physical activity is a big reason why. Use the following to help your child be more physically active.

Encouraging Physical Activity

All children need to do some physical activity every day. If your child is overweight, you may need to help your child get moving. Your goal should be to turn exercise into a lifelong habit.

What you can do

- ☐ **Encourage your child** to set a goal of doing some kind of exercise each day, even if it's walking for only a few minutes at a time.

- ☐ **Make sure your child has things to play with** that are right for his or her age, from balls to plastic bats, to make exercise fun.

- ☐ **Let your child choose** what to play with at any given time.

A family affair

Spend family time doing physical activities that all of you like. When you do things together, your child will see how important exercise is to you. You'll become her most important role model.

What you can do

- ☐ **Play catch** in the yard or spend time hitting a tennis ball at the neighborhood courts.

- ☐ **Take a family hike** or bike ride.

- ☐ **Go to the park** and throw the football back and forth.

- ☐ **Play tag** in the front yard.

- ☐ **Go to the community pool** for a family swim.

- ☐ **Go to the mall and walk** from one end to the other (without spending any time at the food court).

- ☐ **Do household chores together,** such as cleaning, raking leaves, or waxing the car.

Peer group activities

Most children can get involved in organized sports such as Little League; martial arts; or soccer, basketball, hockey, or football leagues. Team sports are fun and the perfect fit for many children. However, some children may feel self-conscious about playing team sports and are much more comfortable getting their exercise in other ways.

What you can do

- ☐ **Let your child choose** something that he or she enjoys, and encourage your child to make it a regular part of life.

- ☐ **Limit TV watching** or time spent on the computer or playing video games to no more than 2 hours a day. Children younger than 2 should not have any screen time.

- ☐ **Try to find activities that fit the family's budget** and schedule and give your child several choices.

- ☐ **Help your child choose** activities that focus on participation, not competition.

- ☐ **Don't forget the lifetime sports** that can last for decades, including golf, tennis, skating, and skiing.

Remember

Regular activity not only burns calories but also strengthens the cardiovascular system, builds strong bones and muscles, and increases flexibility. It can also relieve stress, teach teamwork and sportsmanship, boost self-esteem, and improve a person's overall sense of well-being.

Belief, Assessment, Lifestyle, Activity, Nutrition, Child, Environment

Adapted from American Academy of Pediatrics. *A Parent's Guide to Childhood Obesity: A Road Map to Health.* Hassink SG, ed. Elk Grove Village, IL: American Academy of Pediatrics; 2006
The information contained in this publication should not be used as a substitute for the medical care and advice of your pediatrician. There may be variations in treatment that your pediatrician may recommend based on individual facts and circumstances.

FAMILY MEALS

Eating together as a family is a great way to

- Help your child learn healthy eating habits.
- Model healthy eating for your child.
- Spend valuable time together as a family.

Read on to find out how regular family meals can make a difference in your child's life.

The power of family

Helping your child lose weight should be a family project. You can't expect your child to change his or her eating habits alone while others in the family continue to reach for candy and ice cream.

What you can do

☐ **Get your entire family on board** and support the weight loss efforts of your child.

☐ **Be sure everyone in the family models** healthy eating behaviors.

☐ **Avoid making your child feel singled out** and isolated. It will make your child resentful and increase the chances of failure.

☐ **Explain that the entire family,** whether the person has a weight problem or not, is going to work at getting healthier.

☐ **Turn mealtime into family time** whenever possible.

Structured eating

When you have a child trying to lose weight, you need to pay particular attention to mealtimes. They should be firmly structured, not only for your child, but for the entire family.

What you can do

☐ **Have set times for meals.** If your child knows that dinner is going to be served at 6:00 pm, he or she will be less likely to start searching for a snack at 5:30 pm. If dinner is served at a different time every night, your child might grab a snack rather than risk having to wait 2 or 3 hours to eat.

☐ **Offer your family 3 well-balanced meals each day.** Avoid skipping meals. If your child skips a meal, he or she will become overly hungry, setting the stage for overeating.

☐ **Offer your child 1 to 2 healthy snacks** per day. Discourage grazing (when your child has access to and grabs food all day long).

☐ **Prepare meals that are balanced** and have portion sizes that are right for your child's age.

☐ **Provide** at least 1 fruit or vegetable with every meal.

☐ **Let your child help** choose what will be on the menu. Encourage and praise your child for making healthy food choices.

Mealtime as family time

In too many homes, families rarely sit down for a meal together. Having regular meals together as a family is an important way for families to grow closer. Family meals give everyone the chance to talk about their day. They are also an opportunity for you to keep an eye on what your child is eating.

What you can do

☐ **Try to have as many meals together** as a family as possible.

☐ **Set a no-TV rule** during family meals. The TV is a disruption that you should avoid while you're eating.

☐ **Keep meals pleasant** and focus on the positives. Celebrate your child's successes and offer praise for his or her efforts.

Remember

Children learn more about good food choices and healthy nutrition when family members join one another for meals. Research also shows that kids eat more vegetables and fruits and less fried foods and sugary drinks when they eat with the entire family.

Belief, **A**ssessment, **L**ifestyle, **A**ctivity, **N**utrition, **C**hild, **E**nvironment

Adapted from American Academy of Pediatrics. *A Parent's Guide to Childhood Obesity: A Road Map to Health.* Hassink SG, ed. Elk Grove Village, IL: American Academy of Pediatrics; 2006
The information contained in this publication should not be used as a substitute for the medical care and advice of your pediatrician. There may be variations in treatment that your pediatrician may recommend based on individual facts and circumstances.

THE FIRST 2 YEARS: FOCUS ON GOOD NUTRITION

If you're worried that your young child is overweight or becoming obese, you might be thinking about feeding him or her only low-fat foods. Here's the bottom line—do not restrict your child's dietary fat and calories in the first 2 years of life. Read on to find out why.

Fat is important

The first 2 years of life are critical for normal development of the brain and body. Dietary fat not only helps in that development but also provides energy and helps the body absorb certain vitamins.

What you can do

☐ **For the first year of life,** babies should drink only breast milk or formula, not cow's milk.

☐ **After age 1 year,** offer your child whole milk to ensure his or her diet includes enough fat.

☐ **After age 2 years,** you can switch from whole milk to fat-free milk. You can make this easier on your family by gradually changing from whole milk to 2%, then to 1% milk. You might even try mixing them together to make the changes even easier for your family.

Using formula correctly

Formula is designed to provide about 20 calories per ounce and includes the proper amount of fat to ensure healthy growth.

What you can do

☐ **When preparing formula,** be sure to follow the instructions carefully.

☐ **Be sure to add the correct amount of water.** If you add too much water, you can interfere with your baby's normal physical growth and brain development.

How much fat is enough?

During the first 2 years, about half of your child's calories should come from fat. After age 2, you can modify your child's diet gradually until dietary fat makes up about one-third of the total calories.

What you can do

☐ **Establish healthy eating habits early** by giving your child well-balanced meals and snacks.

☐ **Focus on good nutrition,** not reducing calories.

☐ **Discourage grazing** (this is when your child has access to and grabs food all day long).

☐ **Offer your child meals** that have a balance of fats, protein, carbohydrates, vitamins, and minerals and include foods from the major food groups each day.

☐ **Limit sweets.**

☐ **Steer away from sugary drinks and fast food;** these are "empty" calories that interfere with healthy eating and contribute to excess weight.

Remember

Healthy eating for the first 2 years of your child's life should focus on good nutrition, not calories. Do not limit the amount of dietary fat on your toddler's plate. Instead, help your child form healthy eating habits by giving well-balanced meals and snacks.

Belief, **A**ssessment, **L**ifestyle, **A**ctivity, **N**utrition, **C**hild, **E**nvironment

Adapted from American Academy of Pediatrics. *A Parent's Guide to Childhood Obesity: A Road Map to Health.* Hassink SG, ed. Elk Grove Village, IL: American Academy of Pediatrics; 2006
The information contained in this publication should not be used as a substitute for the medical care and advice of your pediatrician. There may be variations in treatment that your pediatrician may recommend based on individual facts and circumstances.

FOOD AND TV: NOT A HEALTHY MIX

TV is an important part of our lives—it entertains us and has much to teach. But too much TV and food advertising can make eating right very difficult. Limiting TV time can help your child stay on the path to healthy living. Here's how.

TV and babies

Studies have shown that excessive TV watching is associated with obesity and overweight in children. The best way to avoid this is to limit how much TV your baby watches.

What you can do

☐ **Do not place your baby in front of the TV.** TV isn't appropriate for children younger than 2 years because it takes time away from real interactions with you and other family members.

☐ **Avoid using the TV as a babysitter.** Instead, look for ways to interact with your child face to face.

Where the American Academy of Pediatrics stands

In the first 2 years of life, your child's brain and body are growing and developing very quickly. During this time, it is important that your child have real interactions with people and not sit idly in front of the TV.

For that reason, the American Academy of Pediatrics currently recommends that TV not be watched by children 2 years and younger. For older children, TV watching (of educational, nonviolent programming) should be limited to no more than 1 to 2 hours a day.

TV and the family meal

There is plenty of unconscious eating that can take place in front of the TV. It's easy for kids to simply eat their way from one program to the next. Distracted by the TV, they'll often eat long beyond when they're full. The result? Weight gain.

What you can do

☐ **Set a no-TV rule** during meals.

☐ **Serve your meals** at the dining room or kitchen table with other family members as often as possible. Mealtime is an important time for family conversations and sharing the day's experiences without the TV getting in the way.

TV and obesity

Here's another important reason to limit your child's TV watching: the steady stream of ads for high-sugar, high-fat foods aimed directly at children. Studies have shown that children who watch a lot of TV have a greater likelihood of becoming obese. The commercials targeted at children are one of the reasons why.

What you can do

☐ **Do not allow** children younger than 2 years to watch TV.

☐ **Limit TV watching** (as well as video and computer game playing) to 1 to 2 hours a day for older children.

☐ **Talk about the ads** your child sees on TV and explain how they encourage unhealthy eating.

☐ **Stay strong** when your child begs for the latest food or candy shown on TV. Explain why you think it's not healthy for him or her.

Remember

Even if your child doesn't eat in front of the TV, you still need to restrict his or her TV watching. A daily limit of TV viewing and playing computer or video games should not exceed 1 to 2 hours.

Belief, **A**ssessment, **L**ifestyle, **A**ctivity, **N**utrition, **C**hild, **E**nvironment

Adapted from American Academy of Pediatrics. *A Parent's Guide to Childhood Obesity: A Road Map to Health.* Hassink SG, ed. Elk Grove Village, IL: American Academy of Pediatrics; 2006
The information contained in this publication should not be used as a substitute for the medical care and advice of your pediatrician. There may be variations in treatment that your pediatrician may recommend based on individual facts and circumstances.

FRUITS AND VEGETABLES: HOW TO GET MORE EVERY DAY

We all know that eating fruits and vegetables is important. But how do you get kids to eat more of these foods? The following tips might help.

What to include

Adding fruits and vegetables to your child's meals is not as difficult as you may think.

What you can do

☐ **Use fruits and vegetables as snacks.**

☐ **Serve salads more often.** Teach your child what an appropriate amount of salad dressing is and how it can be ordered on the side at restaurants.

☐ **Try out child-friendly vegetarian recipes** for spaghetti, lasagna, chili, or other foods using vegetables instead of meat.

☐ **Include** one green leafy or yellow vegetable for vitamin A such as spinach, broccoli, winter squash, greens, or carrots.

☐ **Include** one vitamin C–rich fruit, vegetable, or juice, such as citrus juices, orange, grapefruit, strawberries, melon, tomato, and broccoli.

☐ **Include a fruit or vegetable as part of every meal or snack.** For example, you could put fruit on cereal, add a piece of fruit or small salad to your child's lunch, use vegetables and dip for an after-school snack, or add a vegetable or two you want to try to the family's dinner.

☐ **Be a role model**—eat more fruits and vegetables yourself.

How much is enough?

Be sure your child is getting the recommended amount of fruits and vegetables each day.

What you can do

☐ **Visit MyPlate at www.myplate.gov** to find out how much of each food group your child should be getting.

☐ **When shopping** for food, start in the area of the store where they keep fresh fruits and vegetables. Stock up. That way you know you always have some on hand to serve your child.

☐ **Avoid buying high-calorie foods** such as chips, cookies, and candy bars. Your child may not ask for these treats if they are not in sight.

☐ **Limit or eliminate how much fruit juice** you give your child and make sure it is 100% juice, not juice "drinks."

☐ **Eat as a family** whenever possible. Research shows that kids eat more vegetables and fruits and less fried foods and sugary drinks when they eat with the entire family.

Remember

By choosing health-promoting foods, you can establish good nutritional habits in your child that will last for the rest of his or her life.

Belief, Assessment, Lifestyle, Activity, Nutrition, Child, Environment

---

Fruit and vegetable choking hazards

Children don't fully develop the grinding motion involved in chewing until they're about 4 years old. Until that time, stick with fruits and vegetables that are small and easy to chew and avoid those that might be swallowed whole and get stuck in your toddler's windpipe, such as

- Raw carrots
- Raw celery
- Whole grapes
- Raw cherries with pits

Adapted from American Academy of Pediatrics. *A Parent's Guide to Childhood Obesity: A Road Map to Health.* Hassink SG, ed. Elk Grove Village, IL: American Academy of Pediatrics; 2006
The information contained in this publication should not be used as a substitute for the medical care and advice of your pediatrician. There may be variations in treatment that your pediatrician may recommend based on individual facts and circumstances.

Are you worried about your child's weight? Have you felt helpless as your child gained 2, 5, or 10 extra pounds a year—one year after the next? Maybe you've tried putting your child on a diet, only to be met with frustration and failure. The good news is you can help your child. If you and your child are ready to start on the path to good health, the following tips might help.

Where to start

An important place to start is with your pediatrician. The doctor has the tools and the expertise to help you on this journey.

What you can do

☐ **Talk with your pediatrician** about where your child falls on the growth charts. Growth charts show how your child compares with peers. Does your child fall within the normal range of height and weight for his or her age?

☐ **Find out what your child's body mass index (BMI) is.** BMI is a calculation of your child's body weight relative to height. It's an important way to determine whether your child is overweight. **Use this formula** or visit www.cdc.gov to measure your child's BMI.

- Multiply weight (in pounds) by 703.
  Example: 110 pounds × 703 = 77,330 (A)

- Multiply height (in inches) by itself.
  Example: 48 inches × 48 = 2,304 (B)

- Divide A by B. This will give you the BMI score.
  Example: 77,330 ÷ 2,304 = 33.56

☐ **Talk with your pediatrician** to find out if your child's BMI indicates he or she is at risk of being overweight or already is overweight.

☐ **Get a sense of your child's current weight, nutrition, and activity level** and where you'd like him or her to be headed. Talk to your pediatrician about how best to meet those goals.

You are not alone

Parents often feel guilty and blame themselves for their children's extra weight. But obesity is a problem that's bigger than one child, parent, or family. It affects boys and girls of all ages, races, ethnic groups, and socioeconomic classes.

What you can do

☐ **Don't feel you have to deal with this by yourself.** Your pediatrician cares about your child's health and can help you and your child on this journey.

☐ **Get your entire family on board** and support the weight loss efforts of your obese child. Be sure everyone in the family models healthy eating behaviors.

☐ **Talk with others** in your child's life about supporting these efforts. This includes relatives, friends, school, and child care providers. Your child is more likely to succeed if everyone is offering support.

Remember

You and your child can succeed. It may not be easy, but you have already taken the first step. Getting the information and skills you need to help your child adopt good nutrition and activity habits will ease the journey to good health.

Belief, **A**ssessment, **L**ifestyle, **A**ctivity, **N**utrition, **C**hild, **E**nvironment

Adapted from American Academy of Pediatrics. *A Parent's Guide to Childhood Obesity: A Road Map to Health.* Hassink SG, ed. Elk Grove Village, IL: American Academy of Pediatrics; 2006
The information contained in this publication should not be used as a substitute for the medical care and advice of your pediatrician. There may be variations in treatment that your pediatrician may recommend based on individual facts and circumstances.

HUNGRY OR JUST BORED?

Children (as well as adults) often use food for reasons other than to satisfy hunger. Children often eat in response to their emotions and feelings. If your child seems hungry all the time, use the following tips to get a better idea of what is really going on.

What triggers hunger?

If your child is eating 3 well-balanced meals and 1 snack a day but still claims to be hungry, there may be other reasons beyond hunger that make him or her want to eat.

What you can do

Ask yourself the following questions:

- ☐ **Does your child sometimes reach for food** when experiencing any of the following?

  - Boredom
  - Depression
  - Stress
  - Frustration
  - Insecurity
  - Loneliness
  - Fatigue
  - Resentment
  - Anger
  - Happiness

- ☐ **Does your child eat at times other than regular mealtimes** and snacks? Is your child munching at every opportunity?

- ☐ **Do you reward your child with food** (does an A on a test sometimes lead to a trip to the ice cream shop)? This can inadvertently contribute to your child's obesity.

- ☐ **When your child is doing things right, do you tell him or her?** Words of approval can boost a child's self-esteem. They can also help keep a child motivated to continue making the right decisions for health and weight.

- ☐ **How are you speaking to your child?** Is it mostly negative? Is it often critical? It's hard for anyone, including children, to make changes in that kind of environment.

Healthy alternatives

If you suspect your child is eating out of boredom, you may need to steer him or her toward other activities as a distraction.

What you can do

- ☐ **Make sure your child is eating 3 well-balanced meals and 1 snack a day.** This will prevent feelings of hunger between meals.

- ☐ **Help your child choose** other things to do instead of eating, such as

  - Walking the dog
  - Running through the sprinklers
  - Playing a game of badminton
  - Kicking a soccer ball
  - Painting a picture
  - Going in-line skating
  - Dancing
  - Planting a flower in the garden
  - Flying a kite
  - Joining you for a walk through the mall (without stopping at the ice cream shop)

- ☐ **Offer healthy snacks** such as raw vegetables, fruit, light microwave popcorn, vegetable soup, sugar-free gelatin, and fruit snacks. Snacks such as chips and candy bars have empty calories that will not make your child feel full.

- ☐ **You pick the snack.** When children are allowed to pick their own snacks, they often make unhealthy choices. Talk to your child about why healthy snacks are important. Come up with a list of snacks that you can both agree on and have them on hand.

Remember

Your own relationship with food and weight, dating back to your childhood, can influence the way you parent your own overweight child. One of your biggest challenges is to determine whether your child is eating for the right reasons.

Belief, **A**ssessment, **L**ifestyle, **A**ctivity, **N**utrition, **C**hild, **E**nvironment

Adapted from American Academy of Pediatrics. *A Parent's Guide to Childhood Obesity: A Road Map to Health.* Hassink SG, ed. Elk Grove Village, IL: American Academy of Pediatrics; 2006
The information contained in this publication should not be used as a substitute for the medical care and advice of your pediatrician. There may be variations in treatment that your pediatrician may recommend based on individual facts and circumstances.

MANAGING SETBACKS AND DETOURS ON THE WAY TO HEALTHY EATING AND ACTIVITY

No matter how strongly your child tries to gain control over food and activity choices, he or she will likely have some backsliding from time to time. When you meet a few roadblocks on the journey to better health, the following tips might help.

Stay positive

Mistakes will happen. Maybe your child will overeat for a few days in a row. Maybe your child will sneak some junk food when you are not looking. But focusing on the mistake is not usually helpful.

What you can do

☐ **Try not to view mistakes as total failure.** Instead, think of them as minor stumbling blocks, which is exactly what they are.

☐ **Don't let disappointment be a reason to give up.** Remind your child of all the successes achieved so far.

☐ **Think about what went wrong** and how you can help your child avoid it happening again.

☐ **Avoid scolding your child** or other family members for these inevitable detours. Remember that none of us are perfect. Stay optimistic and return your attention to healthier living.

Team effort

No one likes to feel alone. Your child will feel much better knowing that there are others who are there to help when the going gets rough.

What you can do

☐ **Reassure your child** that you are there for support and want to help in any way you can.

☐ **Let your child help figure out what went wrong** and work together on how to prevent it from happening again.

☐ **Let your child in on meal planning,** food shopping and preparation, and family activity planning. This will help him or her learn to make good decisions from your example.

Identify the problem

Give some thought to what might be the problem. You'd be surprised at how often parents and children know that something isn't going right, but never take the time to evaluate what's really happening.

What you can do

☐ **Write down what your child is eating** and what his or her activity level is. This can help you identify specific problem areas and why they might be taking place.

☐ **Try to figure out** if the setbacks happen at certain times. For example, does Grandma bring sweets every time she visits? Did you run out of time to make dinner and stop at a fast-food restaurant?

☐ **As a family, return to your commitment** to eating healthy.

☐ **Keep monitoring your child's progress** in the weeks and months ahead. Make sure he doesn't fall back into old habits.

Remember

Learning how to make good decisions about nutrition and activity is important. Help your child understand that it's a process that takes time. The journey will not always be easy. There may be plenty of obstacles along the way that could temporarily derail your child from the path toward better health.

Belief, **A**ssessment, **L**ifestyle, **A**ctivity, **N**utrition, **C**hild, **E**nvironment

Adapted from American Academy of Pediatrics. *A Parent's Guide to Childhood Obesity: A Road Map to Health.* Hassink SG, ed. Elk Grove Village, IL: American Academy of Pediatrics; 2006
The information contained in this publication should not be used as a substitute for the medical care and advice of your pediatrician. There may be variations in treatment that your pediatrician may recommend based on individual facts and circumstances.

SETTING GOALS

If you've ever tried to lose weight, you know how hard it is. Being overweight is no less challenging for children. But your child can succeed. If you and your child are ready to start on the road to better health, the following tips may be helpful.

Start small

Weight loss is a journey. And like every other road on which we travel, there may be bumps and detours along the way.

What you can do

☐ **Don't expect instant results.** That's just not realistic and will only set you and your child up for disappointment.

☐ **Help your child make small changes** at first. These small steps can lead to bigger steps that are more likely to be kept up over time.

☐ **Start with the basics.** Help your child choose healthier foods and cut down on high-fat or sugary snacks.

☐ **Have your child do some kind of physical activity every day,** even if it's only for a few minutes initially.

Family goals

There are many ways in which you and other family members can help your child succeed in losing weight.

What you can do

☐ **Become a role model.** That means getting out the door and being active yourself, perhaps along with your child.

☐ **Be supportive,** not critical in how you help your child make good decisions about eating and being active. Be sure other family members follow this as well.

☐ **Keep only those foods in the house** that fit into your child's nutritional plan. Even if other family members do not need to lose weight, they can still benefit from healthier eating.

☐ **Eat meals together** as a family whenever possible and away from the TV; help your child choose appropriate portion sizes.

Remember

The changes that will help your child manage his or her weight today could also keep a serious illness from developing later. Modeling good eating habits and setting daily physical activity goals will serve your child well for the rest of his or her life.

Belief, **A**ssessment, **L**ifestyle, **A**ctivity, **N**utrition, **C**hild, **E**nvironment

Adapted from American Academy of Pediatrics. *A Parent's Guide to Childhood Obesity: A Road Map to Health.* Hassink SG, ed. Elk Grove Village, IL: American Academy of Pediatrics; 2006
The information contained in this publication should not be used as a substitute for the medical care and advice of your pediatrician. There may be variations in treatment that your pediatrician may recommend based on individual facts and circumstances.

SNEAKING FOOD

Plenty of children sneak food, often believing (or hoping) that they'll never get caught. In most families, sneaking food doesn't go undetected for long. If your child sneaks food, the following tips may help.

Why kids sneak food

It's important to understand why a child might feel the need to sneak food. Sometimes children find emotions simply too hard to handle, and they find food soothing and comforting. Other times, children might be feeling anxious, stressed, bored, or sad.

What you can do

☐ **Explain that you know** your child is sneaking food. Encourage your child to talk to you about why. Let your child do most of the talking and really listen to what he or she has to say.

☐ **Reassure your child** that you love him or her and that you will do anything you can to help with the problem.

Ask; don't sneak

Rather than simply telling your child, "Don't sneak!" encourage your child to ask for food when wanted. Set up a reward system to encourage your child to stop sneaking.

What you should do

☐ **For a young child,** provide a sticker or star as a reward each time he or she asks you for something to eat. Other ideas are to read an extra bedtime story or give points the child can put toward a low-cost toy or school supplies.

☐ **For an older child,** set up a point system and let the child build up points for a ticket to the movies, a day at the skating rink or zoo, or a DVD or video game rental.

☐ **Suggest other things to do** instead of eating, such as going for a bike ride, going for a walk, playing with friends, or exercising to a workout video.

Remember

It is very important to help your child adopt healthy eating and activity habits that can last a lifetime. By taking steps like serving your child appropriate foods and encouraging physical activity every day, any weight concerns that exist now will become less of a problem as your child gets older.

Belief, **A**ssessment, **L**ifestyle, **A**ctivity, **N**utrition, **C**hild, **E**nvironment

Adapted from American Academy of Pediatrics. *A Parent's Guide to Childhood Obesity: A Road Map to Health.* Hassink SG, ed. Elk Grove Village, IL: American Academy of Pediatrics; 2006
The information contained in this publication should not be used as a substitute for the medical care and advice of your pediatrician. There may be variations in treatment that your pediatrician may recommend based on individual facts and circumstances.

WHAT ABOUT JUICE?

Fruit is one of the 5 food groups and an important part of every child's diet. Offering fruit juice is an easy way for kids to get the recommended amount of fruit in their diets. But too much juice can have its problems. If your child drinks juice, the following tips may be helpful to you.

How much is OK?

Because juice tastes good, it's easy to give your child too much. Too much juice in a child's diet is linked to obesity. It can also cause diarrhea, poor nutrition, and tooth decay.

What you can do

- ☐ **Do not give juice to infants** younger than 6 months.

- ☐ **Give only 4 to 6 oz** of fruit juice per day to children between the ages of 1 to 6 years.

- ☐ **Give only 8 to 12 oz** of fruit juice per day to children between the ages of 7 to 18 years.

- ☐ **Give juice only to infants who can drink from a cup;** never give it in a bottle.

- ☐ **Do not allow your child to carry** a cup or box of juice around throughout the day.

How can you tell it's juice?

It's not always easy to tell fruit juice from fruit "drinks." However, the information should be on the label if you know what to look for.

What you can do

- ☐ **Look for the word "juice"** on the label. It can't be called juice if it's not 100% fruit juice.

- ☐ **Avoid products that are called "drinks," "beverages," or "cocktails."** They do not contain 100% real fruit juice. If you do buy these products for your child, look for ones with the highest percentage of juice. This information is on the label.

- ☐ **Read the ingredients** on the label. Juice drinks often add sweeteners and artificial flavors.

Alternatives to juice

Like adults, children need variety in their diets. Instead of relying on juice as your child's only drink, consider other drinks as well.

What you can do

- ☐ **Offer your child water.** Water is a healthy drink for children of all ages. To make drinking water more interesting to your child, try adding a slice of lemon or lime.

- ☐ **Offer your child low-fat milk** rather than juice.

- ☐ **Try a piece of fruit instead of juice.** Although a 6-oz glass of fruit juice equals 1 fruit serving, a piece of whole fruit, such as an apple, is healthier. Fruit provides more fiber than fruit juice.

Remember

The nutritional choices you make for your child today will help determine his or her health not only now but in the future. If you make an effort to feed your child primarily healthy meals, drinks, and snacks, you have a much better chance of helping him or her attain a healthy weight.

Belief, **A**ssessment, **L**ifestyle, **A**ctivity, **N**utrition, **C**hild, **E**nvironment

Adapted from American Academy of Pediatrics. *A Parent's Guide to Childhood Obesity: A Road Map to Health.* Hassink SG, ed. Elk Grove Village, IL: American Academy of Pediatrics; 2006
The information contained in this publication should not be used as a substitute for the medical care and advice of your pediatrician. There may be variations in treatment that your pediatrician may recommend based on individual facts and circumstances.

A.2

Growth Charts

Index

Boys

Girls

Birth to 24 months: Boys
Head circumference-for-age and
Weight-for-length percentiles

NAME _____

RECORD # _____

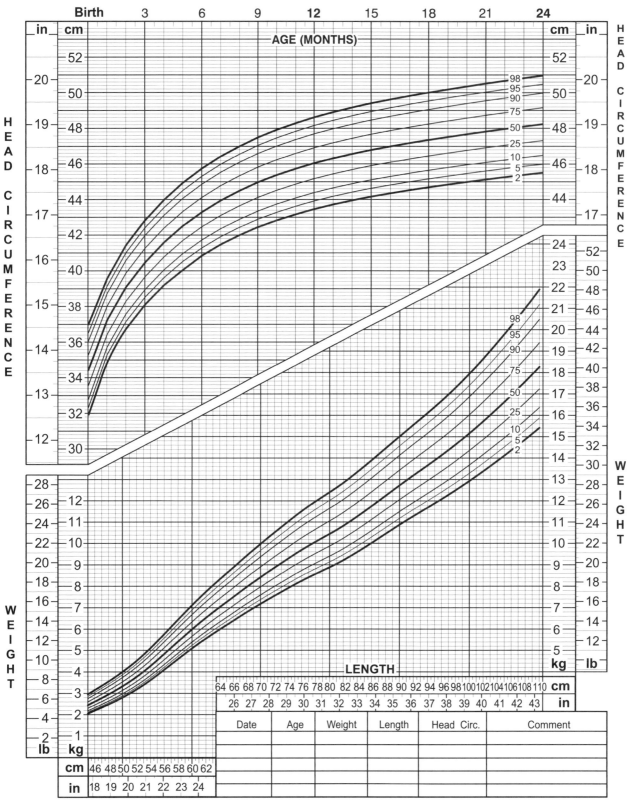

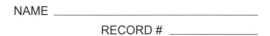

Published by the Centers for Disease Control and Prevention, November 1, 2009
SOURCE: WHO Child Growth Standards (http://www.who.int/childgrowth/en)

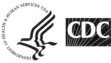

2 to 20 years: Boys
Body mass index-for-age percentiles

NAME _____

RECORD # _____

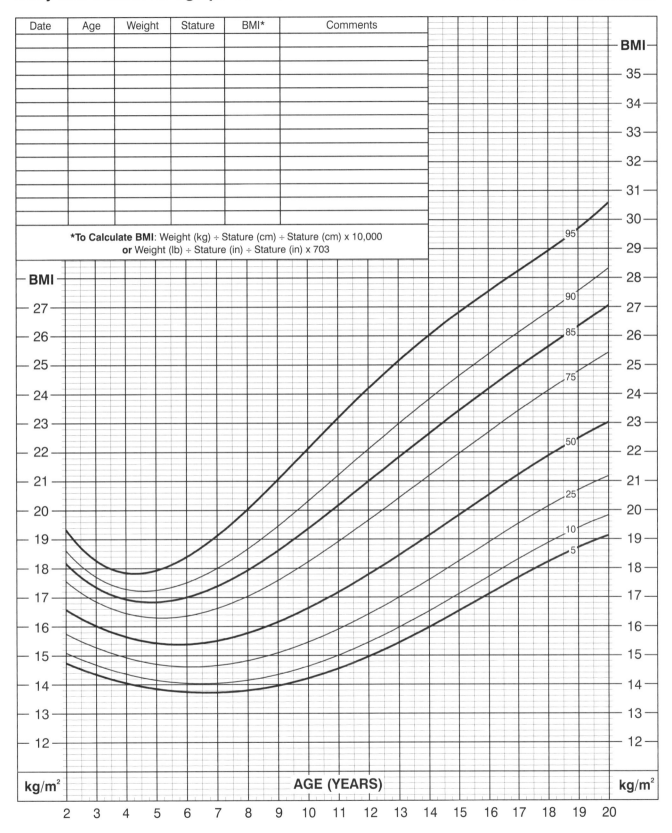

Date	Age	Weight	Stature	BMI*	Comments

*To Calculate BMI: Weight (kg) ÷ Stature (cm) ÷ Stature (cm) x 10,000
or Weight (lb) ÷ Stature (in) ÷ Stature (in) x 703

AGE (YEARS)

kg/m²

BMI

Published May 30, 2000 (modified 10/16/00).
SOURCE: Developed by the National Center for Health Statistics in collaboration with
the National Center for Chronic Disease Prevention and Health Promotion (2000).
http://www.cdc.gov/growthcharts

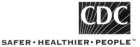

SAFER • HEALTHIER • PEOPLE™

Birth to 24 months: Girls
Head circumference-for-age and
Weight-for-length percentiles

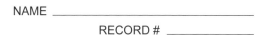

NAME _____

RECORD # _____

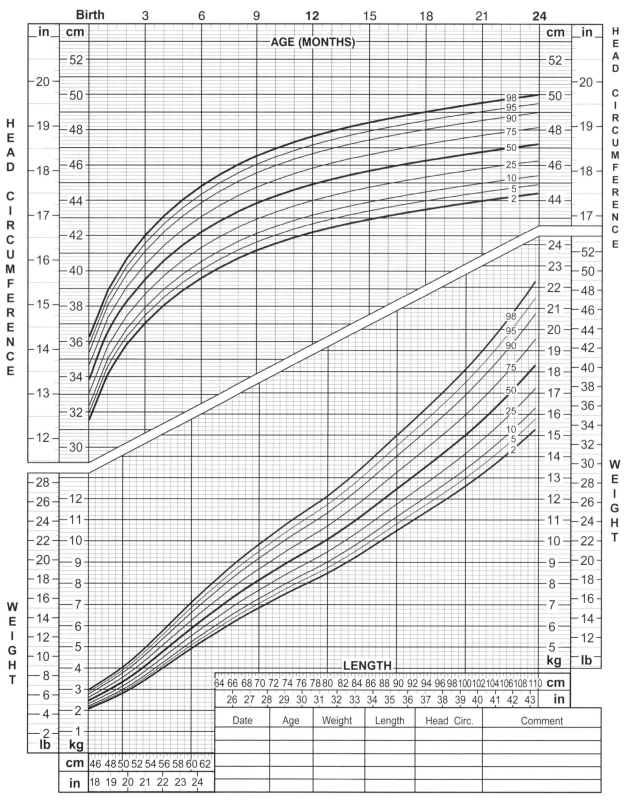

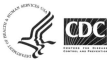

Published by the Centers for Disease Control and Prevention, November 1, 2009
SOURCE: WHO Child Growth Standards (http://www.who.int/childgrowth/en)

2 to 20 years: Girls
Body mass index-for-age percentiles

NAME _____

RECORD # _____

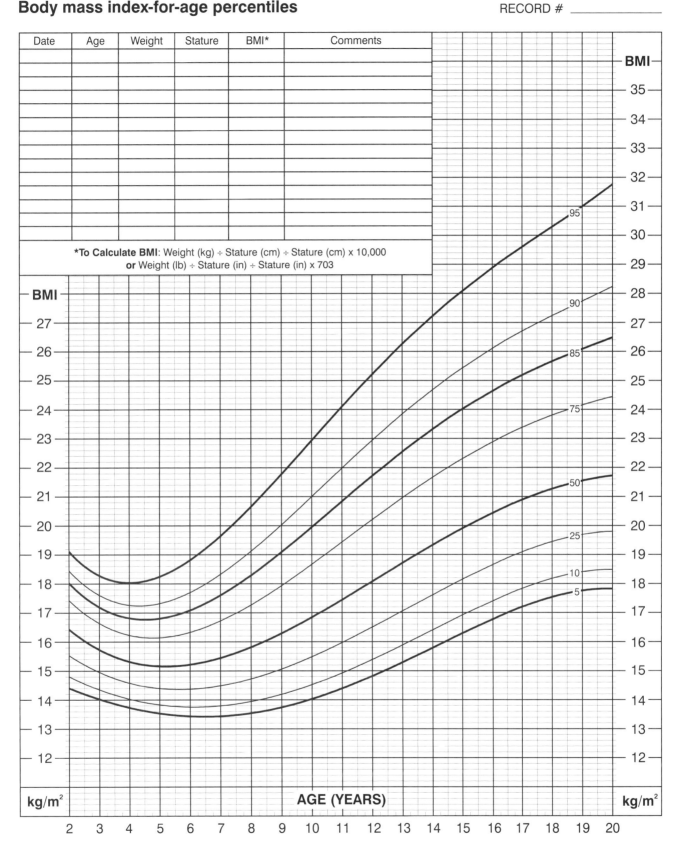

Date	Age	Weight	Stature	BMI*	Comments

*To Calculate BMI: Weight (kg) ÷ Stature (cm) ÷ Stature (cm) x 10,000
or Weight (lb) ÷ Stature (in) ÷ Stature (in) x 703

BMI

BMI

AGE (YEARS)

kg/m²

kg/m²

Published May 30, 2000 (modified 10/16/00).
SOURCE: Developed by the National Center for Health Statistics in collaboration with
the National Center for Chronic Disease Prevention and Health Promotion (2000).
http://www.cdc.gov/growthcharts

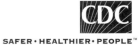

SAFER · HEALTHIER · PEOPLE™

A.3 Feeding Guide for Children

Feeding Guide for Children

Food	2 to 3 (1000–1400 kcal) Portion Size	2 to 3 (1000–1400 kcal) Daily Amounts	4 to 6 (1200–1800 kcal) Portion Size	4 to 6 (1200–1800 kcal) Daily Amounts	7 to 12 (1400–2000 kcal) Portion Size	7 to 12 (1400–2000 kcal) Daily Amounts	Comments
Low-fat milk and dairy	½ cup (4 oz)	2 ½ cups	½–¾ cup (4–6 oz)	2 ½–3 cups	½–1 cup (4–8 oz)	2 ½–3 cups	The following may be substituted for ½ cup fluid milk: ½ oz natural cheese, 1 oz processed cheese, ½ cup low fat yogurt, 2 ½ T nonfat dry milk.
Meat, fish, poultry or equivalent	1–2 oz (2–3 T)	2–4 oz	12 oz (4–6 T)	3–5 oz	2 oz	4–5 ½ oz	The following may be substituted for 1 oz meat, fish, or poultry: 1 egg, 1 T peanut butter, ¼ cup cooked beans or peas.
Vegetables and fruit							
Vegetables Cooked, Raw[a]	2–3 T Few pieces	1 ½ cup	4–6 T Few pieces	1 ½–2 ½ cups	¼–½ cup Several pieces	1 ½–2 ½ cups	Include dark green (1 cup per week) and orange vegetables (3 cups per week) for vitamin A, such as carrots, spinach, broccoli, winter squash, or greens. Limit starchy vegetables (potatoes) to 3 ½ cups weekly.
Fruit Raw, Canned, Juice	½–1 small 2–3 T 3–4 oz	1 ½ cup	½–1 small 4–6 T 4 oz	1–1 ½ cups	1 medium ¼–½ cup 4 oz	1 ½–2 cups	Include one vitamin C-rich fruit, vegetable, or juice, such as citrus juices, orange, grapefruit, strawberries, melon, tomato, or broccoli.
Grain products Whole grain or enriched bread Cooked cereal Dry cereal	½–1 slice ¼–½ cup ½–1 cup	3–5 oz 1 ½–2½ oz whole grain	1 slice ½ cup 1 cup	4–6 oz	1 slice ½–1cup 1 cup	5–6 oz	The following may be substituted for 1 slice of bread: ½ cup spaghetti, macaroni, noodles, or rice; 5 saltines; ½ English muffin or bagel; 1 tortilla; corn grits; or posole. Make ½ of grain intake *whole grains*.
Oils		4 tsp		4–5 tsp		4–6 tsp	Choose soft margarines. Avoid *trans* fats. Use liquid vegetable oils rather than solid fats.

Adapted from ChooseMyPlate at http://www.choosemyplate.gov/ and the 2010 Dietary Guidelines for Americans.

[a] Do not give to young children until they can chew well.

American Academy of Pediatrics Committee on Nutrition. Feeding the Child and Adolescent. In: Kleinman RE, Greer FR, eds. *Pediatric Nutrition.* 7th ed. Elk Grove Village, IL: American Academy of Pediatrics; 2014:153

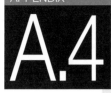
Index

ENVIRONMENTAL FACTORS

The following assessment will help you understand the environmental influences associated with your child's weight problem.

What Problems Exist Today (Home, School)?

Are there problems in your child's school/child care environment? _____

Are snacks healthy and portions controlled? _____

Is there time for outdoor play/recess? _____

Is there regular physical education at school? _____

Is there more than 1 to 2 hours of screen time (TV, computer)? _____

The Community Environment

Are there safe playgrounds and places to play outside in the neighborhood? _____

Are there after-school programs nearby that provide activity alternatives? _____

Are there opportunities to play sports/games at community centers? _____

Is it safe for your child to walk to school, activities, and friends' houses? _____

The Home Environment

Does the family have regularly scheduled TV/computer time? _____

Do family members regularly engage in physical activity together? _____

Is there an indoor and outdoor play space for the children? _____

Are there indoor activities your child can do at home instead of watching TV or using the computer? _____

Family Behavior

With family members in mind (including you, your spouse, and your child's siblings and grandparents), which of them

Overeats regularly _____

_____

Binges on food _____

_____

Rushes through meals _____

_____

Insists on keeping high-calorie snacks in the house _____

_____

Eats while watching TV _____

_____

Eats frequently at fast-food restaurants _____

Overeats to calm anxiety _____

Gets little or no physical activity each day _____

Your Child's Behavior

Does your child demonstrate the following behaviors that can contribute to an obesity problem?
(Answer yes or no.)

☐ Yes ☐ No	Other family members Overeats regularly	
☐ Yes ☐ No	Binges on food	
☐ Yes ☐ No	Rushes through meals	
☐ Yes ☐ No	Chooses high-calorie snacks	
☐ Yes ☐ No	Selects high-sugar drinks	
☐ Yes ☐ No	Eats while watching TV	
☐ Yes ☐ No	Eats frequently at fast-food restaurants	
☐ Yes ☐ No	Overeats to calm anxiety	
☐ Yes ☐ No	Gets little or no physical activity each day	

☐ Yes ☐ No Sneaks or hides food

☐ Yes ☐ No Seems hungry all the time

☐ Yes ☐ No Gets upset when you try to limit portions or snacks

☐ Yes ☐ No Watches TV/uses the computer more than 1 hour per day

☐ Yes ☐ No Gets own food or snacks

☐ Yes ☐ No Eats alone

☐ Yes ☐ No Drinks a lot of sweetened beverages

YOUR CHILD'S GENETICS AND FAMILY HISTORY

How Does Family History Currently Influence Your Child's Health?

Let's look more closely at your own family. In the tables that follow, place a check mark beside the conditions and diseases of each family member. The more check marks you make, the greater your child's risk is developing the serious diseases associated with excess weight.

	Mother	Father	Sibling 1	Sibling 2	Sibling 3
Obese/overweight	☐	☐	☐	☐	☐
High blood pressure	☐	☐	☐	☐	☐
High cholesterol	☐	☐	☐	☐	☐
High triglyceride level	☐	☐	☐	☐	☐
Diabetes	☐	☐	☐	☐	☐
Heart disease	☐	☐	☐	☐	☐
Asthma	☐	☐	☐	☐	☐
Joint pain	☐	☐	☐	☐	☐
Sleep apnea	☐	☐	☐	☐	☐
Liver disease	☐	☐	☐	☐	☐
Other	☐	☐	☐	☐	☐

Next, fill out a similar chart for your child's grandparents. Which of the following conditions apply to your youngster's grandfathers and grandmothers?

	Maternal		Paternal	
	Grandmother	Grandfather	Grandmother	Grandfather
Obese/overweight	☐	☐	☐	☐
High blood pressure	☐	☐	☐	☐
High cholesterol	☐	☐	☐	☐
High triglyceride level	☐	☐	☐	☐
Diabetes	☐	☐	☐	☐
Heart disease	☐	☐	☐	☐
Asthma	☐	☐	☐	☐
Sleep apnea	☐	☐	☐	☐
Liver disease	☐	☐	☐	☐
Joint pain	☐	☐	☐	☐
Other	☐	☐	☐	☐

HOW IS YOUR CHILD EATING NOW?

To help produce lasting improvements in a child's weight, many parents find it helpful to keep a food diary to monitor exactly what the child is eating. Toward that end, use this worksheet for the next 4 days to record what your child eats, from the time he or she awakens to the time he or she goes to sleep.

Foods Eaten Today (enter date): _____

Under each meal and snack write down *what* and *how much* your child ate.

Breakfast _____

Mid-morning Snack _____

Lunch _____

Afternoon Snack _____

Juice or Soda _____

Dinner _____

Late-night Snack _____

Foods Eaten Today (enter date): _____

Under each meal and snack write down *what* and *how much* your child ate.

Breakfast _____

Mid-morning Snack _____

Lunch _____

Afternoon Snack _____

Juice or Soda _____

Dinner _____

Late-night Snack _____

Foods Eaten Today (enter date): _____

Under each meal and snack write down *what* and *how much* your child ate.

Breakfast _____

Mid-morning Snack _____

Lunch _____

Afternoon Snack _____

Juice or Soda _____

Dinner _____

Late-night Snack _____

Foods Eaten Today (enter date): _____

Under each meal and snack write down *what* and *how much* your child ate.

Breakfast _____

Mid-morning Snack _____

Lunch _____

Afternoon Snack _____

Juice or Soda _____

Dinner _____

Late-night Snack _____

HOW WILL YOU AND YOUR CHILD GET THERE?

Let's be more specific about the goals for your youngster.

As you get started, what short-term goals do you and your child have?

_____

_____

Specifically, how does your family plan to eat healthier, meal by meal?

_____

_____

Specifically, how does your family plan to become more active, day by day?

_____

_____

What other short-term and intermediate goals do you and your child have?

_____

_____

Do you think that making behavioral changes associated with these goals will be easy or difficult?

_____

_____

Who is going to go with you on this weight loss journey? Who can help you and your child achieve your goals? (Check all that apply.)

☐ Other family members	☐ Siblings	☐ Friends	☐ Parent groups	☑ Your pediatrician
☐ Spouse	☐ Grandparents	☐ School	☐ Child care staff	☐ Others

What information do you need to help you achieve these goals? (Check all that apply.)

☐ More knowledge of proper nutrition

☐ Help with activity alternatives

☐ Skills to help your child and family make healthy changes

☐ Information about age-appropriate diet and activity

☐ Information about the health consequences of obesity

WHERE DO YOU AND YOUR CHILD WANT TO GO?

With this worksheet, you'll begin to look toward your child's future.

What are your child's health goals relative to his or her weight? (These should be health goals, rather than being related primarily to weight.)

Is there a health problem associated with your child's weight that you'd like to improve or correct?

- ☐ Lower cholesterol level
- ☐ Lower blood pressure
- ☐ Improve blood sugar glucose level
- ☐ Be able to run or be physically active and keep up with friends without becoming winded so quickly

Are there eating behaviors you would like to help your child improve?

(Check all that apply.)

- ☐ Overeating at meals
- ☐ Eating too many snacks
- ☐ Making unhealthy food choices
- ☐ Eating at night
- ☐ Eating in front of the TV
- ☐ Eating too many fast-food meals
- ☐ Making very limited diet choices

Are there activity behaviors you would like to help your child improve?

(Check all that apply.)

- ☐ Limiting TV/computer use
- ☐ Being more motivated to be active
- ☐ Participating in more peer group activities
- ☐ Others: _____

What are the long-term goals that you and your child have relative to your child's weight? (Check all that apply.)

- ☐ Improving your child's overall health
- ☐ Decreasing the chances that your child will be an overweight/obese adult
- ☐ Increasing your child's self-esteem
- ☐ Reducing family conflict around food and activity
- ☐ Decreasing teasing

ASSESSING YOUR HOME ENVIRONMENT

Let's continue the journey toward helping your child manage his or her weight by pausing at this checkpoint to make another assessment. This time, you'll evaluate the following components of this part of the road trip toward controlling your child's obesity:

- Your home environment
- Your parenting role within this environment
- Areas in which improvements may be needed

What Is Currently Happening at Home?

In answering the following questions, you'll get a clearer sense of what is taking place in your home environment that may play a role in your child's health.

Does your family mostly eat well-balanced meals? During a typical week, how many well-balanced meals are prepared in the home?

Breakfast _____ Lunch _____ Dinner _____

On average, how many times a week does the family eat fast-food meals that are brought into the home or eaten at restaurants?

_____

Who does the grocery shopping in your family? _____

Do other family members (eg, parents, children) contribute to the decisions on what will be purchased in the supermarket?

If so, who? Is most of the food brought into the home healthy? _____

Who is giving your child snacks at home (or elsewhere)?

- ☐ Parent(s)   ☐ Other family members

- ☐ Other children   ☐ Child care staff

Does your child and/or family use food

- ☐ As a reward?   ☐ For comfort?   ☐ To relieve boredom?

Is your child physically active every day? _____

How much time does your child spend in physical activities each day? _____

How many hours do family members spend watching TV or using the computer every day? _____

How many TVs/computers do you have in the house? _____

Do family members have TVs/computers in their bedrooms? _____

Does your child have a TV/computer in his or her bedroom? _____

Who sets limits on your child's TV/computer use? _____

How many hours does your child watch TV or play computer or video games during a typical day? _____

What Is Going Well in Your Household?

Based on your previous answers, what areas are you pleased with in your home life that contribute to your child's health? Specifically, check off what is going well in your household.

☐ Well-balanced meals

☐ Healthy snacking

☐ Limited fast-food meals

☐ Regular participation in physical activity

☐ Limited TV watching and video or computer games

Use this space to elaborate on any of the above:

_____

_____

What Problems Exist in Your Household?

What problem areas are present in your home environment that may need changing or improving? (Check all that apply.)

☐ Poor food/meal selection

☐ Poor snack food choices

☐ Too many fast-food meals

☐ Not enough physical activity or time outdoors

☐ Too much computer, TV, or video game time

Others:

_____

_____

What Change(s) Do You Need to Make, and How Will You Make Them?

As the next step in your journey toward better health, identify the specific obstacles that are contributing to your household problems. Which of the following apply to you and your family?

☐ Family preferences (eg, unhealthy favorite foods)

☐ Not enough available time (to prepare meals, for physical activity)

☐ Not enough money

☐ Not enough time spent outdoors

☐ No safe places to play

☐ Your child won't go to activities or play outside

☐ Other _____

Next, select a single, specific change that you'd like to work on with your child and the rest of the family (eg, improving the snacks available in your house and chosen by your family).

_____

_____

To make this change possible, identify who can support you in this process. In addition to you and your child, who else can go on this journey with you and help your child reach this goal?

☐ Your spouse

☐ Your other children

☐ Grandparents

☐ Others

Now, use the following space to create a plan to make possible the change you've chosen.

_____

_____

In the past, how has your child reacted and how did you respond to your child when you tried to make changes (eg, did you give in to your child's complaints or demands)?

_____

_____

What could you do differently this time? How can you change your own actions to produce more positive results?

_____

_____

From a parenting point of view, is there anything else standing in the way of making healthier changes in your home environment?

_____

_____

_____

_____

YOUR CHILD AND HIS OR HER WEIGHT

For this assessment, answer the following questions about your youngster:

How does your child feel about his or her weight? (Explain.)

_____

Does your child worry about how much he or she weighs?

_____

What kinds of things concern your child?

_____

Does your child worry about taking gym class at school?

_____

Does your child worry about keeping up with other children on the playground?

_____

Is your child concerned about being teased?

_____

Is your child worried about how he or she looks in clothes?

_____

Is your child concerned about his or her health?

_____

Other concerns:

_____

How do you feel about your child's weight?

_____

Are you concerned about your child being teased by peers?

_____

Are you anxious about the short- and long-term consequences of your child's weight gain and eating behaviors?

_____

Other worries:

_____

WHERE DOES YOUR CHILD STAND?

What's Currently Happening With Physical Activity?

Let's take a few moments to determine how your child is currently faring in terms of physical activity. The answers to the following questions will help you identify how much time your child spends in structured and unstructured activities and areas in which your child may need to improve.

How many days a week does your child participate in physical education (PE) classes at school? _____

On those days, approximately how many minutes does your child spend moving or doing activity (as opposed to standing around) in those PE classes?

_____

How many days a week does your child play outdoors?

_____

About how many minutes (or hours) does your child spend playing outdoors on a typical weekday? _____

On a typical Saturday or Sunday? _____

What structured physical activities does your child participate in (eg, a youth sports team or organized activities at an after-school program)?

_____

In a typical week, how many minutes (or hours) does your child spend in these structured activities? _____

On average, how many hours a day does your child watch TV or play video or computer games? _____

Does your child often snack while in front of the TV or computer screen? _____

What outdoor physical activities does your child enjoy doing?

_____

_____

What other outdoor physical activities would you like to introduce to your child?

_____

_____

What Is Going Well?

Use the answers to the previous questions to determine those areas in which your child is already doing well incorporating physical activity in his or her life. In the following space, write down the ways in which your child is active:

_____

_____

_____

What Changes Need to Be Made?

Next, take a few minutes to determine areas in which your child needs to improve. For example:

Does your child need to spend more time playing outdoors? _____

Would your child benefit from participating in youth sports or other organized activities? Would your child get more benefit and be more successful with activities in a small group or with his or her family?

_____

Does your child need to spend less time in front of the TV or computer or playing video games? _____

Choose a way in which your child can become more active, and write down a strategy for incorporating that activity into his or her life. For example, you may believe your child is watching too much TV after school and explore after-school activities at the local YMCA or Boys & Girls Clubs of America. Or you may find that your child is more comfortable increasing activity with a family member by taking a walk or shooting some hoops with a sibling.

_____

_____

What additional improvements would you like to help your child make in his or her efforts to become more active?

_____

_____

_____

CONQUERING SETBACKS

Has your child experienced a lapse in his or her progress toward better health? If a setback does take place, use this worksheet to help both of you understand and overcome the obstacles that may have tripped your child up. Remember, when trying to work through a setback, it's important to partner with your pediatrician.

What's Currently Happening?

What setback has occurred in your child's life that has interfered with his or her weight loss efforts?

_____

_____

Did it happen just once, or repeatedly? _____ Is it still going on? _____

Why do you think this backsliding has occurred? Is there an event, a person, or a behavior that has contributed to the problem?

_____

_____

What Changes Need to Be Made, and How Will You Make Them?

In the following space, write down a specific area in which a setback has occurred and where you and your child would like to make a change.

_____

_____

Are there obstacles that you and your youngster need to deal with effectively to ensure success in preventing this setback from recurring in the future?

_____

_____

What specific steps can you and your youngster take to make this change and minimize the risk of future setbacks?

_____

_____

Who can support you and your child in making these changes?

_____

_____

EVALUATING SNACKING BEHAVIORS

In this worksheet, we'll look at your child's snacking and ways in which problems can be effectively managed as the family navigates its way toward a healthier life.

What's Currently Happening With Snacking?

Are there certain times of day when your child snacks? _____

Does your child appear to snack because he or she is genuinely hungry? _____

Does your child make mostly healthy choices when he or she reaches for snacks? _____

If so, what kinds of healthy snacks does your child choose?

_____

What Problems Exist With Snacking?

Does your child sometimes select snacks that provide poor nutrition? _____
If so, what kinds of snacks does your child tend to choose?

_____

Does your child's urge to snack, and do the snacking choices your child makes, seem to be affected by his or her mood or external events to which your child is reacting (eg, stressful situations, particular times of the day)?

_____

What Changes Need to Be Made, and How Will You Make Them?

What obstacles are interfering with your child snacking on healthy foods and appropriate portion sizes?

_____

Select a problem area related to snacking with which your child is having difficulty (eg, snacking excessively when watching TV or doing homework). You and your child should create a specific plan for attacking this problem. Write down this approach here.

_____

_____

Who can support you in making this change?

_____

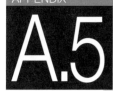

Responding to Common Parental Concerns

Adapted from *A Parent's Guide to Childhood Obesity: A Road Map to Health,* the following are questions or statements commonly posed by parents during clinical visits. So often, the questions or statements are in the format of, "Yes…but." For example, *"Yes,* my child should exercise more, *but* there's just no time," or *"Yes,* I'd like to get the cookies out of our house, *but* what should I tell the other kids who still want cookies here?"

Reviewing these questions or statements and their responses may assist health care professionals in addressing parental concerns.

"Yes, I'd like to give my kids more fruits and vegetables, but fresh produce is too expensive!"

Fresh fruits and vegetables may be more affordable than you think, particularly if you buy them when they're in season. When in season, they'll be much more reasonably priced than at other times of the year. Also, compare the costs of produce to other foods that you may already be buying for your child. For example, processed foods—from cookies to potato chips—not only are more expensive but certainly aren't as nutritious as fresh fruits and vegetables.

A number of studies have confirmed that fresh produce is more affordable than you might think. In 2004 the US Department of Agriculture analyzed and released data from household food purchases made in 1999, including multiple types of fruits and vegetables. The researchers concluded that the average American can purchase 4 servings of vegetables and 3 servings of fruits for just 64 cents a day. If this figure were adjusted to today's costs, the price might be an average of less than a dollar a day. No matter how you analyze the numbers, that's a great deal.

By the way, the same study found that two-thirds of all fresh fruits and more than half of all fresh vegetables are less costly than processed versions of the same produce.

"Yes, I'd prefer to feed a variety of vegetables to my child, but he absolutely hates vegetables. The only 'vegetables' he'll eat are French fries. That's it!"

As a parent, your job is to provide your child with well-balanced meals, including a variety of vegetables. Once the food is on the plate in front of the child, he or she may choose whether to eat it. Sure, it can be frustrating when kids push the plate away and refuse to even try something new, but be persistent. The good news is that over time, most children will develop a taste for enough healthy foods—even some vegetables—to be eating a balanced diet.

Some children may be more agreeable to consuming vegetables if you ask them to help you in the kitchen while you're preparing meals. They may be more receptive if you add vegetables to a pasta dish or put them in soups or meat loaf. Some youngsters prefer raw vegetables over cooked, and they'll often snack on cherry tomatoes or cut-up vegetables with yogurt dip. When eating in restaurants, accompany children on trips through the salad bar; expose them to vegetables they may never have tried at home.

Meanwhile, continue to serve as a role model. If your child sees you eating vegetables, he or she is more likely to try them. Have your child get used to the idea that vegetables are part of every lunch and dinner. Remember your child will need to have at least 1 serving of fruits and vegetables with every meal and snack to meet the recommended 5 servings a day.

"Yes, I know my child shouldn't have dessert with dinner every night or sweetened juices whenever he wants them, but I feel terrible if he complains about feeling deprived."

Don't lose sight of why you're making these dietary changes. As a parent, your child's health must be a top priority, and that may require making some adjustments in what your child eats and the amount of physical activity he or she gets.

Of course, you don't want your youngster to feel deprived, and there's no need for you to completely eliminate all of his or her favorite desserts. However, save those treats, such as rich ice cream or chocolate chip cookies, for special occasions and serve appropriate portion sizes when you do. At the same time, introduce your child to healthier desserts, such as a dish of strawberries or a piece of angel food cake.

When beverages are concerned, rely more often on low-fat milk or water rather than sugar-laden soft drinks or juices. Before long, your child will stop demanding the high-calorie, high-fat treats once craved.

"Yes, I'm willing to get unhealthy foods out of the house, but other adults in the home haven't come onboard yet. They tell me that they've been drinking sugary soft drinks all their lives, and they're not willing to give them up."

If other adults in the home insist on keeping high-fat snacks or high-calorie drinks in the cupboard or refrigerator, those kinds of temptations aren't fair to your child. To support your youngster's efforts to lose weight, it's essential that the entire family get involved. The family needs to sit down and discuss the implications of continuing to live a lifestyle of poor eating choices. If the others still can't be convinced of the potential consequences of doing their own things, perhaps your pediatrician can talk to them. With your youngster's health at stake, your pediatrician may be able to motivate the others to give some ground. If they need to have sugary soft drinks, ask them to indulge at work and leave those kinds of snacks out of the house.

"Yes, my own mother seems to understand how important it is for my child to lose weight, but she still thinks it's a grandmother's prerogative to give my child candy whenever we visit. How can I convince her to get rid of that candy dish?"

The answer to this question is not much different than the previous one about others in the home having an attachment to soft drinks. You need to talk to your child's grandmother about the health risks your youngster faces unless he or she eats more nutritiously, one meal and one snack after another. As accustomed as Grandma may be to baking cookies when the grandchildren visit, you can probably appeal to her strong desire to give your child the best possible chance of living a healthy life. Let Grandma know about the nutritious food choices she can have available for the next family visit (see the patient handout, "Avoiding Food Traps").

"Yes, I realize that when the family goes out to dinner, we should stay away from fast-food restaurants most of the time, but whenever we drive by one of those places, my child pleads with me to stop."

It's fine to eat at fast-food restaurants once in a while. Because of their high-fat fare, though, don't make it a habit. Try to encourage lower-fat options at fast-food restaurants.

When you visit these types of restaurants, order carefully for the family, finding choices to keep your child happy without sabotaging efforts to eat healthier. Whenever possible, for example, select a grilled chicken sandwich without any dressing for your youngster. If your child insists on a hamburger, choose the smaller size, not the supersized double burger that looks like it could feed the entire family. Order a salad with low-fat dressing that your child can eat as part of the meal.

Rather than overrelying on fast-food restaurants, choose to eat at sit-down family restaurants more frequently and look for healthy options on the menu. Split a dinner between the two of you. You will save money and eat healthier!

"Yes, snacking before bedtime may not be a good idea for my child while he's trying to lose weight, but when I was growing up, my mother always gave us cookies and milk before we went to bed. It's just something that I feel comfortable doing, and it would be hard to do things differently."

Habits may be difficult to break, but for the well-being of your child, you need to make some adjustments. Nothing's inherently wrong with a bedtime snack, but you may need to adjust the kinds of snacks you're offering your youngster.

In general, try to limit the number of snacks to 2 per day. For those late-night munchies, make choices that contribute to overall healthy eating. You might turn to

- Air-popped popcorn rather than high-fat cheeses on crackers
- Frozen yogurt instead of ice cream
- Baked tortilla chips rather than potato chips
- Graham crackers (and milk) instead of chocolate chip cookies
- A piece of fruit rather than sugary cereal

"Yes, I understand that healthy eating is the best way for my child to lose weight, but I sometimes think that he could benefit from a little kick start, and the latest fad diets promise fast results. What's wrong with following one of these diets for a few weeks to get him off to a good start?"

Most people have lost weight at some point in their lives—but then gained it all back. They know that fad diets don't work, at least not over the long term, but the alluring promises on magazine covers and book jackets are often too tempting to resist.

Unfortunately, fad diets can be dangerous. They often emphasize a single food or food group, and they can be particularly risky for growing children for whom balanced nutrition is extremely important.

You need to put your child's health and well-being first. Don't be persuaded by promises of overnight weight loss. Instead, stick with a plan for good nutrition and physical activity. Your child's weight loss will be gradual and safe and have the best chance for permanent success.

"Yes, I feel that I can control what my child eats at home, but when he's at child care, I have no control over what the child care provider gives him. He's served whatever the other kids eat."

Express your concerns to the child care staff. Even if the facility serves identical meals to all the children, make some suggestions for fine-tuning the menu in the direction of healthier foods. The staff may turn out to be much more flexible than you expected and might be willing to bend to your requests, perhaps serving your youngster a turkey sandwich and small salad for lunch instead of a hamburger and French fries.

If you're sensing some reluctance on their part, offer to pack your child's lunch and/or snacks to make sure that the foods being eaten are supportive of the family's commitment to more nutritious eating.

"Yes, I'd love to sign my child up for a fitness program at the Y, but we just can't afford it."

Kids can enjoy the benefits of physical activity without busting the family budget. Play is the major way kids can increase their activity. You don't need costly exercise equipment like treadmills, nor do you have to enroll them in classes with expensive sign-up fees. Outdoor play in a safe area can be a major help to increasing physical activity.

There are plenty of activities that won't cause financial stress (see the patient handout, "Everyone Get Fit"). Walking, for example, is one of the best forms of exercise, and it doesn't require any special equipment, other than a good pair of walking shoes. If the entire family gets involved, your overweight child is more likely to be motivated to walk regularly. In fact, the best forms of physical activity are family activities. Keep them fun, and your child won't feel that he or she is missing out on the formal program at the Y.

"Yes, my child knows that he needs to become more physically active, but he has so much homework, plus piano lessons after school, and there's just no time for exercise."

So many of today's kids lead very busy lives. It seems as though their planned activities start immediately after school and continue until well after nightfall. If you think about it, there's probably some time in your child's afternoon and evening, even just 15 or 20 minutes, when he could fit in some physical activity.

Remember, activity needs to become a priority in your child's life. That means that exercise wins out over video games or surfing the Web almost every time. After school, can your child play catch with the neighborhood kids in the park down the block or work out to an exercise video?

Frankly, there aren't too many kids who don't have a few minutes to spare each day for squeezing in some physical activity. Physical activity promotes motor and mental development and is essential for developing coordination.

"Yes, my child should be getting more physical activity, but in our neighborhood, I just don't think it's safe for him to be playing outdoors."

There are plenty of ways for your child to stay active other than playing in your front yard or on the neighborhood playground. Consider participating in a swimming program at the Boys & Girls Clubs of America or joining a karate class. Your child can also stay active indoors at home by dancing, spinning a hula hoop, jumping rope, or doing chores like straightening up the bedroom.

"Yes, eating right and being active makes sense, but my teenager has so much weight to lose that we've been talking about weight loss surgery. Is that something we should consider?"

Although the overwhelming majority of bariatric surgeries are being performed in adults, a relatively small number of teenagers have undergone the procedure. However, this is major surgery, and the decision to have the operation should not be made hastily.

Weight loss surgery is advisable only for extremely overweight adolescents for whom more conservative weight loss measures haven't worked, particularly if they also have developed serious obesity-related medical conditions such as high blood pressure, diabetes, and sleep apnea.

Your pediatrician can provide an initial assessment of whether your teenager might be a candidate for surgery. If the pediatrician refers you for a consultation to a weight loss surgeon, make sure that there is a team available to help assess your teens and the family's readiness for surgery. The team should include at least a pediatrician, surgeon, psychologist, nutritionist, exercise trainer, and social worker. You and your teenager will have the opportunity to discuss the potential benefits of the operation, plus get your questions answered about the complications sometimes associated with the operation, such as infections, bleeding, blood clots, vitamin deficiencies, and weight regain.

A.6 Obesity and Related Comorbidities Coding Fact Sheet for Primary Care Pediatricians

Although coding for the care of children with obesity and related comorbidities is relatively straightforward, ensuring that appropriate reimbursement is received for such services is a more complicated matter. Some insurance carriers will deny claims submitted with "obesity" *International Classification of Diseases, 9th Revision, Clinical Modification (ICD-9-CM)* codes (eg, **278.00),** essentially carving out obesity-related care from the scope of benefits. Therefore, coding for obesity services is fundamentally a two-tiered system in which the first tier requires health care professionals to submit claims using appropriate codes and the second tier involves the practice-level issues of denial management and contract negotiation.

This coding fact sheet provides a guide to coding for obesity-related health care services. Strategies and a template letter for pediatric practices to handle carrier denials and contractual issues are given in "Denial Management and Contract Negotiation for Obesity Services" (Appendix A.7).

Procedure Codes
Current Procedural Terminology (CPT®) Codes

Body Fat Composition Testing

There is no separate *Current Procedural Terminology (CPT®)* code for body fat composition testing. This service would be included in the examination component of the evaluation and management (E/M) code reported.

Calorimetry

94690	Oxygen uptake, expired gas analysis; rest, indirect (separate procedure)
	or
94799	Unlisted pulmonary service or procedure [Note: Special report required.]

Glucose Monitoring

95250	Ambulatory continuous glucose monitoring of interstitial tissue fluid via a subcutaneous sensor for up to 72 hours; sensor placement, hookup, calibration of monitor, patient training, removal of sensor, and printout of recording
95251	Ambulatory continuous glucose monitoring of interstitial tissue fluid via a subcutaneous sensor for up to 72 hours; interpretation and report

Routine Venipuncture

36415	Collection of venous blood by venipuncture
36416	Collection of capillary blood specimen (eg, finger, heel, ear stick)

Venipuncture Necessitating Physician's Skill

36406	Venipuncture, younger than 3 years, necessitating physician's or other qualified healthcare professional's skill, not to be used for routine venipuncture; other vein
36410	Venipuncture, 3 years or older, necessitating physician's other qualified healthcare professional's skill (separate procedure), for diagnostic or therapeutic purposes (not to be used for routine venipuncture)

Digestive System Surgery Codes

43644	Laparoscopy, surgical, gastric restrictive procedure; with gastric bypass and Roux-en-Y gastroenterostomy (Roux limb 150 cm or less)
43645	Laparoscopy, surgical, gastric restrictive procedure; with gastric bypass and small intestine reconstruction to limit absorption
43842	Gastric restrictive procedure, without gastric bypass, for morbid obesity; vertical-banded gastroplasty

43843   Gastric restrictive procedure, without gastric bypass, for morbid obesity; other than vertical-banded gastroplasty

43845   Gastric restrictive procedure with partial gastrectomy, pylorus-preserving duodenoileostomy and ileoileostomy (50 to 100 cm common channel) to limit absorption (biliopancreatic diversion with duodenal switch)

43846   Gastric restrictive procedure, with gastric bypass for morbid obesity; with short limb (150 cm or less) Roux-en-Y gastroenterostomy

43847   Gastric restrictive procedure, with gastric bypass for morbid obesity; with small intestine reconstruction to limit absorption

43848   Revision, open, of gastric restrictive procedure for morbid obesity; other than adjustable gastric band (separate procedure)

Health and Behavior Assessment/Intervention Codes

These codes cannot be reported by a physician, nor can they be reported on the same day as preventive medicine counseling codes **(99401–99412).**

96150   Health and behavior assessment (eg, health-focused clinical interview, behavioral observations, psychophysiologic monitoring, health-oriented questionnaires), each 15 minutes face-to-face with the patient; initial assessment

96151   Health and behavior assessment (eg, health-focused clinical interview, behavioral observations, psychophysiologic monitoring, health-oriented questionnaires), each 15 minutes face-to-face with the patient; reassessment

The focus of the assessment is not on mental health but on the biopsychosocial factors important to physical health problems and treatments.

96152   Health and behavior intervention, each 15 minutes, face-to-face; individual

96153   Health and behavior intervention, each 15 minutes, face-to-face; group (2 or more patients)

96154   Health and behavior intervention, each 15 minutes, face-to-face; family (with patient present)

96155   Health and behavior intervention, each 15 minutes, face-to-face; family (without patient present)

The focus of the intervention is to improve the patient's health and well-being using cognitive, behavioral, social, and/or psychophysiologic procedures designed to ameliorate the specific obesity-related problems.

Medical Nutrition Therapy Codes

These codes cannot be reported by a physician.

97802   Medical nutrition therapy; initial assessment and intervention, individual, face-to-face with patient, each 15 minutes

97803   Medical nutrition therapy; reassessment and intervention, individual, face-to-face with the patient, each 15 minutes

97804   Medical nutrition therapy; group (2 or more individuals), each 30 minutes

Healthcare Common Procedural Coding System (HCPCS)

Level II Procedure and Supply Codes

Current Procedural Terminology codes are also known as Healthcare Common Procedure Coding System (HCPCS) Level I codes. HCPCS also contains Level II codes. Level II codes (commonly referred to as HCPCS ["hick-picks"] codes) are national codes that are included as part of the Health Insurance Portability and Accountability Act of 1996 (HIPAA) standard procedural transaction coding set along with *CPT* codes.

Healthcare Common Procedure Coding System Level II codes were developed to fill gaps in the *CPT* nomenclature. Although they are reported in the same way as *CPT* codes, they consist of 1 alphabetic character (A–V) followed by 4 digits. In the past, insurance carriers did not uniformly recognize HCPCS Level II codes. However, with the advent of HIPAA, carrier software systems must now be able to recognize all HCPCS Level I (*CPT*) and Level II codes.

HCPCS Education and Counseling Codes

S9445 Patient education, not otherwise classified, nonphysician provider, individual, per session

S9446 Patient education, not otherwise classified, nonphysician provider, group, per session

S9449 Weight management classes, nonphysician provider, per session

S9451 Exercise class, nonphysician provider, per session

S9452 Nutrition class, nonphysician provider, per session

S9454 Stress management class, nonphysician provider, per session

S9455 Diabetic management program, group session

S9460 Diabetic management program, nurse visit

S9465 Diabetic management program, dietitian visit

S9470 Nutritional counseling, dietitian visit

Diagnosis Codes

International Classification of Diseases, Ninth Revision, Clinical Modification (ICD-9-CM) Codes

Circulatory System

401.9 Essential hypertension; unspecified

429.3 Cardiomegaly

Congenital Anomalies

758.0 Down syndrome

759.81 Prader-Willi syndrome

759.83 Fragile X syndrome

759.89 Other specified anomalies (Laurence-Moon-Biedl syndrome)

Digestive System

530.81 Esophageal reflux

564.00 Constipation, unspecified

571.8 Other chronic nonalcoholic liver disease

Endocrine, Nutritional, Metabolic

244.8 Other specified acquired hypothyroidism

244.9 Unspecified hypothyroidism

250.00 Diabetes mellitus without mention of complication, type II or unspecified type, not stated as uncontrolled

250.02 Diabetes mellitus without mention of complication, type II or unspecified type, uncontrolled

253.8 Other disorders of the pituitary and other syndromes of diencephalohypophysial origin

255.8 Other specified disorders of adrenal glands

256.4 Polycystic ovaries

259.1 Precocious sexual development and puberty, not elsewhere specified

259.9 Unspecified endocrine disorder

272.0 Pure hypercholesterolemia

272.1 Pure hyperglyceridemia

272.2 Mixed hyperlipidemia

272.4 Other and unspecified hyperlipidemia

272.9 Unspecified disorder of lipoid metabolism

277.7 Dysmetabolic syndrome X/metabolic syndrome (Use additional codes for associated manifestation, such as: obesity [278.00–278.03])

278.00 Obesity, unspecified

278.01 Morbid obesity

278.02 Overweight

278.1 Localized adiposity

278.8 Other hyperalimentation

Genitourinary System

611.1 Hypertrophy of the breast

Mental Disorders

300.00	Anxiety state, unspecified
300.02	Generalized anxiety disorder
300.4	Dysthymic disorder
307.50	Eating disorder, unspecified
307.51	Bulimia nervosa
307.59	Other disorders of eating
308.3	Other acute reactions to stress
308.9	Unspecified acute reaction to stress
311	Depressive disorder, not elsewhere classified
313.1	Misery and unhappiness disorder
313.81	Oppositional defiant disorder

Musculoskeletal System and Connective Tissue

732.4	Juvenile osteochondrosis of lower extremity, excluding foot

Nervous System and Sense Organs

327.23	Obstructive sleep apnea (adult) (pediatric)
348.2	Benign intracranial hypertension

Skin and Subcutaneous Tissue

701.2	Acquired acanthosis nigricans

Symptoms, Signs, and Ill-Defined Conditions

780.51	Insomnia with sleep apnea, unspecified
780.53	Hypersomnia with sleep apnea, unspecified
780.54	Hypersomnia, unspecified
780.57	Unspecified sleep apnea
780.59	Sleep disturbance; other
780.71	Chronic fatigue syndrome
780.79	Other malaise and fatigue
783.1	Abnormal weight gain
783.3	Feeding difficulties and mismanagement
783.40	Lack of normal physiological development, unspecified
783.43	Short stature
783.5	Polydipsia
783.6	Polyphagia
783.9	Other symptoms concerning nutrition, metabolism, and development
786.05	Shortness of breath
789.1	Hepatomegaly
790.22	Impaired glucose tolerance test (oral)
790.29	Other abnormal glucose; prediabetes not otherwise specified
790.4	Nonspecific elevation of levels of transaminase or lactic acid dehydrogenase (LDH)
790.6	Other abnormal blood chemistry (hyperglycemia)

Other

Note: The *ICD-9-CM* codes that follow are used to deal with occasions in which circumstances other than a disease or injury are recorded as diagnoses or problems. Some carriers may request supporting documentation for the reporting of V codes.

V18.0	Family history of diabetes mellitus
V18.19	Family history of other endocrine and metabolic diseases
V49.89	Other specified conditions influencing health status
V58.67	Long-term (current) use of insulin
V58.69	Long-term (current) use of other medications
V61.01	Family disruption due to family member on military deployment
V61.02	Family disruption due to return of family member from military deployment
V61.03	Family disruption due to divorce or legal separation
V61.04	Family disruption due to parent-child estrangement
V61.05	Family disruption due to child in welfare custody
V61.06	Family disruption due to child in foster care or in care of non-parental family member
V61.07	Family disruption due to death of family member
V61.08	Family disruption due to other extended absence of family member
V61.09	Other family disruption
V61.20	Counseling for parent-child problem, unspecified

V61.29 Parent-child problems; other

V61.49 Health problems with family; other

V61.8 Health problems within family; other specified family circumstances

V61.9 Health problems within family; unspecified family circumstances

V62.81 Interpersonal problems, not elsewhere classified

V62.89 Other psychological or physical stress not elsewhere classified; other

V62.9 Unspecified psychosocial circumstance

V65.19 Other person consulting on behalf of another person

V65.3 Dietary surveillance and counseling

V65.41 Exercise counseling

V65.49 Other specified counseling

V69.0 Lack of physical exercise

V69.1 Inappropriate diet and eating habits

V69.8 Other problems relating to lifestyle; self-damaging behavior

V69.9 Problem related to lifestyle, unspecified

V85.51 Body mass index, pediatric, less than 5th percentile for age

V85.52 Body mass index, pediatric, 5th percentile to less than 85th percentile for age

V85.53 Body mass index, pediatric, 85th percentile to less than 95th percentile for age

V85.54 Body mass index, pediatric, greater than or equal to 95th percentile for age

For more information on coding, contact the AAP Division of Health Care Finance and Quality Improvement at aapcodinghotline@aap.org.

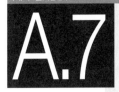

Denial Management and Contract Negotiation for Obesity Services

The current private carrier coverage environment for obesity services is mixed. Private carriers may have health plans that do not cover obesity-related services under the medical plan; they may be carved out of the benefits package completely or part of disease management programs.

The key is to determine the level of coverage by the health plan for obesity evaluation and treatment. If the health plan denies an appropriately coded service for obesity,

- Determine the nature of the denial to determine the appropriate follow-up.
- Review the carrier's denial letter or explanation of benefits (EOB) for the reason for the denial. The most commonly provided reasons are *bundling* of services, it is a *carve-out* from the medical plan benefits, or it is a *noncovered* service.
  - **Bundling.** Obesity evaluation and treatment services may be bundled with the evaluation and management (E/M) services by the carrier. The *Current Procedural Terminology (CPT®)* codes listed in Appendix A.6 represent separately identifiable services and should be reported as such. Although there is no legal mandate requiring private carriers to adhere to *CPT* guidelines, it is considered a good faith gesture for them to do so, given that the guidelines are the current standard within organized medicine. All inappropriate bundling of services should be appealed by the pediatric practice to the carrier.
  - **Carve-out.** Some carriers may carve out obesity-related services from the provider network to a smaller specialty network or disease management program. The pediatrician may consider contacting the carrier to determine the extent of the carve-out and to what degree coverage and payment are available for obesity-related services. As a contractual issue between the health plan and pediatric practice, the pediatrician may discuss with the carrier becoming part of the network or disease management program.
  - **Noncovered service.** Carriers may have different levels of health plan benefits, and the family may be covered by a health plan with limited benefits coverage that does not provide any benefits coverage for obesity-related services. In these situations, the family would be

financially responsible for services provided to evaluate and treat obesity.

Strategies to Enhance Coverage

In addressing issues with carriers, strategies include *filing appeals* and *negotiating contractual provisions*. A sample letter to send to carriers addressing bundling and carve-outs is included in Appendix A.8.

- Filing appeals. Pediatric practices can follow these general guidelines when appealing claim denials or partially paid claims (excerpted from "Appealing claim denials can improve the bottom line." *AAP News.* 2004;24:257):
  1. Review all carrier EOBs. Compare the billed amount and *CPT* codes with the EOBs to determine the level of discounts, denials, inappropriate carrier recoding, or partial payments.
  2. Make sure the claim was prepared properly, all information is correct, and documentation supports the *CPT* codes. Once assured the denial was not caused by an error on the practice's part, proceed with the appeal.
  3. Send appeals in writing and to the right person—look up the contact person in the contract or call the carrier and explain the situation and what is coming so they can be on the lookout. If you are not satisfied with the response, contact the plan's medical director.
  4. Send the appeal by certified mail to verify receipt by the health plan.
  5. List the member's name, carrier identification number, and claim number on all documentation.
  6. State your case in objective and factual terms. Identify the result you want and provide medical justification and *CPT* coding guidelines to support your case (keep in mind, most claim processors do not have a medical or coding background, so be clear and specific). Sample appeal letters that can be used as templates are available on the American Academy of Pediatrics (AAP) Web site on the Private Payer Advocacy page (http://www.aap.org/en-us/professional-resources/practice-support/financing-and-payment/Pages/Private-Payer-Advocacy.aspx).

7. Suggest how denials can be avoided in the future, particularly if they are a recurring problem.

8. Monitor for a response. If the carrier does not respond within the time frame specified in your initial appeal, follow up with a second letter.

9. Create a spreadsheet to track appeals to each carrier so at contract renewal time, you can determine whether to continue to work with that carrier and identify items to modify in the contract.

10. Each health plan should have a written statement explaining the procedures required for first- and second-level appeals. If services are not excluded in the contract and the practice has correctly coded and properly documented them, continue to appeal. Should further action be required, contact the state department of insurance or, depending on the state in which you practice, the state department of banking and insurance or health. Most states have prompt pay laws. If a managed care organization violates the prompt pay law, the physician may be eligible for interest payments on the amount owed, depending on state law.

11. If a claim is denied and the health plan informs that it is a noncovered service or the plan member's responsibility, bill the plan member and include a copy of the EOB and denial with the bill.

12. Contact your AAP chapter to keep it aware of your issues. Some chapters have pediatric councils that meet regularly with health plan medical directors and Medicaid representatives to address coverage issues. Use the AAP Hassle Factor Form to report problems with payers. (Some chapters have made the Hassle Factor Form available on their Web sites; it also can be accessed at http://www2.aap.org/moc/reimburse/hasslefactor/HassleForm.cfm.)

■ Negotiating contractual provisions. In contacts with health plans to discuss contractual issues, the keys are to

1. Address this issue with the person who has the authority to make decisions about payment. The carrier provider representative may not have the decision-making authority in this type of matter.

2. Focus the argument on how this is cost-effective to the family and health plan, as well as how it relates to quality care (provide documentation supporting your position).

3. Frame your position on how it affects the quality of care, cost-effectiveness, and patient satisfaction. Carriers are very conscious of quality issues, how a proposed change will affect overall expenses and

efficiency, and market share. The carrier's current policy may not cover obesity-related services and the carrier needs to be made aware of the effect on the patient, family, pediatrician, and carrier.

4. Consider notifying the family and employer because they may bring pressure on the carrier and employer to expand health plan coverage.

American Academy of Pediatrics Activities

Some chapters have created pediatric councils that meet with carrier medical directors to discuss pediatric issues. American Academy of Pediatrics members may contact their chapters to report issues related to coverage for obesity with carriers. Members may also report carrier issues using the AAP Hassle Factor Form, available on the AAP Web site under Practice Support > Financing and Payment > Private Payer Advocacy (http://www2.aap.org/moc/reimburse/hasslefactor/HassleForm.cfm).

The AAP Private Payer Advocacy Advisory Committee (PPAAC) and the Provisional Section on Obesity are addressing coverage and payment issues for primary care pediatricians and other health professionals, including carve-outs, health plan provider networks, and coverage and compensation for prevention, evaluation, and treatment. PPAAC continues to develop strategies and resources to help pediatric practices advocate for enhanced coverage and compensation for obesity-related services, which are available to AAP members at http://www.aap.org/en-us/professional-resources/practice-support/financing-and-payment/Pages/Private-Payer-Advocacy.aspx. Refer to the joint AMA/CDC "Recommendations for Treatment of Child and Adolescent Overweight and Obesity" (http://www2.aap.org/obesity/policystatements.html), endorsed by the AAP, as well as the AAP "Prevention of Pediatric Overweight and Obesity" policy statement (aappolicy.aappublications.org/cgi/content/full/pediatrics; 112/2/424) for recommendations for health care professionals on the clinical assessment, prevention, and treatment of obesity.

For more information on private payer advocacy, contact lterranova@aap.org.

A.8 American Academy of Pediatrics Policy Statements

Index

Active Healthy Living: Prevention of Childhood Obesity Through Increased Physical Activity

Council on Sports Medicine and Fitness and Council on School Health

Organizational Principles to Guide and
Define the Child Health Care System and/or
Improve the Health of All Children

ABSTRACT

The current epidemic of inactivity and the associated epidemic of obesity are being driven by multiple factors (societal, technologic, industrial, commercial, financial) and must be addressed likewise on several fronts. Foremost among these are the expansion of school physical education, dissuading children from pursuing sedentary activities, providing suitable role models for physical activity, and making activity-promoting changes in the environment. This statement outlines ways that pediatric health care providers and public health officials can encourage, monitor, and advocate for increased physical activity for children and teenagers.

INTRODUCTION

IN 1997, THE World Health Organization declared obesity a global epidemic with major health implications.[1] According to the 1999–2000 National Health and Nutrition Examination Survey (www.cdc.gov/nchs/nhanes.htm), the prevalence of overweight or obesity in children and youth in the United States is over 15%, a value that has tripled since the 1960s.[2] The health implications of this epidemic are profound. Insulin resistance, type 2 diabetes mellitus, hypertension, obstructive sleep apnea, nonalcoholic steatohepatitis, poor self-esteem, and a lower health-related quality of life are among the comorbidities seen more commonly in affected children and youth than in their unaffected counterparts.[3–7] In addition, up to 80% of obese youth continue this trend into adulthood.[8,9] Adult obesity is associated with higher rates of hypertension, dyslipidemia, and insulin resistance, which are risk factors for coronary artery disease, the leading cause of death in North America.[10]

Assessment of Overweight

Ideally, methods of measuring body fat should be accurate, inexpensive, and easy to use; have small measurement error; and be well documented with published reference values. Direct measures of body composition, such as underwater weighing, magnetic resonance imaging, computed axial tomography, and dual-energy radiograph absorptiometry, provide an estimate of total body fat mass. These techniques, however, are used mainly in tertiary care centers for research purposes. Anthropometric measures of relative fatness may be inexpensive and easy to use but rely on the skill of the measurer, and their relative accuracy must be validated against a "gold-standard" measure of adiposity. Such indirect methods of

www.pediatrics.org/cgi/doi/10.1542/
peds.2006-0472

doi:10.1542/peds.2006-0472

All policy statements from the American
Academy of Pediatrics automatically
expire 5 years after publication unless
reaffirmed, revised, or retired at or
before that time.

Key Words
healthy living, physical activity, obesity,
overweight, advocacy, children, youth

Abbreviations
PE—physical education
AAP—American Academy of Pediatrics

PEDIATRICS (ISSN Numbers: Print, 0031-4005;
Online, 1098-4275). Copyright © 2006 by the
American Academy of Pediatrics

estimating body composition include measuring weight and weight for height, body mass index (BMI), waist circumference, skinfold thickness, and ponderal index.[11] Of these, perhaps the most convenient is BMI, which can be calculated according to the following formulas (www.cdc.gov/growthcharts):

BMI = weight (kg)/(height) (m²) or

BMI = weight (kg)/height (cm)/height (cm) × 10 000

BMI = weight (lb)/height (in)/height (in) × 703

BMI varies with age and gender. It typically increases during the first months of life, decreases after the first year, and increases again around 6 years of age.[11] A specific BMI value, therefore, should be evaluated against age- and gender-specific reference values. In the United States, such reference charts based on early 1970s survey data of children 2 to 20 years of age are readily available for clinical use.[12] Children and youth with a BMI greater than the 95th percentile are classified as overweight or obese, and those between the 85th and 95th percentiles are designated at risk of overweight.[13] Although BMI tends to underestimate overweight in tall individuals and overestimate overweight in short individuals and those with high lean body mass (ie, athletes), it generally correlates well with more precise measures of adiposity in individuals with BMI in the 95th percentile or greater.[14]

Factors Contributing to Obesity

Some children have medical conditions associated with obesity and/or require pharmacologic treatments resulting in significant weight gain. Others (1%–2% of obese children) have underlying genetic conditions such as Down, Prader-Willi, or Bardet-Biedle syndrome, which can be associated with obesity. Rarely, single-gene disorders, including congenital leptin deficiency and defects in the melanocortin 4 receptor, cause morbid childhood obesity.

Observations in twin, sibling, and family studies suggest that children are more likely to be overweight if relatives are similarly affected and that heritability may play a role in as many as 25% to 85% of cases. However, to suggest that only genetic factors have caused the recent global epidemic of childhood obesity would not be realistic. It is more likely that most of the world's population carries a combination of genes that may have evolved to cope with food scarcity. In obesogenic environments in which calorie-dense foods are readily available and low-energy expenditure is commonplace, this genetic predisposition would be maladaptive and could lead to an obese population.[11]

Nutritional factors contributing to the increase in obesity rates include, in no particular order, (1) insufficient infant breastfeeding, (2) a reduction in cereal fiber, fruit, and vegetable intake by children and youth, and (3) the excessive consumption of oversized fast foods and soda, which are encouraged by fast-food advertising during children's television programming and a greater availability of fast foods and sugar-containing beverages in school vending machines.[15,16] Although nutritional issues have a significant role to play, this statement focuses on factors associated with decreased energy expenditure, namely excessive sedentary behaviors and lack of adequate physical activity.

Children and youth are more sedentary than ever with the widespread availability of television, videos, computers, and video games. Data from the 1988–1994 National Health and Nutrition Examination Survey indicated that 26% of American children (up to 33% of Mexican American and 43% of non-Hispanic black children) watched at least 4 hours of television per day, and these children were less likely to participate in vigorous physical activity. They also had greater BMIs and skinfold measurements than those who watched <2 hours of television per day.[17]

Not only are the rates of sedentary activities rising, but participation in physical activity is not optimal. In a 2002 Youth Media Campaign Longitudinal Survey, 4500 children 9 to 13 years of age and their parents were polled about physical activity levels outside of school hours. The report indicated that 61.5% of 9- to 13-year-olds did not participate in any organized physical activities and 22.6% did not partake in nonorganized physical activity during nonschool hours.[18]

Youth at Risk of Decreased Physical Activity

Particular individuals at increased risk of having low levels of physical activity have been identified and include children who are from ethnic minorities (especially girls) in the preadolescent/adolescent age groups, children living in poverty, children with disabilities, children residing in apartments or public housing, and children living in neighborhoods where outdoor physical activity is restricted by climate, safety concerns, or lack of facilities.[19,20] According to the Centers for Disease Control and Prevention (www.cdc.gov/nccdphp/sgr/adoles.htm), inactivity is twice as common among females (14%) as males (7%) and among black females (21%) as white females (12%). In a meta-analysis that evaluated physical activity and cardiorespiratory fitness, 6- to 7-year-olds were more active in moderate to vigorous physical activity (46 minutes/day) compared with 10- to 16-year-olds (16–45 minutes/day). Boys were approximately 20% more active than girls, and mean activity levels decreased with age by 2.7% per year in boys compared with 7.4% per year in girls.[21] Many reasons are stated for the general lack of physical activity among children and youth. These reasons include inactive role models (eg, parents and other caregivers), competing demands/time pressures, unsafe environments, lack of recreation facilities or insufficient funds to begin recreation programs, and inadequate access to quality daily physical education (PE).

Physical Activity in Schools

Children and youth spend most of their waking hours at school, so the availability of regular physical activity in that setting is critical. Although the *Healthy People 2010* report recommends increasing the amount of daily PE for all students in a larger proportion of US schools, such changes do not seem to be forthcoming.[19] In 2000, a school health policies and program study[22] looked at a nationally representative sample of private and public schools and found that only 8% of American elementary schools, 6.4% of middle schools, and 5.8% of high schools with existing PE requirements provided daily PE classes for all grades for the entire year. In addition, although approximately 80% of states have policies calling for students to participate in PE in all schools, 40% of elementary schools, 52% of middle schools, and 60% of high schools allow exemption from PE classes, particularly for students with permanent physical disabilities and those having religious reasons.[22] The National Association of State Boards of Education recommends 150 minutes per week of PE for elementary students and 225 minutes per week for middle and high school students.[23] Unfortunately, these requirements are not being implemented. In a study of 814 third-grade students from 10 different US data-collection sites, the mean duration of PE was 33 minutes twice a week, with only 25 minutes per week at a moderate to vigorous intensity level.[24] In addition, 1991–2003 Youth Risk Behavior Surveillance data showed that although the percentage of high school students enrolled in PE class remained constant (48.9%–55.7%), the percentage of students with daily PE attendance decreased from 41.6% in 1991 to 25.4% in 1995 and remained stable thereafter (25.4%–28.4%).[25]

Management of the Obese Child

The successful treatment of obesity in the pediatric age group has been somewhat obscure to date. Studies have shown that younger children seem to respond better to treatment than adolescents and adults.[11,26] Reasons given for this include greater motivation, more influence of the family on behavioral change, and the ability to take advantage of longitudinal growth, which allows children to "grow into their weight." Treatment programs that include nutritional intervention in combination with exercise have higher success rates than diet modification alone. Indeed, a research program that included dietary modification, exercise, and family-based behavioral modification demonstrated enhanced weight loss and better maintenance of lost weight over 5 years.[27] Successful activity-related interventions include a reduction in sedentary behavior and an increase in energy expenditure. Improvements in BMI have been shown to occur when television viewing is restricted.[28] In this regard, the American Academy of Pediatrics (AAP) recommends no more than 2 hours of quality television programming per day for children older than 2 years.[29] Lifestyle-related physical activity, as opposed to calisthenics or programmed aerobic exercise, seems to be more important for sustained weight loss.[30] Such treatment programs should be individually tailored to each child, and their success should be measured not just in terms of weight loss but also in terms of the effects of the programs on associated morbidities.

Health Benefits of Physical Activity

Regular physical activity is important in weight reduction and improving insulin sensitivity in youth with type 2 diabetes.[31] Aerobic exercise has been shown in a prospective randomized, controlled study of 64 children (9–11 years old) with hypertension to reduce systolic and diastolic blood pressure over 8 months.[32] Resistance training (eg, weight lifting) after aerobic exercise seems to prevent the return of blood pressure to preintervention levels in hypertensive adolescents.[33] Weight loss through moderate aerobic exercise has been shown to reduce the hyperinsulinemia, hepatomegaly, and liver enzyme elevation seen in patients with steatohepatitis.[6,34] Regular physical activity is also beneficial psychologically for all youth regardless of weight. It is associated with an increase in self-esteem and self-concept and a decrease in anxiety and depression.[35]

Prevention of Overweight in Children and Youth

Given the challenges of reversing existing obesity in the pediatric population, preventive tactics are likely to be the key to success. Unfortunately, controlled prevention trials have been somewhat disappointing to date. In a systematic Cochrane Database review,[36] 3 of 4 long-term studies combining dietary education with physical activity showed no difference in overweight, and 1 long-term physical activity intervention study showed a slight reduction in overweight. However, the randomized control design may not be ideal for the study of most health-promotion interventions. This is because these are typically population-based programs, which tend to be complex, are delivered over long periods of time, and present some difficulties in controlling all variables.[11] Solution-oriented research, which evaluates promising interventions, often in a quasi-experimental manner, may be more appropriate in the long run.[37] It is unlikely, however, that any single strategy will be sufficient to reverse current trends in pediatric obesity. Success is more likely to be achieved by the implementation of sustainable, economically viable, culturally acceptable active-living policies that can be integrated into multiple sectors of society.

Increasing Physical Activity Levels in Children and Youth

Physical activity needs to be promoted at home, in the community, and at school, but school is perhaps the most encompassing way for all children to benefit. As of June 2005, there is a new opportunity for pediatricians to get involved with school districts. Section 204 of the Child Nutrition and WIC [Supplemental Nutrition Program for Women, Infants, and Children] Reauthorization Act of 2004 (Public Law 108–265) requires that every school receiving funding through the National School Lunch and/or Breakfast Program develop a local wellness policy that promotes the health of students, with a particular emphasis on addressing the problem of childhood obesity. By the 2006–2007 school year, each school or school district is required to set goals for healthy nutrition, physical activity, and other strategies to promote student wellness. Parents, students, school personnel, and members of the community are required to be involved in the policy development. Pediatricians can take advantage of this requirement to get involved. In light of the school wellness policy, many schools are looking to modify their present PE programs to improve their physical activity standards.

In past years, PE classes used calisthenics and sport-specific skill acquisition to promote fitness. This approach did not meet the needs of all students, such as those with obesity or physical disabilities. PE curricula and instruction should emphasize the knowledge, attitudes, and motor and behavioral skills required to adopt and maintain lifelong habits of physical activity.[38] Cross-sectional school-based studies have shown modest correlation between physical activity and lower BMI, although long-term follow-up data are lacking. In an observational study of 9751 kindergarten students, an increase in PE instruction time was associated with a significant reduction in BMI among overweight girls.[39] Project SPARK (Sports, Play, and Active Recreation for Kids Curriculum) looked at increasing physical activity through modified PE and classroom-based teaching on health and skill fitness. Physical activity levels increased during PE classes, and fitness levels in girls improved as a result.[40] It is interesting to note that, despite a significant increase in PE class time, there was no interference with academic attainment, and some achievement test results improved. A recent review of the literature suggests that school-based physical activity programs may modestly enhance academic performance in the short-term, but additional research is required to establish any long-term improvements. There does not seem to be sufficient evidence to suggest that daily physical activity detracts from academic success.[41]

An increase in school PE participation alone is not likely to be sufficient to reverse the childhood obesity epidemic. A 2-year study of elementary students showed that those who had enhanced physical activity education as well as modified PE classes to increase lifestyle aerobic activity increased their physical activity inside the classroom, but lower levels were noted outside the classroom in their leisure time, and no improvements on fitness testing or body fat percentage were seen.[42] The PLAY (Promoting Lifestyle Activity for Youth) program, which encourages the accumulation of 30 to 60 minutes of moderate to vigorous physical activity daily beyond school time and during regular school hours outside of PE classes, has been shown to increase the physical activity levels of children, especially girls.[43] Children can increase their physical activity levels in many other ways during school and nonschool hours, including active transportation, unorganized outdoor free play, personal fitness and recreational activities, and organized sports. Parents of children in organized sports should be encouraged to stimulate their children to be physically active on days when they are not participating in these sports and not rely solely on the sports to provide all their away-from-school physical activity. This should include participation in physical activities with the entire family. Communities designed with green spaces and biking trails help provide families the means to enjoy such active lifestyles.

During late childhood and adolescence, strength training may be additionally beneficial. Youth taking part in this type of exercise may gain strength, improve sport performance, and derive long-term health benefits.[44] Obese children often prefer strength training because it does not require agility or aerobic ability, and the benefits become apparent within as little as 2 to 3 weeks. Because of their added body mass, overweight participants also tend to be stronger than their peers, giving them a relative psychological advantage. Recent studies have shown that obese students are more compliant and increase their free fat mass when weight training is added to aerobic exercise or a standardized energy-reduction diet.[45,46]

Recommended physical activity levels for children and youth vary somewhat in different countries. The Centers for Disease Control and Prevention and the United Kingdom Health Education Authority recommend that children and youth accumulate at least 60 minutes daily of moderate to vigorous physical activity in a variety of enjoyable individual and group activities.[47,48] Health Canada guidelines recommend increasing physical activity above the current level by at least 30 minutes (10 minutes vigorous) and reducing sedentary activity by the same amount per day. Each month, physical activity should be increased and sedentary behavior should be decreased by 15 minutes until at least 90 minutes more active time and 90 minutes less inactive time are accumulated (www.paguide.com). The Canadian Paediatric Society has endorsed these recommendations and emphasizes a wide variety of activities as part of recreation, transportation, chores, work, and planned exercise to encourage lifestyle changes that may last a lifetime.[49]

Age-Appropriate Recommendations for Physical Activity

Clinicians should encourage parents to limit sedentary activity and make physical activity and sport recommendations to parents and caregivers that are consistent with the developmental level of the child.[50] The following are guidelines from the AAP for different age groups.

Infants and Toddlers

There is insufficient evidence to recommend exercise programs or classes for infants and toddlers as a means of promoting increased physical activity or preventing obesity in later years. The AAP has recommended that children younger than 2 years not watch any television. The AAP suggests that parents be encouraged to provide a safe, nurturing, and minimally structured play environment for their infant.[51] Infants and toddlers should also be allowed to develop enjoyment of outdoor physical activity and unstructured exploration under the supervision of a responsible adult caregiver. Such activities include walking in the neighborhood, unorganized free play outdoors, and walking through a park or zoo.

Preschool-Aged Children (4–6 Years)

Free play should be encouraged with emphasis on fun, playfulness, exploration, and experimentation while being mindful of safety and proper supervision. Preschool-aged children should take part in unorganized play, preferably on flat surfaces with few variables and instruction limited to a show-and-tell format. Appropriate activities might include running, swimming, tumbling, throwing, and catching. Preschoolers should also begin walking tolerable distances with family members. In addition, parents should reduce sedentary transportation by car and stroller and, as applies to all age groups, limit screen time to <2 hours per day.

Elementary School–Aged Children (6–9 Years)

In this age group, children improve their motor skills, visual tracking, and balance. Parents should continue to encourage free play involving more sophisticated movement patterns with emphasis on fundamental skill acquisition. These children should be encouraged to walk, dance, or jump rope and may enjoy playing miniature golf. There is little difference between the sexes in weight, height, endurance, and motor skill development at this age; thus, co-ed participation is not contraindicated. Organized sports (soccer, baseball) may be initiated, but they should have flexible rules and short instruction time, allow free time in practices, and focus on enjoyment rather than competition. These children have a limited ability to learn team strategy.

Middle School–Aged Children (10–12 Years)

Preferred physical activities that focus on enjoyment with family members and friends should be encouraged as with previous groups. Emphasis on skill development and increasing focus on tactics and strategy as well as factors promoting continued participation are needed. Fully developed visual tracking, balance, and motor skills are typical in late childhood. Middle school–aged children are better able to process verbal instruction and integrate information from multiple sources so that participation in complex sports (football, basketball, ice hockey) is more feasible. Puberty may begin at different rates, making some individuals bigger and stronger than others. Basing placement in contact and collision sports on maturity rather than chronologic age may result in less risk of injury and enhanced chance of success, especially for those at lower Tanner stages. Weight training may be initiated, provided that the program is well supervised, that small free weights are used with high repetitions (15–20), that proper technique is demonstrated, and that shorter sets using heavier weights and maximum lifts (squat lifts, clean and jerk, dead lifts) are avoided.[44]

Adolescents

Adolescents are highly social and influenced by their peers. Identifying activities that are of interest to the adolescent, especially those that are fun and include friends, is crucial for long-term participation. Physical activities may include personal fitness preferences (eg, dance, yoga, running), active transportation (walking, cycling), household chores, and competitive and noncompetitive sports. Ideally, enrollment in competitive contact and collision sports should be based on size and ability instead of chronologic age. Weight training may continue, and as the individual reaches physical maturity (Tanner stage 5), longer sets using heavier weights and fewer repetitions may be safely pursued while continuing to stress the importance of proper technique.

Office-Based Physical Activity Assessment

An accurate assessment of an individual child's physical activity level by history or questionnaire is difficult and fraught with methodologic problems. It may be easier for parents to recall the number of times per week their child plays outside for at least 30 minutes than to estimate the average daily minutes spent in physical activity. In addition, asking parents about the number of hours per day their child spends in front of a television, video game, or computer screen may be simpler to quantify and track than time spent in active play. Pedometers may also be helpful, because they provide a simple and more objective method of measuring activity, are inexpensive, and have a "gadget appeal" among youngsters. It has been recommend that adults accumulate 10 000 steps per day to follow a healthy lifestyle.[52] Requirements are less clearly defined in children, but guidelines range from 11 000 to 12 000 steps per day for girls and 13 000 to 15 000 steps per day for boys.[53,54]

CONCLUSIONS

The prevalence of pediatric obesity has reached epidemic proportions. It is unlikely that the medical profession alone will be able to solve this serious health problem. The promotion of decreased caloric intake and increased energy expenditure will need to take place within all aspects of society. Among the most difficult but most important challenges for society are making exercise alternatives as attractive, exciting, and enjoyable as video games for children, convincing school boards that PE and other school-based physical activity opportunities are as important to long-term productivity as are academics, changing both supplier and consumer attitudes about food selection and portion sizes, and reengineering living environments to promote physical activity.

RECOMMENDATIONS

Research has shown the importance of social, physical, and cultural environments in determining the extent to which people are able to be active in all facets of daily life, including work, education, family life, and leisure.[55] Creating active school communities is an ideal way to ensure that children and youth adopt active, healthy lifestyles. These communities require a collaborative framework between families, schools, community recreation leaders, and health care professionals. Physicians can be instrumental in the development of active school communities by advocating for policy changes at the community, state, and national levels that support healthy nutrition, reducing sedentary time, and increasing physical activity levels while providing education and health supervision about regular physical activity and reduced sedentary time to families in their practices.

ADVOCACY

In addition to promoting healthy nutrition recommendations suggested by the AAP Committee on Nutrition, physicians and health care professionals and their national organizations should advocate for:

- Social marketing that promotes increased physical activity.

- The appropriate allocation of funding for quality research in the prevention of childhood obesity.

- The development and implementation of a school wellness counsel on which local physician representation is encouraged.

- A school curriculum that teaches children and youth the health benefits of regular physical activity.

- Comprehensive community sport and recreation programs that allow for community and school facilities to be open after hours and make physical activities available to all children and youth at reasonable costs; access to recreation facilities should be equally available to both sexes.

- The reinstatement of compulsory, quality, daily PE classes in all schools (kindergarten through grade 12) taught by qualified, trained educators. The curricula should emphasize enjoyable participation in physical activity that helps students develop the knowledge, attitudes, motor skills, behavioral skills, and confidence required to adopt and maintain healthy active lifestyles. These classes should allow participation by all children regardless of ability, illness, injury, and developmental disability, including those with obesity and those who are disinterested in traditional competitive team sports. Commitment of adequate resources for program funding, trained PE personnel, safe equipment, and facilities is also recommended.

- The provision of a variety of physical activity opportunities in addition to PE, including the protection of children's recess time and the requirement of extracurricular physical activity programs and nonstructured physical activity before, during, and after school hours, that address the needs and interests of all students.

- The reduction of environmental barriers to an active lifestyle through the construction of safe recreational facilities, parks, playgrounds, bicycle paths, sidewalks, and crosswalks.

PROMOTING A HEALTHY LIFESTYLE

Physicians and health care professionals should promote active healthy living within each family unit by:

- Serving as role models through the adoption of an active lifestyle.

- Inquiring about nutritional intake, calculating and plotting BMI, identifying obesity-related comorbidities, and promoting healthy eating as suggested by the AAP Committee on Nutrition.

- Documenting the number of hours per day spent on sedentary activities and limiting screen (television, video game, and computer) time according to AAP guidelines.

- Determining physical activity levels of the child and family members at regular health care visits.

- Tabulating the amount of physical activity the child or youth does each day at home, school, or child care as part of transportation, work, recreation, and unorganized sports, which should include determining the actual minutes of PE and recess-related physical activity achieved at school each week. In addition, the number of times per week spent in outdoor play for at least 30 minutes and/or the number of daily steps achieved (monitored by using a pedometer) should be documented. Specific involvement in organized sports and dance also should be noted.

- Encouraging children and adolescents to be physically active for at least 60 minutes per day, which does not need to be acquired in a continuous fashion but rather may be accumulated by using smaller increments. Events should be of moderate intensity and include a wide variety of activities as part of sports, recreation, transportation, chores, work, planned exercise, and school-based PE classes. These activities should be primarily unstructured and fun if they are to achieve best compliance.

- Identifying any barriers the child, youth, or parent might have against increasing physical activity, which might include lack of time, competing interests, perceived lack of motor skills, and fear of injury on the part of the child. Parents might be additionally concerned about financial and safety issues. Efforts must then be made to work with the family to educate them regarding the importance of lifelong physical activity and to identify potential strategies to overcome some of their barriers.

- Recommending that parents become good role models by increasing their own level of physical activity. Parents should also incorporate physical activities that family members of all ages and abilities can do together. They should encourage children to play outside as much as possible. Safety should be promoted by the use of appropriate protective equipment (bicycle helmets, life jackets, etc).

- Advising parents to support their children and youth in developmentally and age-appropriate sports and recreational activities. The child's favorite types of physical activity should be a priority. These might best occur in the school setting during extracurricular activities, in which parents/grandparents can take part as leaders and coaches.

- Suggesting that overweight children partake in activities that take advantage of their tall stature and muscle strength, such as water-based sports and strength training, rather than those that require weight bearing (eg, jumping, jogging).

- Recommending that parents of overweight children and youth play a supporting, accepting, and encouraging role in returning them to healthier lifestyles to increase self-esteem.

- Encouraging youth to promote physical activities for their peers and become role models and leaders for younger students.

COUNCIL ON SPORTS MEDICINE AND FITNESS, 2005–2006

Teri M. McCambridge, MD, Chairperson
David T. Bernhardt, MD
Joel S. Brenner, MD, MPH
Joseph A. Congeni, MD
*Jorge E. Gomez, MD
Andrew J.M. Gregory, MD
Douglas B. Gregory, MD
Bernard A. Griesemer, MD
Frederick E. Reed, MD
Stephen G. Rice, MD, PhD
Eric W. Small, MD
Paul R. Stricker, MD

LIAISONS

*Claire LeBlanc, MD
    Canadian Paediatric Society
James Raynor, MS, ATC
    National Athletic Trainers Association

STAFF

Jeanne Christensen Lindros, MPH

COUNCIL ON SCHOOL HEALTH, 2005–2006

Barbara L. Frankowski, MD, MPH, Chairperson
Rani S. Gereige, MD, MPH
Linda M. Grant, MD, MPH
Daniel Hyman, MD
Harold Magalnick, MD
Cynthia J. Mears, DO
George J. Monteverdi, MD
*Robert D. Murray, MD
Evan G. Pattishall III, MD
Michele M. Roland, MD
Thomas L. Young, MD

LIAISONS

Nancy LaCursia, PhD
    American School Health Association
Mary Vernon-Smiley, MD, MPH
    Centers for Disease Control and Prevention
Donna Mazyck, MS, RN
    National Association of School Nurses
Robin Wallace, MD
    Independent School Health Association

STAFF

Su Li, MPA

*Lead authors

REFERENCES

1. World Health Organization. *Obesity: Preventing and Managing the Global Epidemic. Report of a WHO Consultation on Obesity, 3–5 June 1997, Geneva.* Geneva, Switzerland: World Health Organization; 2001. WHO/NUT/NCD 98.1
2. Ogden CL, Carroll MD, Flegal KM. Epidemiologic trends in overweight and obesity. *Endocrinol Metab Clin North Am.* 2003; 32:741–760, vii

3. Rosenbloom AL. Increasing incidence of type 2 diabetes in children and adolescents: treatment considerations. *Paediatr Drugs.* 2002;4:209–221

4. Sorof JM, Lai D, Turner J, Poffenbarger T, Portman RJ. Overweight, ethnicity, and the prevalence of hypertension in school-aged children. *Pediatrics.* 2004;113:475–482

5. Wing YK, Hui SH, Pak WM, et al. A controlled study of sleep related disordered breathing in obese children. *Arch Dis Child.* 2003;88:1043–1047

6. Rashid M, Roberts EA. Nonalcoholic steatohepatitis in children. *J Pediatr Gastroenterol Nutr.* 2000;30:48–53

7. Schwimmer JB, Burwinkle TM, Varni JW. Health-related quality of life of severely obese children and adolescents. *JAMA.* 2003;289:1813–1819

8. Whitaker RC, Wright JA, Pepe MS, Seidel KD, Dietz WH. Predicting obesity in young adulthood from childhood and parental obesity. *N Engl J Med.* 1997;337:869–873

9. Guo SS, Chumlea WC. Tracking of body mass index in children in relation to overweight in adulthood. *Am J Clin Nutr.* 1999;70(1 pt 2):145S–148S

10. Belay B, Belamarich P, Racine AD. Pediatric precursors of adult atherosclerosis. *Pediatr Rev.* 2004;25:4–16

11. Lobstein T, Baur L, Uauy R. Obesity in children and young people: a crisis in public health. *Obesity Rev.* 2004;5(suppl 1):4–104

12. Kuczmarski RJ, Ogden CL, Grummer-Strawn LM, et al. CDC growth charts: United States. *Adv Data.* 2000;(314):1–28

13. Himes JH, Dietz WH. Guidelines for overweight in adolescent preventive services: recommendations from an expert committee. The Expert Committee on Clinical Guidelines for Overweight in Adolescent Preventive Services. *Am J Clin Nutr.* 1994;59:307–316

14. Sardinha LB, Going SB, Teixeira PJ, Lohman TG. Receiver operating characteristic analysis of body mass index, triceps skinfold thickness, and arm girth for obesity screening in children and adolescents. *Am J Clin Nutr.* 1999;70:1090–1095

15. Krebs NF, Jacobson MS; American Academy of Pediatrics, Committee on Nutrition. Prevention of pediatric overweight and obesity. *Pediatrics.* 2003;112:424–430

16. American Academy of Pediatrics, Committee on School Health. Soft drinks in schools. *Pediatrics.* 2004;113:152–154

17. Andersen RE, Crespo CJ, Bartlett SJ, Cheskin LJ, Pratt M. Relationship of physical activity and television watching with body weight and level of fatness among children: results from the Third National Health and Nutrition Examination Survey. *JAMA.* 1998;279:938–942

18. Centers for Disease Control and Prevention. Physical activity levels among children aged 9–13 years: United States, 2002. *MMWR Morb Mortal Wkly Rep.* 2003;52:785–788

19. US Department of Health and Human Services. *Healthy People 2010: Understanding and Improving Health.* 2nd ed. Washington, DC: US Department of Health and Human Services; 2001

20. Raine KD. *Overweights and Obesity in Canada: A Population Health Perspective.* Ottawa, Ontario, Canada: Canadian Institute for Health Information; 2004. Available at: http://secure.cihi.ca/cihiweb/products/CPHIOverweightandObesityAugust2004_e.pdf. Accessed March 30, 2005

21. Sallis JF. Epidemiology of physical activity and fitness in children and adolescents. *Crit Rev Food Sci Nutr.* 1993;33:403–408

22. Burgeson CR, Wechsler H, Brener ND, Young JC, Spain CG. Physical education and activity: results from the School Health Policies and Programs Study 2000. *J Sch Health.* 2001;71:279–293

23. National Association of State Boards of Education. *Fit, Healthy, and Ready to Learn: A School Health Policy Guide.* Alexandria, VA: National Association of State Boards of Education; 2000

24. Nader PR. Frequency and intensity of activity of third-grade children in physical education. National Institute of Child Health and Human Development Study of Early Child Care and Youth Development Network. *Arch Pediatr Adolesc Med.* 2003;157:185–190

25. Grunbaum JA, Kann L, Kinchen S, et al. Youth risk behavior surveillance: United States, 2003 [published corrections appear in *MMWR Morb Mortal Wkly Rep.* 2004;53(24):536 and *MMWR Morb Mortal Wkly Rep.* 2005;54(24):608]. *MMWR Surveill Summ.* 2004;53(2):1–96

26. Summerbell CD, Ashton V, Campbell KJ, Edmonds L, Kelly S, Waters E. Interventions for treating obesity in children. *Cochrane Database Syst Rev.* 2003;(3):CD001872

27. Epstein LH. Methodological issues and ten-year outcomes for obese children. *Ann N Y Acad Sci.* 1993;699:237–249

28. Robinson TN. Reducing children's television viewing to prevent obesity: a randomized controlled trial. *JAMA.* 1999;282:1561–1567

29. American Academy of Pediatrics, Committee on Public Education. Children, adolescents, and television. *Pediatrics.* 2001;107:423–426

30. Epstein LH, Wing RR, Koeske R, Valoski A. A comparison of lifestyle exercise, aerobic exercise, and calisthenics on weight loss in obese children. *Behav Ther.* 1985;16:345–356

31. American Diabetes Association. Type 2 diabetes in children and adolescents. *Pediatrics.* 2000;105:671–680

32. Hansen HS, Froberg K, Hyldebrandt N, Nielsen JR. A controlled study of eight months of physical training and reduction of blood pressure in children: the Odense schoolchild study. *BMJ.* 1991;303:682–685

33. Hagberg JM, Ehsani AA, Goldring D, Hernandez A, Sinacore DR, Holloszy JO. Effect of weight training on blood pressure and hemodynamics in hypertensive adolescents. *J Pediatr.* 1984;104:147–151

34. Roberts EA. Nonalcoholic steatohepatitis in children. *Curr Gastroenterol Rep.* 2003;5:253–259

35. Calfas KJ, Taylor WC. Effects of physical activity on psychological variables in adolescents. *Pediatr Exerc Sci.* 1994;6:406–423

36. Campbell K, Waters E, O'Meara S, Kelly S, Summerbell C. Interventions for preventing obesity in children. *Cochrane Database Syst Rev.* 2002;(2):CD001871

37. Robinson TN, Sirard JR. Preventing childhood obesity: a solution-oriented research paradigm. *Am J Prev Med.* 2005;28(2 suppl 2):194–201

38. Centers for Disease Control and Prevention. Youth risk behavior surveillance: National College Health Risk Behavior Survey—United States, 1995. *MMWR CDC Surveill Summ.* 1997;46(6):1–56

39. Datar A, Sturm R. Physical education in elementary school and body mass index: evidence from the Early Childhood Longitudinal Study. *Am J Public Health.* 2004;94:1501–1506

40. Sallis JF, McKenzie TL, Kolody B, Lewis M, Marshall S, Rosengard P. Effects of health-related physical education on academic achievement: project SPARK. *Res Q Exerc Sport.* 1999;70:127–134

41. Taras H. Physical activity and student performance at school. *J Sch Health.* 2005;75:214–218

42. Donnelly JE, Jacobsen DJ, Whatley JE, et al. Nutrition and physical activity program to attenuate obesity and promote physical and metabolic fitness in elementary school children. *Obes Res.* 1996;4:229–243

43. Pangrazi RP, Beighle A, Vehige T, Vack C. Impact of Promoting Lifestyle Activity for Youth (PLAY) on children's physical activity. *J Sch Health.* 2003;73:317–321

44. Bernhardt DT, Gomez J, Johnson MD, et al. Strength training by children and adolescents. *Pediatrics.* 2001;107:1470–1472

45. Sothern MS, Loftin JM, Udall JN, et al. Safety, feasibility, and

efficacy of a resistance training program in preadolescent obese children. *Am J Med Sci.* 2000;319:370–375

46. Schwingshandl J, Sudi K, Eibl B, Wallner S, Borkenstein M. Effect of an individualised training programme during weight reduction on body composition: a randomised trial. *Arch Dis Child.* 1999;81:426–428

47. Strong WB, Malina RM, Blimkie CJ, et al. Evidence based physical activity for school-age youth. *J Pediatr.* 2005;146:732–737

48. Biddle S, Sallis J, Cavill N. Policy framework for young people and health-enhancing physical activity. In: Biddle S, Sallis J, Cavill N, eds. *Young and Active: Young People and Physical Activity.* London, England: Health Education Authority; 1998:3–16

49. Canadian Paediatric Society, Healthy Active Living Committee. Healthy active living for children and youth. *Paediatr Child Health.* 2002;7:339–345

50. Harris SS. Readiness to participate in sports. In: Sullivan JA, Anderson SJ, eds. *Care of the Young Athlete.* Rosemont, IL: American Academy of Orthopaedic Surgeons/American Academy of Pediatrics; 2000:19–24

51. American Academy of Pediatrics, Committee on Sports Medicine and Fitness. Infant exercise programs. *Pediatrics.* 1988;82:800

52. Hatano Y. Use of the pedometer for promoting daily walking exercise. *Int Council Health Phys Ed Rec.* 1993;29:4–8

53. Vincent SD, Pangrazi RP. An examination of the activity patterns of elementary school children. *Pediatr Exerc Sci.* 2002;14:432–441

54. Tudor-Locke C, Pangrazi RP, Corbin CB, et al. BMI-referenced standards for recommended pedometer-determined steps/day in children. *Prev Med.* 2004;38:857–864

55. Health Canada, Population and Public Health Branch, Policy Directorate. *The Population Health Template: Key Elements and Actions That Define a Population Health Approach.* Ottawa, Ontario, Canada: Health Canada; 2001

AMERICAN ACADEMY OF PEDIATRICS

Committee on Public Education

Children, Adolescents, and Television

ABSTRACT. This statement describes the possible negative health effects of television viewing on children and adolescents, such as violent or aggressive behavior, substance use, sexual activity, obesity, poor body image, and decreased school performance. In addition to the television ratings system and the v-chip (electronic device to block programming), media education is an effective approach to mitigating these potential problems. The American Academy of Pediatrics offers a list of recommendations on this issue for pediatricians and for parents, the federal government, and the entertainment industry.

ABBREVIATIONS. AAP, American Academy of Pediatrics; MTV, Music Television; E/I, educational/informational.

For the past 15 years, the American Academy of Pediatrics (AAP) has expressed its concerns about the amount of time children and adolescents spend viewing television and the content of what they view.[1] According to recent Nielsen Media Research data, the average child or adolescent watches an average of nearly 3 hours of television per day.[2] This figure does not include time spent watching videotapes or playing video games[3] (a 1999 study found that children spend an average of 6 hours 32 minutes per day with various media combined).[4] By the time the average person reaches age 70, he or she will have spent the equivalent of 7 to 10 years watching television.[5] One recent study found that 32% of 2- to 7-year-olds and 65% of 8- to 18-year-olds have television sets in their bedrooms.[4] Time spent with various media may displace other more active and meaningful pursuits, such as reading, exercising, or playing with friends.

Although there are potential benefits from viewing some television shows, such as the promotion of positive aspects of social behavior (eg, sharing, manners, and cooperation), many negative health effects also can result. Children and adolescents are particularly vulnerable to the messages conveyed through television, which influence their perceptions and behaviors.[6] Many younger children cannot discriminate between what they see and what is real. Research has shown primary negative health effects on violence and aggressive behavior[7–12]; sexuality[7,13–15]; academic performance[16]; body concept and self-im-

age[17–19]; nutrition, dieting, and obesity[17,20,21]; and substance use and abuse patterns.[7]

In the scientific literature on media violence, the connection of media violence to real-life aggressive behavior and violence has been substantiated.[8–12] As much as 10% to 20% of real-life violence may be attributable to media violence.[22] The recently completed 3-year National Television Violence Study found the following: 1) nearly two thirds of all programming contains violence; 2) children's shows contain the most violence; 3) portrayals of violence are usually glamorized; and 4) perpetrators often go unpunished.[23] A recent comprehensive analysis of music videos found that nearly one fourth of all Music Television (MTV) videos portray overt violence and depict weapon carrying.[24] Research has shown that even television news can traumatize children or lead to nightmares.[25] In a random survey of parents with children in kindergarten through sixth grade, 37% reported that their child had been frightened or upset by a television story in the preceding year.[26]

According to a recent content analysis, mainstream television programming contains large numbers of references to cigarettes, alcohol, and illicit drugs.[27] One fourth of all MTV videos contain alcohol or tobacco use.[28] A longitudinal study found a positive correlation between television and music video viewing and alcohol consumption among teens.[29] Finally, content analyses show that children and teenagers continue to be bombarded with sexual imagery and innuendoes in programming and advertising.[14,30,31] To date, there are no data available to substantiate the behavioral impact of this exposure.[31]

The new television ratings system and the v-chip are tools that can help protect children from potentially harmful content. All new television sets with screens measuring 13 inches or greater contain a v-chip that enables parents to program televisions to block out any shows that they deem inappropriate for their children.[32] To block out television shows, parents must use the television ratings system, which has age and content descriptors for violence, sexual situations, suggestive dialogue, and adult language. Although the ratings system and the v-chip can assist parents, ongoing evaluation is necessary to ensure that these tools are as effective as possible.[33–35] For example, the ratings should be applied uniformly and listed in television guides, newspapers, and journals so parents know what they mean.

Besides the v-chip, there are other means of protecting children from what is on television. Evidence

The recommendations in this statement do not indicate an exclusive course of treatment or serve as a standard of medical care. Variations, taking into account individual circumstances, may be appropriate.
PEDIATRICS (ISSN 0031 4005). Copyright © 2001 by the American Academy of Pediatrics.

now shows that media education can help mitigate the harmful effects of media violence[36–40] and alcohol advertising[41,42] on children and adolescents. Media education programs have been included in the school curricula beginning in early elementary school in many states across the United States.[43]

Furthermore, continued support of the Children's Television Act of 1990[44] and additional regulations made in 1996[45] will help to ensure the airing of television programs specifically designated for children. The act requires broadcasters to air educational and informational programming for children at least 3 hours per week and to limit the amount of advertising time allowed during children's programming. The shows must be labeled E/I (for educational and informational) on the television screen.

RECOMMENDATIONS

The following recommendations are given for pediatricians and other health care professionals:

1. Remain knowledgeable about the effects of television, including violent and aggressive behavior, obesity, poor body concept and self-image, substance use, and early sexual activity, by becoming involved in the AAP *Media Matters* campaign.[46] Educate patients and their parents about these effects.
2. Use the AAP *Media History* form[46] to help parents recognize the extent of their children's media consumption.
3. Work with local schools to implement comprehensive media-education programs that deal with important public health issues.[36]
4. Serve as good role models by using television appropriately and by implementing reading programs using volunteer readers in waiting rooms and hospital inpatient units.
5. Become involved in the AAP's Media Resource Team (contact the Division of Public Education), and learn how to work effectively with writers, directors, and producers to make media more appropriate for children and adolescents. Contact networks and producers of television programs with concerns about the content of specific shows and episodes.
6. Ensure that appropriate entertainment options are available for hospitalized children and adolescents. Work with child life staff to assemble a screening committee that selects programs for closed circuit broadcast or a video library. Develop institution-specific, formal guidelines based on the established ratings system (which takes profanity, sex, and violence into account), and screen for content containing ethnic and sex role stereotyping. Considerations should also be made to avoid themes hospitalized children might find upsetting, and efforts should be made to enforce the ratings system in the hospital setting.
7. Support the Children's Television Act of 1990 and its 1996 rules by working to ensure that local television stations are in compliance with the act and by urging local newspapers to list ratings and E/I denotations of programs.
8. Monitor the television ratings system for appropriateness and advocate for substantive, content-based ratings in the future.

Pediatricians should recommend the following guidelines for parents:

1. Limit children's total media time (with entertainment media) to no more than 1 to 2 hours of quality programming per day.
2. Remove television sets from children's bedrooms.
3. Discourage television viewing for children younger than 2 years, and encourage more interactive activities that will promote proper brain development, such as talking, playing, singing, and reading together.
4. Monitor the shows children and adolescents are viewing. Most programs should be informational, educational, and nonviolent.
5. View television programs along with children, and discuss the content. Two recent surveys involving a total of nearly 1500 parents found that less than half of parents reported always watching television with their children.[5,47]
6. Use controversial programming as a stepping-off point to initiate discussions about family values, violence, sex and sexuality, and drugs.
7. Use the videocassette recorder wisely to show or record high-quality, educational programming for children.
8. Support efforts to establish comprehensive media-education programs in schools.
9. Encourage alternative entertainment for children, including reading, athletics, hobbies, and creative play.

Pediatricians should lead efforts in their communities to do the following:

1. Form coalitions including libraries, religious organizations, and other community groups to broaden media education beyond the schools.
2. Organize activities promoting media education, such as letter-writing campaigns to local television stations to advocate for better programming for children, and developing local TV turnoff week projects.[48]

Pediatricians should work with the Academy and local chapters to challenge the federal government to do the following:

1. Initiate legislation and rules that would ban alcohol advertising from television.
2. Fund ongoing annual research, such as the National Television Violence Study, and fund more research on the effects of television on children and adolescents, particularly in the area of sex and sexuality.
3. Assemble a *National Institutes of Health Comprehensive Report on Children, Adolescents, and Media* that would bring together all of the current relevant research.
4. Work with the US Department of Education to support the creation and implementation of media-education curricula for school children.

424   CHILDREN, ADOLESCENTS, AND TELEVISION

Pediatricians should work with the Academy and local chapters to challenge the entertainment industry to do the following:

1. Take responsibility for the programming it produces.
2. Adhere to the current television ratings system, and label programs conscientiously.
3. Collaborate with other public health advocates to convene a series of seminars with writers, directors, and producers to discuss ways to make media more appropriate for children and adolescents.
4. Produce more educational programming for children and adolescents, and ensure that the programming it produces is of higher quality, with less content that is gratuitously violent, sexually suggestive, or drug oriented.

COMMITTEE ON PUBLIC EDUCATION, 2000–2001
Miriam E. Bar-on, MD, Chairperson
Daniel D. Broughton, MD
Susan Buttross, MD
Suzanne Corrigan, MD
Alberto Gedissman, MD
M. Rosario González de Rivas, MD
Michael Rich, MD, MPH
Donald L. Shifrin, MD

LIAISONS
Michael Brody, MD
    American Academy of Child and Adolescent
    Psychiatry
Brian Wilcox, PhD
    American Psychological Association

CONSULTANTS
Marjorie Hogan, MD
H. James Holroyd, MD
Linda Reid, MD
S. Norman Sherry, MD
Victor Strasburger, MD

STAFF
Jennifer Stone

REFERENCES

1. American Academy of Pediatrics, Task Force on Children, and Television. Children, adolescents and television. *News and Comment.* December 1984;35:8
2. 1998 Report on Television. New York, NY. Nielsen Media Research; 1998.
3. Mares ML. Children's use of VCRs. *Ann Am Acad Pol Soc Science.* 1998;557:120–131
4. Roberts DF, Foehr UG, Rideout VJ, Brodie, M. *Kids and Media at the New Millennium: A Comprehensive National Analysis of Children's Media Use.* Menlo Park, CA: The Henry J Kaiser Family Foundation Report; 1999
5. Strasburger VC. Children, adolescents, and the media: five crucial issues. *Adolesc Med.* 1993;4:479–493
6. Gerbner G, Gross L, Morgan M, Signorielli N. Growing up with television: the cultivation perspective. In Bryant J, Zillmann D, eds. *Media Effects: Advances in Theory and Research.* Hillsdale, NJ: Lawrence Erlbaum; 1994:17–41
7. Strasburger VC. "Sex, drugs, rock'n'roll," and the media: are the media responsible for adolescent behavior? *Adolesc Med.* 1997;8:403–414
8. Strasburger VC. *Adolescents and the Media: Medical and Psychological Impact.* Thousand Oaks, CA: Sage; 1995
9. Huston AC, Donnerstein E, Fairchild H, et al. *Big World, Small Screen: The Role of Television in American Society.* Lincoln, NE: University of Nebraska Press; 1992
10. Donnerstein E, Linz D. The mass media: a role in injury causation and prevention. *Adolesc Med.* 1995;6:271–284
11. Eron LR. Media violence. *Pediatr Ann.* 1995;24:84–87
12. Willis E, Strasburger VC. Media violence. *Pediatr Clin North Am.* 1998;45:319–331
13. Kunkel D, Cope KM, Farinola WJM, Biely E, Rollin E, Donnerstein E. *Sex on TV: Content and Context.* Menlo Park, CA: The Henry J Kaiser Family Foundation; 1999
14. Huston AC, Wartella E, Donnerstein E. *Measuring, the Effects of Sexual Content in the Media.* Menlo Park, CA: The Henry J Kaiser Family Foundation Report; 1998
15. Brown JD, Greenberg BS, Buerkel-Rothfuss NL. Mass media, sex and sexuality. *Adolesc Med.* 1993;4:511–525
16. Morgan M. Television and school performance. *Adolesc Med.* 1993;4:607–622
17. Harrison K, Cantor J. The relationship between media consumption and eating disorders. *J Commun.* 1997;47:40–67
18. Signorelli N. Sex roles and stereotyping on television. *Adolesc Med.* 1993;4:551–561
19. A Different World. *Children's Perceptions of Race and Class in the Media.* Oakland, CA: Children Now; 1998
20. Andersen RE, Crespo CJ, Bartlett SJ, Cheskin LJ, Pratt M. Relationship of physical activity and television watching with body weight and level of fatness among children: results from the Third National Health and Nutrition Examination Study. *JAMA.* 1998;279:938–942
21. Jeffrey RW, French SA. Epidemic obesity in the United States: are fast foods and television viewing contributing? *Am J Public Health.* 1998;88:277–280
22. Comstock GC, Strasburger VC. Media violence: Q & A. *Adolesc Med.* 1993;4:495–509
23. Federman J, ed. *National Television Violence Study.* Vol 3. Thousand Oaks, CA: Sage; 1998
24. DuRant RH, Rich M, Emans SJ, Rome ES, Allred E, Woods ER. Violence and weapon carrying in music videos: a content analysis. *Arch Pediatr Adolesc Med.* 1997;151:443–448
25. Cantor J. *"Mommy, I'm Scared": How TV and Movies Frighten Children and What We Can Do to Protect Them.* New York, NY: Harcourt Brace; 1998
26. Cantor J, Nathanson AI. Children's fright reactions to television news. *J Commun.* 1996;46:139–152
27. Gerbner G, Ozyegin N. *Alcohol, Tobacco, and Illicit Drugs in Entertainment Television, Commercials, News, "Reality Shows," Movies, and Music Channels.* Princeton, NJ: Robert Wood Johnson Foundation; 1997
28. DuRant RH, Rome ES, Rich M, Allred E, Emans SJ, Woods ER. Tobacco and alcohol use behaviors portrayed in music videos: a content analysis. *Am J Public Health.* 1997;87:1131–1135
29. Robinson TN, Chen HL, Killen JD. Television and music video exposure and risk of adolescent alcohol use. *Pediatrics* [serial online]. 1998;102:e54. Available at: http://www.pediatrics.org/cgi/content/full/102/5/e54. Accessed May 2, 2000.
30. Brown JD, Steele, JR. *Sex and the Mass Media.* Menlo Park, CA: The Henry J Kaiser Family Foundation; 1995
31. Kunkel D, Cope KM, Colvin C. *Sexual Messages on Family Hour Television: Content and Context.* Menlo Park, CA: Henry J Kaiser Family Foundation; 1996
32. Telecommunications Act of., Pub L No. 104–104, 1996.
33. Cantor J. Ratings for program content: the role of research findings. *Ann Am Acad Pol Soc Science.* 1998;557:54–69
34. Kunkel D, Farinola WJM, Cope KM, Donnerstein E et al. *Rating, the TV Ratings: One Year Out. An Assessment of the Television Industry's Use of V-Chip Ratings.* Menlo Park, CA: Henry J Kaiser Family Foundation; 1998
35. *Parents Rate the TV Ratings.* Minneapolis, MN: National Institute on Media and the Family; 1998
36. Potter WJ. *Media Literacy.* Thousand Oaks, CA: Sage; 1998
37. Huesman LR, Eron LD, Klein R, Brice P, Fischer P. Mitigating, the imitation of aggressive behaviors by changing children's attitudes about media violence. *J Pers Soc Psychol.* 1983;44:899–910
38. Gunter B. The question of media violence. In: Bryant J, Zillmann D, eds. Media Effects: Advances in Theory and Research. Hillsdale, NJ: Lawrence Erlbaum; 1994:163–211
39. Kubey RW. Television dependence, diagnosis, and prevention. In: MacBeth TM, ed. *Tuning in to Young Viewers: Social Science Perspectives on Television.* Thousand Oaks, CA: Sage; 1996:221–260
40. Singer DG, Singer JL. Developing critical viewing skills and media literacy in children. In: Jordan AB, Jamieson KH, eds. Children and television. *Ann Am Acad Pol Soc Science.* 1998;557:164–179

41. Austin EW, Johnson KK. Effects of general and alcohol-specific media literacy training on children's decision making about alcohol. *J Health Commun*. 1997;2:17–42

42. Austin EW, Pinkleton BE, Fujioka Y. The role of interpretation processes and parental discussion in the media's effects on adolescents' use of alcohol. *Pediatrics*. 2000;105:343–349

43. Kubey R, Baker F. Has media literacy found a curricular foothold? *Education Week*. 1999;19:38,56

44. Children's Television Act. 47 USC §303a, 303b, 394

45. Revision of Programming Policies for Television Broadcast Stations. Washington, DC. Federal Communications Commission; August 8, 1996. FCC 96–335 (MM Docket 93–48)

46. American Academy of Pediatrics. *Media Matters: A National Media Education Campaign*. Elk Grove Village, IL: American Academy of Pediatrics; 1997

47. Valerio M, Amodio P, Dal Zio M, Vianello A, Zacchello GP. The use of television in 2- to 8-year-old children and the attitude of parents about such use. *Arch Pediatr Adolesc Med*. 1997;151:22–26

48. TV Turnoff Network Web site. Available at: http://www.tvturnoff.org. Accessed December 27, 2000

Policy Statement—Children, Adolescents, Obesity, and the Media

COUNCIL ON COMMUNICATIONS AND MEDIA

KEY WORDS
media, obesity, overweight, screen time, junk food, television

This document is copyrighted and is property of the American
Academy of Pediatrics and its Board of Directors. All authors
have filed conflict of interest statements with the American
Academy of Pediatrics. Any conflicts have been resolved through
a process approved by the Board of Directors. The American
Academy of Pediatrics has neither solicited nor accepted any
commercial involvement in the development of the content of
this publication.

www.pediatrics.org/cgi/doi/10.1542/peds.2011-1066

doi:10.1542/peds.2011-1066

All policy statements from the American Academy of Pediatrics
automatically expire 5 years after publication unless reaffirmed,
revised, or retired at or before that time.

PEDIATRICS (ISSN Numbers: Print, 0031-4005; Online, 1098-4275).

abstract

Obesity has become a worldwide public health problem. Considerable
research has shown that the media contribute to the development of
child and adolescent obesity, although the exact mechanism remains
unclear. Screen time may displace more active pursuits, advertising of
junk food and fast food increases children's requests for those particular foods and products, snacking increases while watching TV or
movies, and late-night screen time may interfere with getting adequate
amounts of sleep, which is a known risk factor for obesity. Sufficient
evidence exists to warrant a ban on junk-food or fast-food advertising
in children's TV programming. Pediatricians need to ask 2 questions
about media use at every well-child or well-adolescent visit: (1) How
much screen time is being spent per day? and (2) Is there a TV set or
Internet connection in the child's bedroom? *Pediatrics* 2011;128:201–
208

INTRODUCTION

Obesity represents a clear and present danger to the health of children
and adolescents. Its prevalence among American youth has doubled in
the past 3 decades,[1] and there are now more overweight and obese
adults in the United States than adults of normal weight.[2] However,
obesity is also a worldwide problem; rates are increasing in nearly
every country.[3,4] It is increasingly clear that the media, particularly TV,
play an important role in the etiology of obesity.[5] As a result, many
countries are now establishing new regulations for advertising to children on TV, and many government health agencies are now issuing
recommendations for parents regarding the amount of time children
spend watching TV.[6] Unfortunately, there are currently no data relating
other media to obesity.

MEDIA AND OBESITY

There are a number of ways that watching TV could be contributing to
obesity: (1) increased sedentary activity and displacement of more
physical pursuits; (2) unhealthy eating practices learned from both the
programming and the advertisements for unhealthy foods; (3) increased snacking behavior while viewing; and (4) interference with
normal sleep patterns. However, most researchers now agree that the
evidence linking excessive TV-viewing and obesity is persuasive.[7–9]
There have been dozens of longitudinal and correlational studies documenting a connection.[9] An increasing number of these studies hold
ethnicity and socioeconomic status—known to be key factors in
obesity—constant and still reveal that TV-viewing is a significant con-

tributor to obesity.[7,10] Results of the longitudinal studies are particularly convincing. For example, a remarkable 30-year study in the United Kingdom found that a higher mean of daily hours of TV viewed on weekends predicted a higher BMI at the age of 30. For each additional hour of TV watched on weekends at age 5, the risk of adult obesity increased by 7%.[11] A group of researchers in Dunedin, New Zealand, followed 1000 subjects from birth to 26 years of age and found that average weeknight TV-viewing between the ages of 5 and 15 years was strongly predictive of adult BMI.[12] In a study of 8000 Scottish children, viewing more than 8 hours of TV per week at age 3 was associated with an increased risk of obesity at age 7.[13] Also, in 8000 Japanese children, more TV-viewing at age 3 resulted in a higher risk of being overweight at age 6.[14] Numerous American studies have had similar findings.[15–23]

The presence of a TV set in a child's bedroom seems to exacerbate the impact of TV-viewing on children's weight status.[24–28] A study of 2343 children aged 9 to 12 years revealed that having a bedroom TV set was a significant risk factor for obesity, independent of physical activity.[24] A cross-sectional study of 2761 parents with young children in New York found that 40% of the 1- to 5-year-olds had a bedroom TV, and those who did were more likely to be overweight or obese.[25] Teenagers with a bedroom TV spent more time watching TV, less time being physically active, ate fewer family meals, had greater consumption of sweetened beverages, and ate fewer vegetables than did teenagers without a bedroom TV.[26]

Recent correlational studies have also found a strong association between time spent watching TV and blood glucose level control in young people with diabetes,[29] type 2 diabetes mellitus,[30]

insulin resistance,[31] metabolic syndrome,[32] hypertension,[33,34] and high cholesterol levels.[35–37] Furthermore, when TV time is diminished, so are measures of adiposity.[38,39]

MECHANISMS

How might time spent with media result in obesity? Contrary to popular opinion, overweight and obesity probably result from small, incremental increases in caloric intake (or increases in sedentary activities).[40] An excess intake of 50 kcal/day (eg, an extra pat of butter) produces a weight gain of 5 lb/year. Drinking a can of soda per day produces a weight gain of 15 lb/year.[41] Nearly 40% of children's caloric intake now comes from solid fat and added sugars, and soda or fruit drinks provide nearly 10% of total calories.[42] Because obesity is caused by an imbalance between energy intake and energy expenditure, screen time may contribute in several different ways.

Displacement of More Active Pursuits

Children spend more time with media than in any other activity except for sleeping—an average of more than 7 hours/day.[43] Many studies have found that physical activity decreases as screen time increases,[44–46] but many other studies have not.[47–49] Children and teenagers who use a lot of media may tend to be more sedentary in general,[7,50] or researchers' measures of physical activity may be too imprecise.[9] Nevertheless, increasing physical activity, decreasing media time, and improving nutritional practices have been shown to prevent the onset of obesity, if not decrease existing obesity as well.[51–55] Some of the newer interactive video games may be useful in this way.[56,57] For example, a study of preteens playing *Dance Revolution* and Nintendo's *Wii Sports* found that energy expenditure was equivalent to moderate-intensity walking.[58]

Unhealthy Eating Habits and Effects of Advertising

Children and teenagers who watch more TV tend to consume more calories or eat higher-fat diets,[59–64] drink more sodas,[65] and eat fewer fruits and vegetables.[66] Some researchers have argued that the viewing of TV while eating suppresses cues of satiety, which leads to overeating.[60] Others believe that viewers are primed to choose unhealthy foods as a consequence of viewing advertisements for foods high in fat, salt, and/or sugar and low in nutritional content ("junk food").[61] On any given day, 30% of American youngsters are eating fast food and consuming an additional 187 kcal (equaling 6 lb/year).[67,68] Fast food is big business: Americans spend more than $110 billion annually on it, which is more than that spent on higher education, computers, or cars.[69] A December 2010 study examined 3039 possible meal combinations at a dozen restaurant chains and found only 12 meals that met nutrition criteria for preschoolers. The same study found that 84% of parents had purchased fast food for their children in the previous week.[70] More than 80% of all advertisements in children's programming are for fast foods or snacks,[71–73] and for every hour that children watch TV, they see an estimated 11 food advertisements.[74] Although exposure to food ads has decreased in the past few years for young children,[73] it has increased for adolescents.[75]

In 2009, the fast-food industry alone spent $4.2 billion on advertising in all media.[70] A study of 50 000 ads from 2003–2004 on 170 top-rated shows found that 98% of food ads seen by children aged 2 to 11 years and nearly 90% of food ads seen by teenagers are for products that are high in fat, sugar, and/or sodium and low in nutritional content (junk food).[76] A newer study of 1638 hours of TV and nearly 9000 food ads found that young people see an average of 12 to 21 food ads per day, for a total of 4400 to 7600 ads per year, yet they see fewer than 165 ads that promote fitness or good nutrition.[77] In 1 study, black children viewed 37% more ads than other youth.[78] New technology is enabling advertisers to reach young children and teenagers with a variety of online interactive techniques.[79–82] A study of the top 5 brands in 8 different food and beverage categories found that all of them had Internet Web sites: 63% had advergames (games used to advertise the product), 50% had cartoon characters, and 58% had a designated children's area.[79] Half of the Web sites urged children to ask their parents to buy the products, yet only 17% contained any nutritional information.[79] Teenagers' cell phones can be targeted by fast-food companies that can offer teenagers a discount on fast food as they walk by a particular restaurant.[81]

Available research results clearly indicate that advertising is effective in getting younger children to request more high-fat/low-nutrition food (junk food) and to attempt to influence their parents.[5,9,83–85] For example, a 2006 study of 827 third-grade children followed for 20 months found that total TV time and total screen media time predicted future requests for advertised foods and drinks.[86] Even brief exposures to TV food ads can influence children as young as preschool age in their food choices.[87] In 1 recent experiment, children consumed 45% more snacks when exposed to food advertising while watching cartoons than advertising for other products.[64] Similarly, children who played an online advergame that marketed healthy foods were more likely to eat healthy snacks than those who played an online advergame that advertised junk food.[82] Perhaps the most convincing study about the impact of advertising involved 63 children who tasted 5 pairs of identical foods (eg, French fries) and beverages (eg, milk) from unbranded packaging versus branded packaging. The results of the experiment revealed that the children strongly preferred the branded food and drinks to the unbranded foods.[88]

To illustrate the power of marketing, compare the commitment of the Robert Wood Johnson Foundation to spend $100 million per year to try to decrease childhood obesity with the fact that the food industry spends more than that every month marketing primarily junk food and fast food to young people.[84,89]

Food is also unhealthily portrayed in most TV programming and movies.[9,84,90,91] A study of the 30 highest-rated programs among 2- to 5-year-olds found that an average child would see more than 500 food references per week, half of which were to empty-calorie or high-fat/sugar/salt foods (D. L. G. Borzekowski, EdD, "Watching What They Eat: A Content Analysis of Televised Food References Reaching Preschool Children," unpublished manuscript, 2001). In an analysis of 100 films from 1991 through 2000, fats and sweets were the most common foods depicted.[91] Hollywood product placements are also being used to influence the food preferences and purchasing patterns of children and adolescents.[92,93] In the 200 movies examined from 1996 to 2005, a total of 1180 brand placements were identified. Candy (26%) and salty snacks (21%) were the most prevalent food brands, sugar-sweetened beverages (76%) were the most prevalent beverage brands, and fast food composed two-thirds of the food retail establishment brand placements.[93]

Effect of Media on Sleep Habits

TV and other media are known to displace or disturb young people's sleep patterns.[5,94,95] A longitudinal study of adolescents in New York found that viewing 3 or more hours/day of TV doubled the risk of difficulty falling asleep compared with adolescents who watch less than 1 hour/day.[96] There is also now evidence that later bedtimes and less sleep may be associated with a greater risk of obesity.[97–101] The mechanism may be that sleep loss leads to increased snacking and consumption of less healthy foods to maintain energy,[102,103] that sleep deprivation leads to fatigue and therefore greater sedentary behavior,[104] or that children who do not get enough sleep have metabolic changes as well.[105]

Stress may also play a role, although there are only a handful of studies that have studied this subject so far. For example, a Scottish study of nearly 1500 4- to 12-year-olds found that heavier TV use produced greater psychological stress in children and that this effect was independent of, but exacerbated by, decreases in exercise.[106]

CONCLUSIONS

Media clearly play an important role in the current epidemic of childhood and adolescent obesity. The sheer number of advertisements that children and adolescents see for junk food and fast food have an effect. So, too, does the shift away from good nutritional practices that increased media screen time seems to create. Any success in dealing with the current epidemic will require a major change in society's recognition of media exposure as a major risk factor for obesity and in young people's media habits and the advertisements to which they are exposed.[107,108]

RECOMMENDATIONS

1. Pediatricians should ask parents and patients 2 key questions about media use: (1) How much time per day does the child or teenager spend with screen media? and (2) Is there a TV set or unrestricted,

unmonitored Internet connection throughout the house, including in the child's bedroom?[109] This recommendation should be incorporated into every well-child visit, as outlined in *Bright Futures*.[110]

2. Pediatricians should encourage parents to discuss food advertising with their children as they monitor children's TV-viewing and teach their children about appropriate nutrition.[111–113]

3. Pediatricians should continue to counsel parents to limit total non-educational screen time to no more than 2 hours/day, to avoid putting TV sets and Internet connections in children's bedrooms, to coview with their children, to limit night-time screen media use to improve children's sleep, and to try strongly to avoid screen exposure for infants under the age of 2 years. In a recent study of 709 7- to 12-year-olds, children who did not adhere to the American Academy of Pediatrics guidelines of less than 2 hours/day of screen time[114] and 11 000 to 13 000 pedometer steps per day were 3 to 4 times more likely to be overweight.[115] Conversely, preschool-aged children who ate dinner with their parents, got adequate sleep, and had limited screen-time hours had a 40% lower prevalence of obesity than those exposed to none of these routines.[116]

4. Pediatricians should work with community groups and schools to implement media education programs in child care centers, schools, and community-based programs such as the YMCA. Such programs that teach children how to understand and interpret advertisements may have the potential to immunize young people against harmful media effects.[117] In addition, programs that educate parents about limiting media

use in general have already been shown to be highly effective.[8,38,39,118,119] Pediatricians should work with their state chapters, the AAP, parent and public health groups, and the White House[120] to do the following:

• Ask Congress, the Federal Trade Commission, and the Federal Communications Commission to implement a ban on junk-food advertising during programming that is viewed predominantly by young children.[84,121,122] Currently, several European countries restrict food advertising aimed at young children.[123] Several food manufacturers have already indicated a willingness to implement such a ban voluntarily,[124,125] but it remains to be seen whether they will follow through.[126–128] For example, children's cereals remain considerably unhealthier than adult cereals; they contain 85% more sugar, 65% less fiber, and 60% more sodium.[129] One-quarter of all food and beverage advertising originates from companies that do not participate in the initiative, and two-thirds of all advertising by companies that do participate is still for food and beverages of low nutritional value.[85] In addition, the food and beverage industry remains steadfastly opposed to any regulation. For example, in 2007, 1 soft drink company spent more than $1.7 million to lobby against marketing restrictions and school nutrition legislation.[130] Two recent studies showed that a ban on fast-food ads would reduce the number of overweight children and adolescents in the United States by an estimated 14% to 18%.[131,132] Just eliminating federal tax deductions for

fast-food ads that target children would reduce childhood obesity by 5% to 7%.[131] On the other hand, advertisements and public service announcements for health foods and healthy nutritional practices should be encouraged. One recent experiment showed that children exposed to attractive advertisements for healthy foods develop significantly more positive attitudes than children shown junk-food ads.[133]

• Ask Congress and the Federal Communications Commission to prohibit interactive advertising involving junk food or fast food to children via digital TV, cell phones, and other media[79–81,121] and to ban payments for product placement in movies. Restoring power to the Federal Trade Commission to more tightly regulate children's advertising could be another way of accomplishing this goal.[84,134,135]

• Ask Congress to fund media research (eg, the Children Media Research and Advancement Act [CAMRA]). More research is specifically needed to determine (1) how heavy media use in children reflects or contributes to psychosocial elements of the child's life, such as stress in the home, (2) how new media technologies may be playing a role in exacerbating exposure to ads or encouraging more sedentary behavior, and (3) which of the above-mentioned mechanisms is most responsible for contributing to obesity and how such mechanisms can be ameliorated.[83,134]

• Encourage the production of more counteradvertising and more prosocial video games[136,137] and Web sites that encourage children to choose healthy foods.[82]

6. Pediatricians should be aware that children with high levels of screen time have higher levels of childhood stress, which puts them at risk not only for obesity but also for a number of stress-associated morbidities (eg, mood disorders, substance abuse, diabetes, cardiovascular disease, asthma).[138] Consequently, displacing screen time with more prosocial or resilience-building activities (eg, exercise, imaginative or social play) is an important approach to addressing a wide array of societal ills including obesity.[139]

LEAD AUTHOR

Victor C. Strasburger, MD

COUNCIL ON COMMUNICATIONS AND MEDIA, 2010–2011

Deborah Ann Mulligan, MD, Chairperson
Tanya Remer Altmann, MD
Ari Brown, MD
Dimitri A. Christakis, MD
Kathleen Clarke-Pearson, MD
Holly Lee Falik, MD
David L. Hill, MD
Marjorie J. Hogan, MD
Alanna Estin Levine, MD
Kathleen G. Nelson, MD
Gwenn S. O'Keeffe, MD

FORMER EXECUTIVE COMMITTEE MEMBERS

Gilbert L. Fuld, MD, Immediate Past Chairperson
Benard P. Dreyer, MD
Regina M. Milteer, MD
Donald L. Shifrin, MD
Victor C. Strasburger, MD

CONTRIBUTOR

Amy Jordan, PhD

LIAISONS

Michael Brody, MD – *American Academy of Child and Adolescent Psychiatry*
Brian Wilcox, PhD – *American Psychological Association*

STAFF

Gina Ley Steiner
Veronica Laude Noland

REFERENCES

1. Skelton JA, Cook SR, Aunger P, Klein JD, Barlow SE. Prevalence and trends of severe obesity among US children and adolescents. *Acad Pediatr.* 2009;9(5):322–329

2. Ogden CL, Carroll MD, McDowell MA, Flegal KM. Obesity among adults in the United States: no statistically significant chance since 2003–2004. *NCHS Data Brief.* 2007; (1):1–8

3. Preidt R. Overweight now a global problem. Available at: http://abcnews.go.com/print?id=4509129. Accessed April 29, 2010

4. Guthold R, Cowan MJ, Autenrieth CS, Kahn L, Riley LM. Physical activity and sedentary behavior among schoolchildren: a 34-country comparison. *J Pediatr.* 2010; 157(1):43–49

5. Jordan AB, Strasburger VC, Kramer-Golinkoff EK, Strasburger VC. Does adolescent media use cause obesity and eating disorders? *Adolesc Med State Art Rev.* 2008;19(3):431–449

6. Kelly B, Halford JC, Boyland EJ, et al. Television food advertising to children: a global perspective. *Am J Public Health.* 2010;100(9):1730–1736

7. Jordan AB. Heavy television viewing and childhood obesity. *J Child Media.* 2007; 1(9):45–54

8. Dennison BA, Edmunds LS. The role of television in childhood obesity. *Progr Pediatr Cardiol.* 2008;25(2):191–197

9. Strasburger VC, Wilson BJ, Jordan AB. *Children, Adolescents, and the Media.* 2nd ed. Thousand Oaks, CA: Sage; 2009

10. Singh GK, Kogan MD, Van Dyck PC, Siahpush M. Racial/ethnic, socioeconomic, and behavioral determinants of childhood and adolescent obesity in the United States: analyzing independent and joint associations. *Ann Epidemiol.* 2008;18(9):682–695

11. Viner RM, Cole TJ. Television viewing in early childhood predicts adult body mass index. *J Pediatr.* 2005;147(4):429–435

12. Hancox RJ, Milne BJ, Poulton R. Association between child and adolescent television viewing and adult health: a longitudinal birth cohort study. *Lancet.* 2004; 364(9430):257–262

13. Reilly JJ, Armstrong J, Dorosty AR, et al; Avon Longitudinal Study of Parents and Children Study Team. Early life risk factors for obesity in childhood: cohort study. *BMJ.* 2005;330(7504):1357

14. Sugimori H, Yoshida K, Izuno T, et al. Analysis of factors that influence body mass index from ages 3 to 6 years: a study based on the Toyama cohort study. *Pediatr Int.* 2004;46(3):302–310

15. Proctor MH, Moore LL, Gao D, et al. Television viewing and change in body fat from preschool to early adolescence: the Framingham Children's Study. *Int J Obes Relat Metab Disord.* 2003;27(7):827–833

16. Kaur H, Choi WS, Mayo MS, Harris KJ. Duration of television watching is associated with increased body mass index. *J Pediatr.* 2003;143(4):506–511

17. Lumeng JC, Rahnama S, Appugliese D, Kaciroti N, Bradley RH. Television exposure and overweight risk in preschoolers. *Arch Pediatr Adolesc Med.* 2006;160(4):417–422

18. O'Brien M, Nader PR, Houts RM, et al. The ecology of childhood overweight: a 12-year longitudinal analysis. *Int J Obes (Lond).* 2007;31(9):1469–1478

19. Henderson VR. Longitudinal associations between television viewing and body mass index among white and black girls. *J Adolesc Health.* 2007;41(6):544–550

20. Boone JE, Gordon-Larsen P, Adair LS, Popkin BM. Screen time and physical activity during adolescence: longitudinal effects on obesity in young adulthood. *Int J Behav Nutr Phys Act.* 2007;4:26. Available at: www.ijbnpa.org/content/4/1/26. Accessed June 19, 2009

21. Davison BA, Marshall SJ, Birch LL. Cross-sectional and longitudinal associations between TV viewing and girls' body mass index, overweight status, and percentage of body fat. *J Pediatr.* 2006;149(1):32–37

22. Danner FW. A national longitudinal study of the association between hours of TV viewing and the trajectory of BMI growth among US children. *J Pediatr Psychol.* 2008;33(10):1100–1107

23. Meyer AM, Evenson KR, Couper DJ, Stevens J, Pereira MA, Heiss G. Television, physical activity, diet, and body weight status: the ARIC cohort. *Int J Behav Nutr Phys Act.* 2008;5(1):68. Available at: www.ijbnpa.org/content/5/1/68. Accessed June 19, 2009

24. Adachi-Mejia AM, Longacre MR, Gibson JJ, Beach ML, Titus-Ernstoff LT, Dalton MA. Children with a TV set in their bedroom at higher risk for being overweight. *Int J Obes (Lond).* 2007;31(4):644–651

25. Dennison BA, Erb TA, Jenkins PL. Television viewing and television in bedroom associated with overweight risk among low-income preschool children. *Pediatrics.* 2002;109(6):1028–1035

26. Barr-Anderson DJ, van den Berg P, Neumark-Sztainer D, Story M. Characteristics associated with older adolescents

who have a television in their bedrooms. *Pediatrics*. 2008;121(4):718–724

27. Delmas C, Platat C, Schweitzer B, Wagner A, Oujaa M, Simon C. Association between television in bedroom and adiposity throughout adolescence. *Obesity*. 2007; 15(10):2495–2503

28. Sisson SB, Broyles ST, Newton RL Jr, Baker BL, Chernausek SD. TVs in the bedrooms of children: does it impact health and behavior? *Prev Med*. 2011;52(2):104–108

29. Margeirsdottir HD, Larsen JR, Brunborg C, Sandvik L, Dahl-Jørgensen K; Norwegian Study Group for Childhood Diabetes. Strong association between time watching television and blood glucose control in children and adolescents with type I diabetes. *Diabetes Care*. 2007;30(6):1567–1570

30. Hu FB, Li TY, Colditz GA, Willett WC, Manson JE. Television watching and other sedentary behaviors in relation to risk of obesity and type 2 diabetes mellitus in women. *JAMA*. 2003;289(14):1785–1791

31. Hardy LL, Denney-Wilson E, Thrift AP, Okely AD, Baur LA. Screen time and metabolic risk factors among adolescents. *Arch Pediatr Adolesc Med*. 2010;164(7):643–649

32. Mark AE, Janssen I. Relationship between screen time and metabolic syndrome in adolescents. *J Public Health (Oxf)*. 2008; 30(2):153–160

33. Pardee PE, Norman GJ, Lustig RH, Preud'homme D, Schwimmer JB. Television viewing and hypertension in obese children. *Am J Prev Med*. 2007;33(6):439–443

34. Martinez-Gomez D, Tucker J, Heelan KA, Welk GJ, Eisenmann JC. Associations between sedentary behavior and blood pressure in children. *Arch Pediatr Adolesc Med*. 2009;163(8):724–730

35. Fung TT, Rimm EB, Spiegelman D, et al. Association between dietary patterns and plasma biomarkers of obesity and cardiovascular disease risk. *Am J Clin Nutr*. 2001; 73(1):61–67

36. Martinez-Gomez D, Rey-López JP, Chillón P, et al; AVENA Study Group. Excessive TV viewing and cardiovascular disease risk factors in adolescents. The AVENA cross-sectional study. *BMC Public Health*. 2010; 10:274

37. Stamatakis E, Hamer M, Dunstan DW. Screen-based entertainment time, all-cause mortality, and cardiovascular events: population-based study with ongoing mortality and hospital events follow-up. *J Am Coll Cardiol*. 2011;57(3):292–299

38. Robinson TN. Reducing children's television viewing to prevent obesity: a random-

ized controlled trial. *JAMA*. 1999;282(16): 1561–1567

39. Epstein LH, Roemmich JN, Robinson JL, et al. A randomized trial of the effects of reducing television viewing and computer use on body mass index in young children. *Arch Pediatr Adolesc Med*. 2008;162(3): 239–245

40. Dietz WH Jr. Television, obesity, and eating disorders. *Adolesc Med*. 1993;4(3): 543–549

41. Apovian CM. Sugar-sweetened soft drinks, obesity, and type 2 diabetes. *JAMA*. 2004; 292(8):978–979

42. Reedy J, Krebs-Smith SM. Dietary sources of energy, solid fats, and added sugars among children and adolescents in the United States. *J Am Diet Assoc*. 2010; 110(10):1477–1484

43. Rideout V. *Generation M2: Media in the Lives of 8- to 18-Year-Olds*. Menlo Park, CA: Kaiser Family Foundation; 2010

44. Nelson MC, Neumark-Sztainer D, Hannan PJ, Sirard JR, Story M. Longitudinal and secular trends in physical activity and sedentary behavior during adolescence. *Pediatrics*. 2006;118(6). Available at: www.pediatrics.org/cgi/content/full/118/6/e1627

45. Hardy LL, Bass SL, Booth ML. Changes in sedentary behavior among adolescent girls: a 2.5-year prospective cohort study. *J Adolesc Health*. 2007;40(2):158–165

46. Sisson SB, Broyles ST, Baker BL, Katzmarzyk PT. Screen time, physical activity, and overweight in U.S. youth: National Survey of Children's Health 2003. *J Adolesc Health*. 2010;47(3):309–311

47. Burdette HL, Whitaker RC. A national study of neighborhood safety, outdoor play, television viewing, and obesity in preschool children. *Pediatrics*. 2005;116(3):657–662

48. Taveras EM, Field AE, Berkey CS, et al. Longitudinal relationship between television viewing and leisure-time physical activity during adolescence. *Pediatrics*. 2007; 119(2). Available at: www.pediatrics.org/cgi/content/full/119/2/e314

49. Melkevik O, Torsheim T, Iannotti RJ, Wold B. Is spending time in screen-based sedentary behaviors associated with less physical activity: a cross national investigation. *Int J Behav Nutr Phys Act*. 2010;7:46

50. Vandewater E, Shim M, Caplovitz A. Linking obesity and activity level with children's television and video game use. *J Adolesc*. 2004;27(1):71–85

51. Epstein LH, Paluch RA, Consalvi A, Riordan K, Scholl T. Effects of manipulating seden-

tary behavior on physical activity and food intake. *J Pediatr*. 2002;140(3):334–339

52. Washington R. One way to decrease an obesogenic environment. *J Pediatr*. 2005; 147(4):417–418

53. Dietz WH. What constitutes successful weight management in adolescents? *Ann Intern Med*. 2006;145(2):145–146

54. Goldfield GS, Mallory R, Parker T, et al. Effects of open-loop feedback on physical activity and television viewing in overweight and obese children: a randomized, controlled trial. *Pediatrics*. 2006;118(1). Available at: www.pediatrics.org/cgi/content/full/118/1/e157

55. Haerens L, Deforche B, Maes L, Stevens V, Cardon G, De Bourdeaudhuij. Body mass effects of a physical activity and healthy food intervention in middle schools. *Obesity*. 2006;14(5):847–854

56. Mellecker RR, McManus AM. Energy expenditure and cardiovascular responses to seated and active gaming in children. *Arch Pediatr Adolesc Med*. 2008;162(9): 886–891

57. Pate RR. Physically active video gaming: an effective strategy for obesity prevention? *Arch Pediatr Adolesc Med*. 2008;162(9): 895–896

58. Graf DL, Pratt LV, Hester CN, Short KR. Playing active video games increases energy expenditure in children. *Pediatrics*. 2009; 124(2):534–540

59. Robinson TN, Killen JD. Ethnic and gender differences in the relationships between television viewing and obesity, physical activity and dietary fat intake. *J Health Educ*. 1995;26(2 suppl):S91–S98

60. Blass EM, Anderson DR, Kirkorian HL, Pempek TA, Price I, Koleini MF. On the road to obesity: television viewing increases intake of high-density foods. *Physiol Behav*. 2006;88(4–5):597–604

61. Zimmerman FJ, Bell JF. Associations of television content type and obesity in children. *Am J Public Health*. 2010;100(2): 334–340

62. Wiecha JL, Peterson KE, Ludwig DS, Kim J, Sobol A, Gortmaker SL. When children eat what they watch: impact of television viewing on dietary intake in youth. *Arch Pediatr Adolesc Med*. 2006;160(4):436–442

63. Barr-Anderson DJ, Larson NI, Nelson MC, Neumark-Sztainer D, Story M. Does television viewing predict dietary intake five years later in high school students and young adults? *Int J Behav Nutr Phys Activity*. 2009;6:7. Available at: www.ijbnpa.org/content/6/1/7. Accessed March 25, 2011

64. Harris JL, Bargh JA, Brownell KD. Priming

effects of television food advertising on eating behavior. *Health Psychol.* 2009; 28(4):404–413

65. Giammattei J, Blix G, Marshak HH, Wollitzer AO, Pettitt DJ. Television watching and soft drink consumption: associations with obesity in 11- to 13-year old schoolchildren. *Arch Pediatr Adolesc Med.* 2003;157(9): 882–886

66. Krebs-Smith S, Cook A, Subar A, Cleveland L, Friday J, Kahle LL. Fruit and vegetable intakes of children and adolescents in the United States. *Arch Pediatr Adolesc Med.* 1996;150(1):81–86

67. Bowman SA, Gortmaker SL, Ebbeling CB, Pereira MA, Ludwig DS. Effects of fast-food consumption on energy intake and diet quality among children in a national household survey. *Pediatrics.* 2004;113(1 pt 1):112–118

68. Brownell KD. Fast food and obesity in children. *Pediatrics.* 2004;113(1 pt 1):132

69. Schlosser E. *Fast Food Nation.* Boston, MA: Houghton Mifflin; 2001

70. Harris JL, Schwartz MB, Brownell KD, et al. *Evaluating Fast Food Nutrition and Marketing to Youth.* New Haven, CT: Yale Rudd Center for Food Policy & Obesity; 2010

71. Harrison K, Marske AL. Nutritional content of foods advertised during the television programs children watch most. *Am J Public Health.* 2005;95(9):1568–1574

72. Powell LM, Szczypka G, Chaloupka FJ, Braunschweig CL. Nutritional content of television food advertisements seen by children and adolescents in the United States. *Pediatrics.* 2007;120(3):576–583

73. Kunkel D, McKinley C, Stitt C. *Food Advertising During Children's Programming: A Two-Year Comparison.* Tucson, AZ: University of Arizona; 2010

74. Stitt C, Kunkel D. Food advertising during children's television programming on broadcast and cable channels. *Health Commun.* 2008;23(6):573–584

75. Powell LM, Szczypka G, Chaloupka FJ. Trends in exposure to television food advertisements among children and adolescents in the United States. *Arch Pediatr Adolesc Med.* 2010;164(9):794–802

76. Powell LM, Szczypka G, Chaloupka FJ. Exposure to food advertising on television among US children. *Arch Pediatr Adolesc Med.* 2007;161(6):553–560

77. Gantz W, Schwartz N, Angelini JR, Rideout V. *Food for Thought: Television Food Advertising to Children in the United States.* Menlo Park, CA: Kaiser Family Foundation; 2007

78. Harris JL, Weinberg ME, Schwartz MB,

Ross C, Ostroff J, Brownell KD. *Trends in Television Food Advertising.* New Haven, CT: Yale Rudd Center for Food Policy & Obesity; 2010

79. Weber K, Story M, Harnack L. Internet food marketing strategies aimed at children and adolescents: a content analysis of food and beverage brand Web sites. *J Am Diet Assoc.* 2006;106(9):1463–1466

80. Moore ES. *It's Child's Play: Advergaming and the Online Marketing of Food to Children.* Menlo Park, CA: Kaiser Family Foundation; 2006

81. Montgomery KC, Chester J. Interactive food and beverage marketing: targeting adolescents in the digital age. *J Adolesc Health.* 2009;45(3 suppl):S18–S29

82. Pempek TA, Calvert SL. Tipping the balance: use of advergames to promote consumption of nutritious foods and beverages by low-income African American children. *Arch Pediatr Adolesc Med.* 2009; 163(7):633–637

83. Institute of Medicine. *Preventing Childhood Obesity: Health in the Balance.* Washington, DC: National Academies Press; 2005

84. Harris JL, Pomeranz JL, Lobstein T, Brownell KD. A crisis in the marketplace: how food marketing contributes to childhood obesity and what can be done. *Annu Rev Public Health.* 2009;30:211–225

85. Kunkel D, McKinley C, Wright P. *The Impact of Industry Self-regulation on the Nutritional Quality of Foods Advertised on Television to Children.* Oakland, CA: Children Now; 2009

86. Chamberlain LJ, Wang Y, Robinson TN. Does children's screen time predict requests for advertised products? *Arch Pediatr Adolesc Med.* 2006;160(4):363–368

87. Borzekowski DLG, Robinson TN. The 30-second effect: an experiment revealing the impact of television commercials on food preferences of preschoolers. *J Am Diet Assoc.* 2001;101(1):42–46

88. Robinson TN, Borzekowski DLG, Matheson DM, Kraemer HC. Effects of fast food branding on young children's taste preferences. *Arch Pediatr Adolesc Med.* 2007; 161(8):792–292

89. Robert Wood Johnson Foundation. *F as in Fat 2009: How Obesity Policies Are Failing in America.* Princeton, NJ: Robert Wood Johnson Foundation; 2009. Available at: http://healthyamericans.org/reports/obesity2009. Accessed April 29, 2010

90. Greenberg BS, Rosaen SF, Worrell TR, Salmon CT, Volkman JE. A portrait of food

and drink in commercial TV series. *Health Commun.* 2009;24(4):295–303

91. Bell R, Berger C, Townsend M. *Portrayals of Nutritional Practices and Exercise Behavior in Popular American Films, 1991–2000.* Davis, CA: Center for Advanced Studies of Nutrition and Social Marketing, University of California-Davis; 2003

92. Eisenberg D. It's an ad, ad, ad world. *Time Magazine.* August 26, 2002:38–42. Available at: www.time.com/time/magazine/article/0,9171,1101020902-344045,00.html. Accessed April 29, 2010

93. Sutherland LS, MacKenzie T, Purvis LA, Dalton M. Prevalence of food and beverage brands in movies, 1996–2005. *Pediatrics.* 2010;125(3):468–474

94. Zimmerman FJ. *Children's Media Use and Sleep Problems: Issues and Unanswered Questions.* Menlo Park, CA: Kaiser Family Foundation; 2008

95. Landhuis CE, Poulton R, Welch D, Hancox RJ. Childhood sleep time and long-term risk for obesity: a 32-year prospective birth cohort study. *Pediatrics.* 2008; 122(5):955–960

96. Johnson JG, Cohen P, Kasen S, First MB, Brook JS. Association between television and sleep problems during adolescence and early adulthood. *Arch Pediatr Adolesc Med.* 2004;158(6):562–568

97. Sekine M, Yamagami T, Handa K, et al. A dose-response relationship between short sleeping hours and childhood obesity: results of the Toyama Birth Cohort Study. *Child Care Health Dev.* 2002;28(2): 163–170

98. Agras W, Hammer L, McNicholas F, Kraemer H. Risk factors for child overweight: a prospective study from birth to 9.5 years. *J Pediatr.* 2004;145(1):20–25

99. Taheri S. The link between short sleep duration and obesity: we should recommend more sleep to prevent obesity. *Arch Dis Child.* 2006;91(11):881–884

100. Bell JF, Zimmerman FJ. Shortened nighttime sleep duration in early life and subsequent childhood obesity. *Arch Pediatr Adolesc Med.* 2010;164(9):840–845

101. Lytle LA, Pasch K, Farbaksh K. Is sleep related to obesity in young adolescents [abstract]? Presented at: Pediatric Academic Societies meeting; May 4, 2010; Vancouver, British Columbia, Canada

102. Wells TT, Cruess DG. Effects of partial sleep deprivation on food consumption and food choice. *Psychol Health.* 2006;21(1):79–86

103. Oliver G, Wardle J. Perceived effects of stress on food choice. *Physiol Behav.* 1999; 66(3):511–515

104. Nelson MC, Gordon-Larsen P. Physical activity and sedentary behavior patterns are associated with selected adolescent health risk behaviors. *Pediatrics*. 2006; 117(4):1281–1290

105. Van Cauter E, Holmback U, Knutson K, et al. Impact of sleep and sleep loss on neuroendocrine and metabolic function. *Horm Res*. 2007;67(suppl 1):2–9

106. Hamer M, Stamatakis E, Mishra G. Psychological distress, television viewing and physical activity in children aged 4 to 12 years. *Pediatrics*. 2009;123(5):1263–1268

107. Jordan AB, Robinson TN. Children, television viewing, and weight status: summary and recommendations from an expert panel meeting. *Ann Am Acad Polit Soc Sci*. 2008;615(1):119–132

108. Brownell KD, Schwartz MB, Puhl RM, Henderson KE, Harris JL. The need for bold action to prevent adolescent obesity. *J Adolesc Health*. 2009;45(3 suppl):S8–S17

109. Strasburger VC. First do no harm: why have parents and pediatricians missed the boat on children and media? *J Pediatr*. 2007;151(4):334–336

110. Hagan JF Jr, Shaw JS, Duncan PM, eds. *Bright Futures: Guidelines for Health Supervision of Infants, Children, and Adolescents*. Elk Grove Village, IL: American Academy of Pediatrics; 2008

111. Harris JL, Bargh JA. Television viewing and unhealthy diet: implications for children and media interventions. *Health Commun*. 2009;24(7):660–673

112. He M, Piche L, Beynon C, Harris S. Screen-related sedentary behaviors: children's and parents' attitudes, motivations, and practices. *J Nutr Educ Behav*. 2010;42(1): 17–25

113. Carlson SA, Fulton JE, Lee SM, Foley JT, Heitzler C, Huhman M. Influence of limit-setting and participation in physical activity on youth screen time. *Pediatrics*. 2010; 126(1). Available at: www.pediatrics.org/cgi/content/full/126/1/e89

114. American Academy of Pediatrics, Committee on Public Education. Media education. *Pediatrics*. 1999;104(2 pt 1):341–343

115. Laurson KR, Eisenmann JC, Welk G, Wickel EE, Gentile DA, Walsh DA. Combined influence of physical activity and screen time recommendations on childhood overweight. *J Pediatr*. 2008;153(2):209–214

116. Anderson SE, Whitaker RC. Household routines and obesity in US preschool-aged children. *Pediatrics*. 2010;125(3):420–428

117. McCannon R. Media literacy/media education. In: Strasburger VC, Wilson BJ, Jordan AJ, eds. *Children, Adolescents, and the Media*. 2nd ed. Thousand Oaks, CA: Sage; 2009: 519–569

118. Gortmaker SL. Innovations to reduce television and computer time and obesity in childhood. *Arch Pediatr Adolesc Med*. 2008;162(3):283–284

119. Escobar-Chaves SL, Markham CM, Addy RC, Greisinger A, Murray NG, Brehm B. The Fun Families Study: intervention to reduce children's TV viewing. *Obesity (Silver Spring)*. 2010;18(suppl 1):S99–S101

120. White House Task Force on Childhood Obesity. *Solving the Problem of Childhood Obesity Within a Generation: Report to the President*. Washington, DC: Executive Office of the President of the United States; 2010. Available at: www.letsmove.gov/sites/letsmove.gov/files/TaskForce_on_Childhood_Obesity_May2010_FullReport.pdf. Accessed January 12, 2011

121. American Academy of Pediatrics, Committee on Communications. Children, adolescents, and advertising [published correction appears in *Pediatrics*. 2007;119(2): 424]. *Pediatrics*. 2006;118(6):2563–2569

122. Pomeranz JL. Television food marketing to children revisited: the Federal Trade Commission has the constitutional and statutory authority to regulate. *J Law Med Ethics*. 2010;38(1):98–116

123. Strasburger VC. Adolescents and the media. In: Rosenfeld W, Fisher M, Alderman E, eds. *Textbook of Adolescent Medicine*. Elk Grove Village, IL: American Academy of Pediatrics; 2011;359–373

124. Gold J. Snickers maker will aim higher. *Albuquerque Journal*. February 7, 2007:B4

125. Union of European Beverages Associations. *International Council of Beverages Associations Adopts Groundbreaking Guidelines on Marketing to Children* [press release]. Brussels, Belgium: Union of European Beverages Associations; May 20, 2008

126. Wilde P. Self-regulation and the response to concerns about food and beverage marketing to children in the United States. *Nutr Rev*. 2009;67(3):155–166

127. Schwartz MB, Ross C, Harris JL, et al. Breakfast cereal industry pledges to self-regulate advertising to youth: will they improve the marketing landscape? *J Public Health Policy*. 2010;31(1):59–73

128. Noah T. Toy story: why self-regulation of children's advertising is a joke. *Slate Magazine*. Available at: www.slate.com/id/2278241. Accessed January 12, 2011

129. Harris JL, Schwartz MB, Brownell KD, et al. *Cereal FACTS: Evaluating the Nutrition Quality and Marketing of Children's Cereals*. New Haven, CT: Rudd Center for Food Policy and Obesity; 2009

130. Associated Press. Coca-cola spent more than $1.7M to lobby. February 21, 2007

131. Chou SY, Rashad I, Grossman M. Fast-food restaurant advertising on television and its influence on childhood obesity. *J Law Econ*. 2008;51(4):599–618

132. Veerman JL, Van Beeck EF, Barendregt JJ, Mackenbach JP. By how much would limiting TV food advertising reduce childhood obesity? *Eur J Public Health*. 2009;19(4): 365–369

133. Dixon HG, Scully ML, Wakefield MA, White VM, Crawford DA. The effects of television advertisements for junk food versus nutritious food on children's food attitudes and preferences. *Soc Sci Med*. 2007;65(7): 1311–1323

134. Larson N, Story M. *Food and Beverage Marketing to Children and Adolescents: What Changes Are Needed to Promote Healthy Eating Habits?* Princeton, NJ: Robert Wood Johnson Foundation; 2008

135. Pertschuk M. The little agency that could. *The Nation*. June 29, 2009:21–22

136. Durant NH. Not just fun and games: harnessing technology to address childhood obesity. *Child Obes*. 2010;6(5):283–284

137. Biddiss E, Irwin J. Active video games to promote physical activity in children and youth: a systematic review. *Arch Pediatr Adolesc Med*. 2010;164(7):664–672

138. Strasburger VC, Jordan AB, Donnerstein E. Health effects of media on children and adolescents. *Pediatrics*. 2010;125(4): 756–767

139. Ginsburg KR; American Academy of Pediatrics, Committee on Communications and Committee on Psychosocial Aspects of Child and Family Health. The importance of play in promoting healthy child development and maintaining strong parent-child bonds. *Pediatrics*. 2007;119(1):182–191

Policy Statement—Children, Adolescents, Obesity, and the Media. *Pediatrics.* **2011;128(1):201–208**

An error occurred in the American Academy of Pediatrics policy statement "Children, Adolescents, Obesity, and the Media" originally published online June 27, 2011 and published in the July 2011 issue of *Pediatrics* (2011;128:201–208; DOI: 10.1542/peds.2011-1066). On page 204, middle column, third line, a new Recommendation No. 5 should have begun at "Pediatricians should work with their state chapters, the AAP, parent and public health groups, and the White House[120] to do the following:" and included all four subsequent bulleted paragraphs. We regret the error.

doi:10.1542/peds.2011-1970

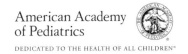

Guidance for the Clinician in
Rendering Pediatric Care

Clinical Report—Identification and Management of Eating Disorders in Children and Adolescents

abstract

The incidence and prevalence of eating disorders in children and adolescents has increased significantly in recent decades, making it essential for pediatricians to consider these disorders in appropriate clinical settings, to evaluate patients suspected of having these disorders, and to manage (or refer) patients in whom eating disorders are diagnosed. This clinical report includes a discussion of diagnostic criteria and outlines the initial evaluation of the patient with disordered eating. Medical complications of eating disorders may affect any organ system, and careful monitoring for these complications is required. The range of treatment options, including pharmacotherapy, is described in this report. Pediatricians are encouraged to advocate for legislation and policies that ensure appropriate services for patients with eating disorders, including medical care, nutritional intervention, mental health treatment, and care coordination. *Pediatrics* 2010;126: 1240–1253

INTRODUCTION

Increases in the incidence and prevalence of anorexia nervosa (AN), bulimia nervosa (BN), and other eating disorders in children and adolescents make it critically important that pediatricians be familiar with early detection and appropriate management of these disorders. Results of epidemiologic studies have indicated that the numbers of children and adolescents with eating disorders increased steadily from the 1950s onward.[1–4] During the past decade, the prevalence of obesity in children and adolescents has also increased dramatically,[5–9] accompanied by further emphasis on dieting and weight loss among children and adolescents.[10–15]

The epidemiology of eating disorders has gradually changed; there is an increasing prevalence of eating disorders in males[16–19] and minority populations in the United States[20–23] as well as in countries in which eating disorders had not been commonly seen.[3,4,24,25] Of particular concern is the increasing prevalence of eating disorders at progressively younger ages.[19,26,27] A recent analysis by the Agency for Healthcare Research and Quality revealed that from 1999 to 2006, hospitalizations for eating disorders increased most sharply—119%—for children younger than 12 years.[19]

It is estimated that approximately 0.5% of adolescent girls in the United States have AN, that approximately 1% to 2% meet diagnostic criteria for BN, and that up to 5% to 10% of all cases of eating disorders occur in males. A large number of people with eating disorders do not meet the strict criteria set forth in the American Psychiatric Association's

David S. Rosen, MD, MPH and THE COMMITTEE ON ADOLESCENCE

KEY WORDS
anorexia nervosa, bulimia nervosa, eating disorders

ABBREVIATIONS
AN—anorexia nervosa
BN—bulimia nervosa
DSM-IV-TR—*Diagnostic and Statistical Manual of Mental Disorders, Fourth Edition Text Revision*
HPA—hypothalamic-pituitary-adrenal
SSRI—selective serotonin-reuptake inhibitor

The guidance in this report does not indicate an exclusive course of treatment or serve as a standard of medical care. Variations, taking into account individual circumstances, may be appropriate.

www.pediatrics.org/cgi/doi/10.1542/peds.2010-2821

doi:10.1542/peds.2010-2821

All clinical reports from the American Academy of Pediatrics automatically expire 5 years after publication unless reaffirmed, revised, or retired at or before that time.

PEDIATRICS (ISSN Numbers: Print, 0031-4005; Online, 1098-4275).

Diagnostic and Statistical Manual of Mental Disorders, Fourth Edition, Text Revision (DSM-IV-TR) for AN or BN and are labeled as having "partial syndromes" or "eating disorder not otherwise specified" (ED NOS).[28] There are many more patients with ED NOS than there are patients with AN or BN; the prevalence is estimated to be between 0.8% and 14%, depending on the definition used.[29] These patients often experience the same physical and psychological consequences as do those who reach the threshold for diagnosis of AN or BN.[28–34] Athletes and performers, particularly those who participate in sports and activities that reward a lean body habitus (eg, gymnastics, running, wrestling, dance, modeling) may be at particular risk of developing partial-syndrome eating disorders.[35,36]

The etiology of eating disorders is multifactorial, and there is increasing evidence from both family and twin studies for a strong genetic component that is shared between AN and BN.[37,38] The mechanism(s) by which genetic factors influence risk have not been elucidated, but various hypotheses have been proposed. Genetic predisposition to various trait disturbances such as behavioral rigidity, perfectionism, or harm avoidance may be more salient than genetic influences on eating, hunger, or satiety.[39–41] Genetic effects seem to be "activated" by puberty,[42–44] and there is strong evidence for genetic-environment interactions.[39,40]

Dieting has also been implicated as a potent proximal risk factor in the development of disordered eating and eating disorders.[45–47] In 1 community-based study, dieters at 5-year follow-up were at significantly higher risk of disordered eating behaviors (eg, vomiting or using diet pills or laxatives) than nondieters and were also at increased risk of obesity.[47] In another large community cohort, dieters were 5 times more likely to develop an

eating disorder and severe dieters were 18 times more likely to develop an eating disorder than nondieters.[48]

Neuroendocrine abnormalities have been implicated in the etiology of eating disorders. Leptin is a circulating hormone produced in adipose tissue and seems to have a significant role in mediating the neuroendocrine effects of AN. Leptin concentrations are sensitive to the acute metabolic effects of decreased intake and energy deficits, and decreased circulating leptin concentrations reflect depleted stores of body fat.[49–51] Physical hyperactivity is a common feature of AN and sometimes manifests as restlessness, athleticism, or compulsive exercise. This hyperactivity also seems to be mediated by leptin.[51]

Physical hyperactivity associated with weight loss seems to occur in animals as well, apparently mediated by hyperactivity of the hypothalamic-pituitary-adrenal (HPA) axis. Syndromes that resemble AN, characterized by food refusal, physical overactivity, and extreme weight loss, occur in pigs, sheep, and goats bred for leanness.[52] Caloric restriction coupled with environmental stress produces animal models for binge-eating.[53] These animals overeat dramatically despite nutritional satiety and normal energy status, which strongly suggests that reward circuits are being activated rather than metabolic needs being satisfied.[43,53]

In community-based studies of adolescents, disturbances of body image and overconcern about body shape are common, although the prevalence of eating disorders remains low.[54] These results reinforce the likelihood of epigenetic effects in which the development of eating disorders reflects the intersection between genetic predisposition, environmental triggers, and personal experience.

SCREENING FOR EATING DISORDERS IN PRACTICE

Primary care providers are in a unique position to detect the onset of eating disorders at the earliest stages and to stop their progression.[32,33] Pediatricians should screen for eating disorders as part of annual health supervision or during preparticipation sports examinations by monitoring weight and height longitudinally and paying careful attention to potential signs and symptoms of disordered eating.

Screening questions about eating patterns and body image should be asked of all preteens and adolescents. The *Bright Futures* guidelines provide examples for addressing this issue with adolescents of different ages.[55] The SCOFF questionnaire, although validated only in adults, can provide a framework for screening (Table 1).[56] Weight, height, and BMI should be determined regularly and plotted on appropriate growth charts. Deviations from normal are easier to identify visually, because nutritional insufficiency may be manifest by falloff in either height or weight percentiles rather than actual weight loss. Growth charts are available for plotting changes in weight, height, and BMI over time and for comparing individual measurements with age-appropriate population norms.

Any evidence of excessive weight concern, inappropriate dieting, or a pattern of weight loss requires further attention, as does primary or secondary

TABLE 1 The SCOFF Questionnaire[56]

1. Do you make yourself **sick** because you feel uncomfortably full?
2. Do you worry you have lost **control** over how much you eat?
3. Have you recently lost **>1 stone** (6.3 kg or 14 lb) in a 3-mo period?
4. Do you believe yourself to be **fat** when others say you are too thin?
5. Would you say that **food** dominates your life?

One point should be given for every "yes" answer; a score of ≥2 indicates a likelihood of AN or BN.

amenorrhea or a failure to achieve appropriate increases in weight or height in growing children. In each of these situations, careful assessment for the possibility of an eating disorder and close monitoring at intervals as frequent as every 1 to 2 weeks may be needed until the situation is clarified. Adolescent girls who seek physician care for weight, shape, or eating concerns have been shown to be at significantly higher risk of a subsequent diagnosis of AN.[57]

A number of studies have shown that most adolescent girls express concerns about being overweight, and many may diet inappropriately.[10–12,14] Most of these children and adolescents do not have an eating disorder. On the other hand, it is known that patients with eating disorders often try to hide their illness, so simple denials by the adolescent do not exclude the possibility of an eating disorder. Obtaining collateral history from a parent may help identify abnormal eating attitudes or behaviors, although parents may, at times, be unaware or in denial as well. When an adolescent is referred to a pediatrician because parents, friends, or school personnel suspect the possibility of an eating disorder, it is likely that disordered eating is present. Pediatricians must, therefore, not be lulled into a false sense of security if the adolescent denies all symptoms. Table 2 outlines questions that are useful in eliciting a history of eating disorders, and Table 3 delineates possible physical findings in children and adolescents with eating disorders.

DSM-IV-TR criteria[28] for the diagnosis of AN and BN are outlined in Table 4. These criteria focus on the weight loss, attitudes and behaviors, and amenorrhea displayed by patients with eating disorders. Limitations of these criteria, especially as they relate to children and adolescents, have been discussed

TABLE 2 History

Specific history
    What is the most you ever weighed? How tall were you then? When was that?
    What is the least you ever weighed in the past year? How tall were you then? When was that?
    What do you think is your healthy weight?
    What would you like to weigh?
    Exercise: how much, how often, level of intensity? How stressed are you if you miss exercising?
    Current eating habits: adequacy of intake, portion sizes, food restrictions, picky eating, fluid intake, ritualized eating habits? Recent vegetarianism? Excessive noncaloric fluid intake?
    24-h diet history?
    Calorie-counting? Fat gram–counting? Carbohydrate-counting?
    Any binge-eating? Frequency? Triggers?
    Purging history?
    Use of diuretics, laxatives, diet pills, or ipecac? Ask about elimination pattern, constipation, diarrhea. Any vomiting? Frequency? Timing in relation to meals?
    Any previous therapy? What kind and how long? What was and was not helpful?
    Symptoms of hyperthyroidism, diabetes, malignancy, infection, inflammatory bowel disease?
  Family history: obesity, eating disorders, depression, other mental illness (especially anxiety disorders and obsessive-compulsive disorder), substance abuse by parents or other family members?
    Menstrual history: age at menarche? Regularity of cycles? Last menstrual period?
    Use of cigarettes, drugs, alcohol?
    Use of anabolic steroids (especially in boys)?
    Use of stimulants?
    Involvement with proanorexia ("pro-ana") or probulimia ("pro-mia") Web sites
    History of physical or sexual abuse?
Review of symptoms
    Dizziness, presyncope, syncope, fatigue?
    Pallor, easy bruising or bleeding?
    Cold intolerance? Cold extremities?
    Palpitations, chest pain, shortness of breath? Exercise intolerance?
    Hair loss, lanugo, dry skin?
    Fullness, bloating, abdominal pain, epigastric burning?
    Vomiting, symptoms of gastroesophageal reflux?
    Change in bowel habits? Diarrhea, constipation, rectal bleeding?
    Weakness, muscle cramps?
    Menstrual irregularities?

TABLE 3 Physical Examination Findings Sometimes Seen in Children and Adolescents With Eating Disorders

Sinus bradycardia; other cardiac arrhythmias
Orthostatic changes in pulse (>20 beats per min) or blood pressure (>10 mm Hg)
Hypothermia
Cachexia; facial wasting
Cardiac murmur (one-third with mitral valve prolapse)
Dull, thinning scalp hair
Sialoadenitis (parotitis most frequently reported)
Angular stomatitis; palatal scratches; oral ulcerations; dental enamel erosions
Dry, sallow skin; lanugo
Bruising/abrasions over the spine related to excessive exercise
Delayed or interrupted pubertal development
Atrophic breasts; atrophic vaginitis (postpubertal)
Russell sign (callous on knuckles from self-induced emesis)
Cold extremities; acrocyanosis; poor perfusion
Carotenemia (orange discoloration of the skin, particularly palms and soles)
Edema of the extremities
Flat or anxious affect

extensively in the literature,[54,58–61] and revisions to these criteria have been proposed for the fifth edition of the manual.[60,61] Alternative schema for the classification of eating disorders in children have been described to better reflect the range of eating issues seen.[58,62]

Younger patients (<13 years of age) with eating disorders are more likely to have premorbid psychopathology (depression, obsessive-compulsive disorder, or other anxiety disorders) and are less likely to have binge/purge behaviors associated with their illness. The predominance of females is far less; among the youngest patients with eating disorders, males and females may be equally affected. Weight loss often occurs at a faster rate than in older patients. Still, studies have shown that more than half

TABLE 4 Diagnosis of AN, BN, and Eating Disorders Not Otherwise Specified, From DSM-IV-TR[28]

AN

1. Refusal to maintain body weight at or above a minimally normal weight for age and height (ie, weight loss that leads to maintenance of body weight 85% of that expected or failure to make expected weight gain during period of growth and leads to a body weight of 85% of that expected).
2. Intense fear of gaining weight or becoming fat, even though underweight
3. Disturbance in the way in which one's body weight or shape is experienced, undue influence of body weight or shape on self-evaluation, or denial of the seriousness of current body weight
4. In postmenarcheal females, amenorrhea (ie, the absence of at least 3 consecutive menstrual cycles)
   Types
   - Restricting type: no regular bingeing or purging (self-induced vomiting or use of laxatives and diuretics)
   - Binge-eating/purging type: regular bingeing or purging behavior

BN

1. Recurrent episodes of binge-eating characterized by (a) eating, in a discrete period of time, an amount of food that is definitely larger than most people would eat in a similar period of time and under similar circumstances and (b) a sense of lack of control over eating during the episode
2. Recurrent inappropriate compensatory behavior to prevent weight gain, such as self-induced vomiting, misuse of laxatives, diuretics, enemas, or other medications; fasting; or excessive exercise
3. The binge-eating and inappropriate compensatory behaviors both occur, on average, at least twice per week for 3 mo
4. Self-evaluation unduly influenced by body shape or weight
5. The disturbance does not occur exclusively during episodes of AN
   Types
   - Purging type: the person has regularly engaged in self-induced vomiting or misuse of laxatives, diuretics, or enemas
   - Nonpurging type: the person has used other inappropriate compensatory behaviors, such as fasting or excessive exercise, but has not regularly engaged in self-induced vomiting or the misuse of laxatives, diuretics, or enemas

Eating disorder not otherwise specified

Disorders of eating that do not meet the criteria for either AN or BN; examples include
- All criteria for AN are met except the patient has regular menses
- All criteria for AN are met except that despite significant weight loss, weight remains in the normal range
- All criteria for BN are met except that binge-eating and inappropriate compensatory behaviors occur less frequently than twice per week or for a duration of <3 mo
- A patient with normal body weight who regularly engages in inappropriate compensatory behavior after eating small amounts of food (eg, self-induced vomiting after eating 2 cookies)

TABLE 5 Differential Diagnosis of Eating Disorders

Gastrointestinal disorders
　Inflammatory bowel disease
　Celiac disease
　Infectious diseases
　Chronic infections (human immunodeficiency virus infection, tuberculosis, others)
Endocrine disorders
　Hyperthyroidism (hypothyroidism)
　Diabetes mellitus
　Other endocrine disorders (eg, hypopituitarism, Addison disease)
Other psychiatric disorders
　Obsessive-compulsive disorder and anxiety disorders
　Substance abuse
Other disorders
　Central nervous system lesions (including malignancies)
　Other cancers
　Superior mesenteric artery syndrome (more commonly a consequence of severe weight loss)

of all children and adolescents with eating disorders may not fully meet all DSM-IV-TR criteria for AN or BN because they do not articulate body-image dissatisfaction or because their inadequate nutrition is manifest by growth failure rather than weight loss to less than 85% of expected weight.[63,64] These patients experience the same medical and psychological consequences of their disorders as do patients who meet criteria for AN or BN. Indeed, because the sequelae of weight loss (or failure to gain weight appropriately) may have even more worrisome implications for younger patients, relaxation of the diagnostic criteria for children and adolescents has been proposed in the development of the fifth edition of the *Diagnostic and Statistical Manual of Mental Disorders* to facilitate earlier diagnosis and treatment.[61]

INITIAL EVALUATION OF THE PATIENT WITH DISORDERED EATING

When screening raises suspicion of an eating disorder, initial evaluation includes establishing the diagnosis, evaluating medical and nutritional status, determining severity, and performing an initial psychosocial evaluation. This comprehensive evaluation is often performed in the pediatric primary care setting, and primary care clinicians who feel competent and comfortable in performing this assessment are encouraged to do so. Others should refer to appropriate medical subspecialists and mental health personnel to ensure that a complete evaluation is performed. A differential diagnosis for the adolescent with symptoms of an eating disorder can be found in Table 5.

Because eating disorders can affect every organ system and the medical complications can be serious or even life-threatening, a comprehensive history should be taken and a comprehensive physical examination should be performed. The most frequently seen medical complications are listed in Table 6 and are detailed in the following section.

Most laboratory results will be normal in patients with eating disorders; however, normal laboratory results do not exclude serious illness or medical instability in these patients. Still, an initial laboratory assessment should include a complete blood cell count; measurement of serum electrolytes, calcium, magnesium, and glucose; liver function tests; urinalysis; and measurement of thyrotropin level. Additional studies (eg, urine pregnancy test, serum luteinizing and follicle-stimulating hormones, serum prolactin, and se-

TABLE 6 Medical Complications That Result From Eating Disorders

General
  Dehydration
  Hypokalemia
  Hypomagnesemia
  Hyponatremia
  Irreversible cardiomyopathy and myositis
    (ipecac toxicity)
  Amenorrhea and menstrual irregularities
  Low bone mineral density; osteoporosis
  Cognitive deficits
  Mood symptoms
  Obsessive/compulsive symptoms
  Suicide
Caloric restriction and weight loss
  Inability to maintain body temperature
  Prolonged corrected QT interval or increased
    QT dispersion (uncommon but may
    predispose patient to sudden death)
  Dysrhythmias (including supraventricular
    beats and ventricular tachycardia, with or
    without exercise)
  Other electrocardiographic abnormalities
  Mitral valve prolapse
  Pericardial effusions
  Delayed gastric emptying and impaired
    gastrointestinal tract motility
  Constipation
  Bloating; postprandial fullness
  Hypoglycemia
  Hypercholesterolemia
  Abnormal liver function test results
  Sterile pyuria
  Anemia, leukopenia; thrombocytopenia
  Sick-euthyroid syndrome
  Growth retardation
  Cortical atrophy
Vomiting-related
  Hypochloremic metabolic alkalosis (vomiting)
  Esophagitis
  Gastroesophageal reflux
  Dental erosions
  Mallory-Weiss tears
  Esophageal or gastric rupture (rare)
  Aspiration pneumonia (rare)
Laxative-related
  Hyperchloremic metabolic acidosis (laxative
    abuse)
  Hyperuricemia
  Hypocalcemia
  Fluid retention (may gain up to 10 lb in 24 h)
    with laxative withdrawal
Refeeding
  Diaphoresis and night sweats
  Polyuria and nocturia
  Peripheral edema
  Refeeding syndrome

rum estradiol) may be indicated for patients with amenorrhea. Bone densitometry, using age-appropriate software, should also be considered for

those with amenorrhea for more than 6 to 12 months. Other studies including erythrocyte-sedimentation rate, screening for celiac disease, or radiographic imaging, such as computed tomography or MRI of the brain or studies of the upper or lower gastrointestinal system, should be considered if there are uncertainties about the diagnosis. An electrocardiogram should be performed for any patient with cardiovascular signs or symptoms, for any patient with electrolyte abnormalities, or for any patient with significant purging or weight loss.

The initial mental health assessment should include an evaluation of the patient's obsession with food and weight, his or her understanding of the diagnosis, and his or her willingness to receive help. The patient's social functioning at home, in school, and with friends should be assessed. Psychiatric comorbidity is common with eating disorders and is often previously undiagnosed.[34,65] The pediatrician should identify other potential psychiatric diagnoses (such as depression, anxiety, or obsessive-compulsive disorder), which may be a cause or consequence of disordered eating. Use of tobacco, alcohol, or illicit drugs or misuse of prescription or over-the-counter medications may also complicate the management of eating disorders. Suicidal ideation and history of physical or sexual abuse or violence should also be assessed. Suicide attempts and completed suicide are relatively common, particularly for patients who have binge/purge or purging behavior and are a major contributor to eating disorder–associated mortality. Death from suicide is 50 times more likely in patients with AN,[66] and 25% to 35% of patients with BN report a history of attempted suicide.[34]

The parents' reaction to the illness should also be assessed. Parental indifference or denial of the problem or inconsistent views about treatment

may affect the course of the illness and recovery.

Determining where and by whom the patient will be treated is an important and practical component of the initial evaluation. Patients with limited nutritional, medical, and psychological dysfunction can be managed in the pediatrician's office in conjunction with outpatient nutrition and mental health support. Patients who are more ill often require more intensive services, ideally delivered by a specialized multidisciplinary team, and sometimes in day-treatment, hospital, or residential settings.

MEDICAL COMPLICATIONS IN PATIENTS WITH EATING DISORDERS

Medical complications associated with eating disorders are listed in Table 5, and details of these complications have been described in many reviews.[32,33,67–74] Significant complications are seen in both outpatients and inpatients.[75] Most of the medical complications of eating disorders resolve with refeeding and/or resolution of purging.[70] However, there is increasing concern that some complications—particularly growth retardation, structural brain changes, and low bone mineral density—may, with time, become irreversible.[72] Malnutrition underlies many of the somatic symptoms seen initially, and these changes are often adaptive to the associated energy deficits. Over time, adaptation fails and signs and symptoms reflect the inability to compensate for inadequate nutrition. Metabolic rate decreases, body temperature can no longer be maintained, and nearly every organ system is compromised.[70,75,76]

Common cardiovascular signs and symptoms include orthostasis with blood pressure and/or pulse changes, bradycardia, and poor peripheral perfusion characterized by cold extremities, delayed capillary refill, and sometimes acrocyanosis. Conduction abnormalities may occur as a result of myocardial atrophy and are thought to be the most common proximal cause of death with AN. Repolarization abnormalities, characterized by QTc prolongation and/or increased QT dispersion, are reported with widely variable prevalence and seem to be more frequent in older patients and with increasing duration of illness.[77] Repolarization abnormalities are potentially life-threatening and should be managed aggressively. Pericardial effusion, a functional mitral valve prolapse, myocardial dysfunction, and emetine (ipecac-related) cardiomyopathy are all seen less frequently. Congestive heart failure can occur during refeeding, particularly in the setting of electrolyte abnormalities.[72,73,78]

Gastrointestinal complaints are common and sometimes precede diagnosis of the eating disorder. Delayed gastric emptying and increased intestinal transit time often contribute to subjective descriptions of bloating and postprandial fullness, which can further compromise nutritional restoration. In patients who vomit, symptoms of gastroesophageal reflux are common, and upper gastrointestinal bleeding sometimes occurs. Severe bleeding secondary to Mallory-Weiss tears of the esophagus is rare. Constipation is common and often difficult to manage. Nutritional strategies, stool softeners, or polyethylene glycol 3350 (Miralax) are the treatments of choice; stimulant laxatives should be avoided. Rectal prolapse sometimes occurs in the setting of constipation and/or laxative abuse. Hepatic transaminase levels are often elevated as a consequence of malnutrition and are not usually indicative of viral hepatitis. Hypertrophy of the salivary glands often occurs and may be a clue to binge-eating and/or vomiting. Esophageal or gastric rupture are catastrophic but rare compli-

cations that usually occur during refeeding.[73]

Fluid and electrolyte abnormalities may occur as a result of purging or with increasing cachexia. Dehydration can be seen in any patient with an eating disorder and can sometimes lead to orthostatic symptoms, presyncope, or syncope. Chronic dehydration and the body's effort to conserve water may induce a pseudohyperaldosteronism, which also leads to hypokalemia. However, significant deficits in total body potassium and the associated risk of arrhythmia may exist even with a normal serum potassium level. Patients with vomiting may have a hypochloremic metabolic alkalosis because of chronic loss of hydrochloric acid. Patients who abuse laxatives may have a hyperchloremic metabolic acidosis related to bicarbonate wasting. Dilutional hyponatremia can be seen in patients who "water load" instead of eating or to misrepresent their weight at outpatient visits. Hypomagnesemia that results from inadequate intake is associated with sudden cardiac death, may interfere with potassium repletion in patients who are hypokalemic, and sometimes contributes to refeeding syndrome.[70] Edema, sometimes significant, may be seen as a result of hypoproteinemia, during refeeding, or in association with laxative abuse.[70]

Endocrine dysfunction is common and includes hypothyroidism, hypercortisolism, and disturbances of the HPA axis, which result in hypogonadotropic hypogonadism, luteal phase abnormalities, and anovulation. Euthyroidsick syndrome (low free thyroxine, normal thyrotropin) is the most common thyroid abnormality and is reversible with refeeding. Supplemental thyroid hormone is not indicated. Activation of the HPA axis has been clearly demonstrated. In addition to its deleterious effects on growth, thyroid function, and the reproductive system, HPA

hyperactivity also contributes to the appetite suppression and physical overactivity that characterize eating disorders.[79] Hypothalamic suppression causing amenorrhea is attributable not only to weight loss but also to physical overactivity, emotional stress, and the metabolic changes associated with acute energy deficits[70,75]; it sometimes precedes weight loss.[70] Hypothalamic secretion of gonadotropins reverts to a prepubertal pattern that reverses with refeeding.[70] Amenorrhea is an important marker for increased risk of low bone mineral density and osteoporosis (discussed in a later paragraph),[80–83] and an intriguing recent report suggested that amenorrhea is also associated with the cognitive impairments seen with AN.[84]

Common skin changes include lanugo, dry scaly skin, and yellow discoloration related to carotenemia. Acrocyanosis can be seen when perfusion is poor. Hair and nail changes are often seen as well, and angular stomatitis may be related to either vomiting or vitamin deficiencies.[70]

Growth retardation, short stature, and pubertal delay may all be seen in prepubertal and peripubertal children and adolescents with eating disorders.[75,85] Many endocrine abnormalities contribute to this growth failure; abnormal thyroid function, abnormal adrenal function, low levels of sex steroids, and uncoupling of growth hormone from insulin-like growth factor 1 (IGF-1) have all been implicated.[72] Catch-up growth has been inconsistently reported in the literature; younger patients may have greater and more permanent effects on growth.[72,86]

Low bone mineral density is a frequent complication of eating disorders in both male and female patients. It is worrisome not only because of the increased risk of pathologic fractures but also because of its potential to be irreversible and compromise skeletal health across the entire life span. The pathophysiology of abnormal bone mineralization in the eating disorders is likely to be multifactorial; proposed mechanisms include deficiencies of gonadal steroids (estrogen and/or testosterone), deficiencies of calcium and vitamin D, reduction in lean muscle mass and its mechanical effects on bone, and excesses of endogenous glucocorticoids related to hyperactivity of the HPA axis. The reversibility of skeletal changes is unclear and probably varies on the basis of disease severity, the timing of illness and recovery, and perhaps genetic factors. Because adolescence is a critical period for bone mineralization, younger patients with AN are at higher risk of skeletal changes than are older patients. Treatment strategies, such as supplemental estrogen, bisphosphonates, calcium, and vitamin D replacement, have not been shown to be consistently effective, are not a substitute for nutritional recovery, and are not recommended for routine use.[72,87,88]

Volume deficits in both gray and white matter of the brain and associated increases in the cerebrospinal fluid space occur with weight loss in AN and are proportional to weight loss. Brain changes may be associated with elevated cortisol concentrations related to HPA-axis dysfunction, analogous to changes now being reported in other psychiatric disorders such as posttraumatic stress disorder.[89] Cognitive impairment has been demonstrated across the wide range of neuropsychological domains but does not seem to be directly proportional to structural brain changes.[84] Functional imaging studies of the brain show decreases in both global and localized brain activity, but it is unknown whether these decreases precede or are a consequence of weight loss or whether they are re-

versible.[90] Normalization of white matter occurs with refeeding; however, gray matter changes seem to persist despite weight recovery.[84,89]

TREATMENT CONTINUUM FOR CHILDREN AND ADOLESCENTS WITH EATING DISORDERS

Most adolescent patients with eating disorders will be treated in outpatient settings. Pediatricians play an important role in the management of these patients, assessing treatment progress, screening for and managing medical complications, and coordinating care with nutrition and mental health colleagues. Some pediatricians in primary care practice will feel comfortable in coordinating care; others will choose to refer some or all patients with eating disorders to those with special expertise. Depending on the availability of local resources, these providers may be a specialty eating disorders program, an adolescent medicine specialist, a psychiatrist, or another mental health provider.[32,91]

Collaborative Outpatient Care

Most children and adolescents with eating disorders will be managed in an outpatient setting by a multidisciplinary team coordinated by a pediatrician or medical subspecialist with expertise in the care of children and adolescents with eating disorders. Pediatricians generally work with nursing, nutrition, and mental health colleagues in provision of the medical, nutrition, and mental health care required by these patients.

It is generally accepted that medical stabilization and nutritional rehabilitation are the most important determinants of short-term outcomes and are essential for correcting cognitive deficits to allow for effective mental health interventions. Components of nutritional rehabilitation required in the management of patients with eating

disorders have been presented in several reviews.[32,33,92–95] In the United States, oral refeeding is clearly the preferred modality for nutritional rehabilitation. However, for patients who are unwilling or unable to eat, supplements or nasogastric feeding may be life-saving.

Meals and snacks generally are reintroduced or improved in a stepwise manner for those with AN, which leads, in most cases, to an eventual intake of 2000 to 3000 kcal (or more) per day and a weight gain of 0.25 to 1 kg per week. Smaller, more frequent meals; increasing the caloric density of foods; and substituting nutrient fluids (eg, fruit juice) for water can sometimes help patients overcome the postprandial fullness and psychological barriers associated with the substantial increase in caloric intake that is required. Patients with abdominal complaints from acquired nutritionally mediated lactase deficiency may benefit from supplemental lactase. Meals are changed to ensure ingestion of 2 to 3 servings of protein per day. Daily fat intake should be slowly shifted toward a goal of 30 to 50 g per day. The stereotypical and obsessional eating habits favored by many patients with eating disorders and the observation that similar levels of weight loss and malnutrition can lead to dramatically different medical consequences suggest that deficiencies of specific micronutrients may share responsibility with protein-calorie malnutrition for the medical consequences in eating disorders.[70] Food variety should be encouraged, and a multivitamin should be recommended. Behavioral interventions are often required to encourage reluctant (and often resistant) patients to meet necessary caloric intake and weight-gain goals.[96–99]

Ranges for treatment goal weight should be individualized and based on age, height, pubertal stage, premorbid weight, and previous growth trajectory. Furthermore, for growing children or adolescents, the goal weight range should be reevaluated at regular intervals (eg, every 3 to 6 months) on the basis of changing age and height. In postmenarcheal girls, resumption of menses provides an objective measure of biological health[100]; in 1 recent study, resumption of menses occurred at a mean BMI percentile of 27; 75% of the girls resumed menstruating once they had achieved and sustained approximately the 40th percentile for BMI.[101] Resumption of menses can also be used to refine the treatment goal weight.

Family-Based ("Maudsley") Therapy

Over the past decade, specialized eating disorder–focused family-based interventions, based on work originally performed at the Maudsley Hospital in London, have gained attention in the treatment of adolescent AN because of promising short-term and long-term outcomes. Although the etiologic underpinnings of this treatment approach have lost much of their support over time (ie, it is no longer believed that eating disorders are caused mainly by family dysfunction), family-based interventions, nevertheless, remain an effective and evidence-based treatment strategy for adolescent AN in both open trials and randomized controlled studies.[102–105] Family-based interventions are typically described as having 3 phases. In the first phase, parents, supported by the therapist, take responsibility to make certain that their adolescent is eating adequately and limiting other pathologic weight-control behaviors. In the second phase, substantial weight recovery has already occurred, and the adolescent is helped to gradually resume responsibility for his or her own eating. In the final phase of treatment, weight has been restored, and the

therapy shifts to address the more general issues of adolescent development and how they may have been derailed by the eating disorder.[102] A manual for providers[106] and a family-support manual[107] are now available. Unfortunately, family-based treatment by experienced providers is not available in all communities. Nevertheless, the essential principles of family-based treatment can still be encouraged by community providers in their work with patients and families.[105] Family-based treatment may not be suitable for all patients; caution has been advised for families in which there is parental psychopathology or hostility toward the affected child, for older patients, or for patients who are the most medically compromised.[102,104] Additional randomized controlled studies of family-based treatment, including studies of long-term outcomes, are still needed. Family-based approaches are now being evaluated for the treatment of BN as well.[108]

Treatment of BN in adolescents has been poorly studied, and there is little evidence to guide treatment recommendations. For adults, BN-focused cognitive behavioral therapy is the treatment of choice. Pharmacotherapy (see "Pharmacotherapy") has been helpful as well.

Day-Treatment Programs

Day-treatment programs (day hospitalization, partial hospitalization) have been developed to provide an intermediate level of care for patients with eating disorders who require more than outpatient care but less than 24-hour hospitalization.[109–112] These programs have been used in an attempt to prevent the need for hospitalization; in some cases, they are used as a "step-down" from inpatient to outpatient care. Day-treatment programs are less costly and more accessible than traditional hospitalization. In addition,

they allow for more family and social support and for recovery to occur in a more naturalistic environment that may be more generalizable.[109] Day treatment typically involves 8 to 10 hours of care (including meals, therapy, groups, and other activities) by a multidisciplinary staff 5 days/week. Evaluation of day-treatment programs has been characterized by small samples and the difficulty in undertaking randomized controlled trials.[113] Still, short-term outcomes have generally been reported to be good.[110,113,114] A recent study that used a range of outcome measures, including BMI and measurement of binge-purge behavior, demonstrated day treatment to be highly effective in the treatment of both restrictive and binge-purge AN and BN. Furthermore, these results were sustained or improved over 18 months of follow-up.[113]

Hospital-Based Treatment

Hospital-based treatment for eating disorders is less common when intensive outpatient or day-treatment programs are available. Hospitalization is much more frequently required for adolescent patients with AN than for patients with BN. Criteria for hospitalization of children and adolescents with eating disorders have been enumerated by the Society for Adolescent Medicine and are listed in Table 7.[32] Similar criteria are endorsed in the American Psychiatric Association's practice guideline for the treatment of patients with eating disorders[33] and by other organizations.[115] These criteria acknowledge that hospitalization may be required because of medical or psychiatric needs or when there is failure of outpatient treatment to achieve medical, nutritional, or psychiatric goals. Unfortunately, many third-party payers in the United States do not adhere to these criteria and make it difficult for some children and adolescents with eating disorders to receive the

TABLE 7 Criteria for Hospital Admission for Children, Adolescents, and Young Adults With Eating Disorders[32]

AN
  <75% ideal body weight or ongoing weight loss despite intensive management
  Refusal to eat
  Body fat < 10%
  Heart rate < 50 beats per min daytime; <45 beats per min nighttime
  Systolic pressure < 90 mm Hg
  Orthostatic changes in pulse (>20 beats per min) or blood pressure (>10 mm Hg)
  Temperature < 96°F
  Arrhythmia
BN
  Syncope
  Serum potassium concentration < 3.2 mmol/L
  Serum chloride concentration < 88 mmol/L
  Esophageal tears
  Cardiac arrhythmias including prolonged QTc
  Hypothermia
  Suicide risk
  Intractable vomiting
  Hematemesis
  Failure to respond to outpatient treatment

recommended level of care.[116,117] Children and adolescents have the best prognosis if their disease is treated rapidly and aggressively (an approach that may not be as effective for adults with a more long-term, protracted course).[91] Hospitalization, when indicated, allows for medical stabilization, adequate weight gain, and establishment of safe and healthy eating habits and improves the prognosis for children and adolescents. Discharge of hospitalized patients too soon often results in medical complications, a worse clinical course, and readmission. In 1 study, patients with AN who were discharged while still underweight had a 50% readmission rate compared with a rate of less than 10% for patients who had reached at least 90% of their recommended average body weight before discharge.[118]

The pediatrician involved in the treatment of hospitalized patients must be prepared to provide nutrition via a nasogastric tube or even intravenously when necessary. In hospitalized male adolescents, supplemental nighttime nasogastric feedings have been shown to significantly increase both weight gain and improvement in BMI compared with oral refeeding alone.[119]

Refeeding syndrome may occur in severely malnourished patients, particularly in the setting of aggressive nutritional rehabilitation. Refeeding syndrome refers to a constellation of metabolic, cardiovascular, neurologic, and hematologic complications primarily related to shifts of phosphate from extracellular to intracellular spaces in the setting of total body phosphorus depletion. The syndrome is most common in hospitalized patients during the first week of hospitalization and patients who are receiving supplemental enteral or parenteral nutrition. Cautious refeeding, careful monitoring of serum electrolyte, magnesium, phosphorus, and glucose levels, and a low threshold for phosphorus supplementation prevent the development of refeeding syndrome.[71,72,120–123] Refeeding syndrome is unusual after the first 2 weeks of nutritional rehabilitation or in patients being treated in the outpatient setting.

Pharmacotherapy

No medications have been approved by the US Food and Drug Administration for the treatment of AN.[124] Pharmacotherapy is sometimes prescribed but is typically targeted at comorbid symptoms of depression and anxiety. Selective serotonin-reuptake inhibitors (SSRIs) are most often used but may not be effective in severely malnourished patients. There is also limited evidence for the use of SSRIs for relapse prevention in AN.[125] In recent case reports and open-label trials, atypical neuroleptic agents, predominantly olanzapine (Zyprexa), have been noted to improve both weight gain and dysfunctional thinking in patients with AN.[126] A recently completed randomized, double-blind, placebo-controlled trial in adults showed a significant increase in weight gain in those who were taking olanzapine and a concomitant decrease in obsessive symptoms, although the effect size was modest.[127] Further evaluation of the effectiveness of these agents is underway, and caution is warranted because of the risk of developing insulin resistance and metabolic syndrome.

In contrast to AN, several pharmacologic agents have been demonstrated to be effective for the treatment of BN. Although only fluoxetine has been approved by the Food and Drug Administration, other SSRIs, serotonin/norepinephrine-reuptake inhibitors (eg, venlafaxine), and tricyclic antidepressants have also been shown to decrease binge-eating and purging in BN.[124,128] Topiramate has been shown to significantly decrease binge-eating and may be an option for patients who do not respond to or are not able to tolerate SSRIs.[129] Other drugs, including naltrexone and ondansetron (Zofran), are being used with some success in BN, although data are lacking to recommend their use more broadly.[130]

Hormonal supplementation, although capable of restoring menstruation, has not been shown to reliably improve bone mineral density and is not a substitute for nutritional rehabilitation and restoration of positive energy balance.

PROGNOSIS

The prognosis of eating disorders in adolescents has varied widely in the literature, and outcomes have depended on methodology, definitions of recovery, and duration of follow-up in the studies reported.[131] Adolescent outcomes are significantly better than the outcomes reported in adults. Longitudinal reports reflect a more optimistic and less hopeless outcome; followed over time, the majority of patients fully recover, and an even larger proportion have a behavioral cure (normal eating, normal weight, and resumption of menses). However, these results accrue only after more than 10 years of follow-up; therefore, patients, their families, and clinicians must be prepared to remain engaged in what may sometimes be a protracted treatment process.[132–134]

Strober et al[132] conducted an important study in which 95 people who had been hospitalized for AN as adolescents were followed for 10 to 15 years. By the end of follow-up, 86.3% had achieved partial or complete recovery, and there were no deaths. However, the median time to partial recovery was 57.4 months, and the median time to full recovery (met by >75% of the study population) was 79.1 months. A study from Germany produced similar findings; at 10-year follow-up, 69% of the patients (including 7 boys) had achieved full recovery, and there were no deaths. Again, however, the course was protracted and the authors pointed out a high rate of residual psychiatric disorders even after full recovery from AN.[135]

Patients with an earlier age of onset seem to have a better prognosis.[85,134] Other characteristics associated with a better prognosis include shorter duration of symptoms and a better parent-child relationship. Purging behavior, physical hyperactivity, more significant weight loss, and disease chronicity are all associated with a less favorable prognosis.[134] Even after recovery, there are high rates of residual psychiatric illness—predominantly depression and anxiety—that persist.[133,136,137] A meta-analysis of 119 AN outcome studies showed little improvement in the success of treatment over the 5 decades reviewed.[133]

Mortality rates for adolescents with both AN and BN are lower than those that have historically been reported.[133,134] In a recent meta-analysis, the mortality rate among adolescents with AN was reported to be 1.8% compared with a mortality rate of 5.9% when adults and adolescents were considered together.[134] Mortality, when it does occur, is most often attributable to the complications of starvation or to suicide.[66]

PEDIATRICIANS' ROLE IN PREVENTION AND ADVOCACY

Efforts to prevent eating disorders can take place both in practice and community settings, such as schools. Primary care pediatricians can help families and children learn to apply the principles of proper nutrition and physical activity and to avoid an unhealthy emphasis on weight and dieting.[138] In addition, pediatricians can screen to detect the early onset of disordered eating and be careful to avoid seemingly innocuous statements (such as "you could stand to lose a little weight") that are sometimes reported by patients to have triggered the onset of their eating disorder. At the community level, there is general agreement that changes in the cultural approaches to weight, dieting, and body image will be required to decrease the growing numbers of children and adolescents at risk of developing eating disorders. This cultural shift is made more challenging by the increasing prevalence of obesity and the competing responsibility to address its health risks as well.[15]

A variety of successful programs for preventing eating pathology have been developed for various settings.[139] The largest effect sizes were seen in programs targeted at high-risk populations, in programs that were interactive rather than didactic, and in programs aimed at older adolescents. Content varied even in the most successful programs, which suggests that a variety of approaches may be effective. Multisession programs were more effective than single-session programs,[140] and there has even been some concern that single-session programs may be counterproductive.[141–146] An important question currently being asked is whether we can work simultaneously toward the prevention of eating disorders and obesity.[15]

Reimbursement issues continue to limit the access of many patients with eating disorders to appropriate services. Availability of mental health services, lack of mental health parity, and service "carve-outs" all have been barriers to patients and families who seek clinically necessary treatment and seem to be disproportionately problematic for patients with eating disorders. Despite evidence of its effectiveness, family-based treatment is not available in many communities. Through advocacy, pediatricians can help support health care reform efforts that will ensure that children and adolescents with eating disorders are able to receive necessary care.

GUIDANCE FOR PEDIATRICIANS

1. Pediatricians need to be knowledgeable about the risk factors and early signs and symptoms of disordered eating and eating disorders.

2. When counseling families on preventing obesity, pediatricians should focus on healthy eating and building self-esteem while still addressing weight concerns. Care needs to be taken not to inadvertently enable excessive dieting, compulsive exercise, or other potentially unhealthy weight-management strategies.

3. Pediatricians should be encouraged to calculate and plot weight, height, and BMI by using age- and gender-appropriate charts and assess menstrual status in girls at annual health supervision visits.

4. Pediatricians should screen patients for disordered eating

and related behaviors and be prepared to intervene when necessary.

5. Pediatricians should monitor or refer patients with eating disorders for medical and nutritional complications.

6. Pediatricians need to be familiar with treatment resources in their communities so that they can coordinate or facilitate multidisciplinary care.

7. Pediatricians can play a role in primary prevention during office visits and through school-based and community interventions with a focus on education, early screening, and advocacy.

8. Pediatricians are encouraged to advocate for legislation and policy changes that ensure appropriate services for patients with eating disorders, including medical care, nutritional intervention, mental health treatment, and care coordination, in settings that are appropriate for the severity of the illness.

LEAD AUTHOR
David S. Rosen, MD, MPH

COMMITTEE ON ADOLESCENCE, 2009–2010
Margaret J. Blythe, MD, Chairperson
Paula K. Braverman, MD
Cora C. Breuner, MD, MPH
David A. Levine, MD
Pamela J. Murray, MD, MPH
Rebecca F. O'Brien, MD
Warren M. Seigel, MD

PAST COMMITTEE MEMBERS
David S. Rosen, MD, MPH
Michelle S. Barratt, MD, MPH
Charles J. Wibbelsman, MD

LIAISONS
Lesley Breech, MD – American College of Obstetricians and Gynecologists
Jorge L. Pinzon, MD – Canadian Paediatric Society
Benjamin Shain, MD, PhD – American Academy of Child and Adolescent Psychiatry

STAFF
Karen Smith
ksmith@aap.org
Mark Del Monte, JD

REFERENCES

1. Whitaker AH. An epidemiological study of anorectic and bulimic symptoms in adolescent girls: implications for pediatricians. *Pediatr Ann.* 1992;21(11):752–759

2. Lucas AR, Beard CM, O'Fallon WM, Kurland LT. 50-year trends in the incidence of anorexia nervosa in Rochester, Minn.: a population-based study. *Am J Psychiatry.* 1991;148(7):917–922

3. Hsu LK. Epidemiology of the eating disorders. *Psychiatr Clin North Am.* 1996;19(4):681–700

4. Dorian BJ, Garfinkel PE. The contributions of epidemiologic studies to the etiology and treatment of the eating disorders. *Psychiatry Ann.* 1999;29:187–192

5. Troiano RP, Flegal KM. Overweight children and adolescents: description, epidemiology, and demographics. *Pediatrics.* 1998;101(3 pt 2):497–504

6. Ogden CL, Carroll MD, Curtin LR, McDowell MA, Tabak CJ, Flegal KM. Prevalence of overweight and obesity in the United States, 1999–2004. *JAMA.* 2006;295(13):1549–1555

7. Ogden CL, Flegal KM, Carroll MD, Johnson CL. Prevalence and trends in overweight among U.S. children and adolescents, 1999–2000. *JAMA.* 2002;288(14):1728–1732

8. Kohn M, Booth M. The worldwide epidemic of obesity in adolescents. *Adolesc Med.* 2003;14(1):1–9

9. Barlow SE; Expert Committee. Expert Committee recommendations regarding the prevention, assessment, and treatment of child and adolescent overweight and obesity. *Pediatrics.* 2007;120(suppl 4):S164–S192

10. Strauss RS. Self-reported weight status and dieting in a cross-sectional sample of young adolescents: National Health and Nutrition Examination Survey III. *Arch Pediatr Adolesc Med.* 1999;153(7):741–747

11. Stein D, Meged S, Bar-Hanin T, Blank S, Elizur A, Weizman A. Partial eating disorders in a community sample of female adolescents. *J Am Acad Child Adolesc Psychiatry.* 1997;36(8):1116–1123

12. Patton GC, Carlin JB, Shao Q, et al. Adolescent dieting: healthy weight control or borderline eating disorder? *J Child Psychol Psychiatry.* 1997;38(3):299–306

13. Field AE, Austin SB, Taylor CB, et al. Relation between dieting and weight change among preadolescents and adolescents. *Pediatrics.* 2003;112(4):900–906

14. Haines J, Neumark-Sztainer D. Prevention of obesity and eating disorders: a consideration of shared risk factors. *Health Educ Res.* 2006;21(6):770–782

15. Neumark-Sztainer D. Preventing obesity and eating disorders in adolescents: what can health providers do? *J Adolesc Health.* 2009;44(3):206–213

16. Dominé F, Berchtold A, Akré C, Michaud PA, Suris JC. Disordered eating behaviors: what about boys? *J Adolesc Health.* 2009;44(2):111–117

17. Carlat DJ, Camargo CA Jr, Herzog DB. Eating disorders in males: a report on 135 patients. *Am J Psychiatry.* 1997;154(8):1127–1132

18. Rosen DS. Eating disorders in adolescent males. *Adolesc Med.* 2003;14(3):677–689

19. Agency for Healthcare Research and Quality. Eating disorders sending more Americans to the hospital. *AHRQ News and Numbers.* April 1, 2009. Available at: www.ahrq.gov/news/nn/nn040109.htm. Accessed May 6, 2010

20. Robinson TN, Killen JD, Litt IF, et al. Ethnicity and body dissatisfaction: are Hispanic and Asian girls at increased risk for eating disorders? *J Adolesc Health.* 1996;19(6):384–393

21. Crago M, Shisslak CM, Estes LS. Eating disturbances among American minority groups: a review. *Int J Eat Disord.* 1996;19(3):239–248

22. Gard MC, Freeman CP. The dismantling of a myth: a review of eating disorders and socioeconomic status. *Int J Eat Disord.* 1996;20(1):1–12

23. Pike KM, Walsh BT. Ethnicity and eating disorders: implications for incidence and treatment. *Psychopharmacol Bull.* 1996;32(2):265–274

24. Lai KY. Anorexia nervosa in Chinese adolescents: does culture make a difference? *J Adolesc.* 2000;23(5):561–568

25. le Grange D, Telch CF, Tibbs J. Eating attitudes and behaviors in 1435 South African Caucasian and non-Caucasian college students. *Am J Psychiatry.* 1998;155(2):250–254

26. Krowchuk DP, Kreiter SR, Woods CR, Sinal SH, DuRant RH. Problem dieting behaviors among young adolescents. *Arch Pediatr Adolesc Med.* 1998;152(9):884–888

27. Field AE, Camargo CA Jr, Taylor CB, et al. Overweight, weight concerns, and bulimic behaviors among girls and boys. *J Am Acad Child Adolesc Psychiatry.* 1999;38(6): 754–760

28. American Psychiatric Association. *Diagnostic and Statistical Manual of Mental Disorders, 4th ed., Text Revision (DSM-IV-TR).* Washington, DC: American Psychiatric Association; 2000

29. Chamay-Weber B, Narring F, Michaud P. Partial eating disorders among adolescents: a review. *J Adolesc Health.* 2005;37(3): 417–427

30. Eddy KY, Celio Doyle A, Hoste RR, Herzog DB, le Grange D. Eating disorder not otherwise specified in adolescents. *J Am Acad Child Adolesc Psychiatry.* 2008;47(2):156–164

31. Steiner H, Lock J. Anorexia nervosa and bulimia nervosa in children and adolescents: a review of the past 10 years. *J Am Acad Child Adolesc Psychiatry.* 1998;37(4):352–359

32. Fisher M, Golden NH, Katzman DK, et al. Eating disorders in adolescents: a background paper. *J Adolesc Health.* 1995; 16(6):420–437

33. American Psychiatric Association. Practice guideline for the treatment of patients with eating disorders (revision). *Am J Psychiatry.* 2006;163(suppl 1):1–54

34. Herpertz-Dahlmann B. Adolescent eating disorders: definitions, symptomatology, epidemiology, and comorbidity. *Child Adolesc Psychiatr Clin N Am.* 2009;18(1):31–47

35. Nichols JF, Rauh MJ, Lawson MJ, Ji M, Barkai H. Prevalence of the female athlete triad syndrome among high school athletes. *Arch Pediatr Adolesc Med.* 2006; 160(2):137–142

36. Sundgot-Borgen J. Eating disorders in female athletes. *Sports Med.* 1994;17(3): 176–188

37. Bulik CM. Exploring the gene-environment nexus in eating disorders. *J Psychiatry Neurosci.* 2005;30(5):335–339

38. Strober M, Freeman R, Lampert C, Diamond J, Kaye W. Controlled family study of anorexia nervosa and bulimia nervosa: evidence of shared liability and transmission of partial syndromes. *Am J Psychiatry.* 2000;157(3):393–401

39. Mazzeo SE, Bulik CM. Environmental and genetic risk factors for eating disorders: what the clinician needs to know. *Child Adolesc Psychiatr Clin N Am.* 2009;18(1): 67–82

40. Hudson JI, Mangweth B, Pope HG, et al. Family study of affective spectrum disorders. *Arch Gen Psychiatry.* 2003;60(2): 170–177

41. Attia E, Walsh BT. Anorexia nervosa. *Am J Psychiatry.* 2007;164(12):1805–1810

42. Klump K, Gobrogge KL, Perkins PS, Thorne D, Sisk CL, Breedlove SM. Preliminary evidence that gonadal hormones organize and activate disordered eating. *Psychol Med.* 2006;36(4):539–546

43. Hagan MM, Chandler PC, Wauford PK, Rybak RJ, Oswald KD. Role of palatable food and hunger as trigger factors in an animal model of stress-induced binge eating. *Int J Eat Disord.* 2003;34(2):183–197

44. Klump KL, McGue M, Iacono WG. Differential heritability of eating attitudes and behaviors in prepubertal versus pubertal twins. *Int J Eat Disord.* 2003;33(3):287–292

45. Striegel-Moore RH, Bulik CM. Risk factors for eating disorders. *Am Psychol.* 2007; 62(3):181–198

46. McKnight Investigators. Risk factors for the onset of eating disorders in adolescent girls: results of the McKnight longitudinal risk factor study. *Am J Psychiatry.* 2003;160(2):248–254

47. Neumark-Sztainer D, Wall M, Guo J, Story M, Haines J, Eisenberg M. Obesity, disordered eating, and eating disorders in a longitudinal study of adolescents: how do dieters fare 5 years later? *J Am Diet Assoc.* 2006;106(4):559–568

48. Patton GC, Selzer R, Coffey C, Carlin JB, Wolfe R. Onset of adolescent eating disorders: population based cohort study over 3 years. *BMJ.* 1999;318(7186): 765–768

49. Monteleone P, DiLieto A, Castaldo E, Maj M. Leptin functioning in eating disorders. *CNS Spectr.* 2004;9(7):523–529

50. Chan JL, Mantzoros CS. Role of leptin in energy deprivation states: normal human physiology and clinical implications for hypothalamic amenorrhea and anorexia nervosa. *Lancet.* 2005;366(9479):74–85

51. Hebebrand J, Muller TD, Holtkamp K, Herpertz-Dahlmann B. The role of leptin in anorexia nervosa: clinical implications. *Mol Psychiatry.* 2007;12(1):23–35

52. Treasure JL, Owen JB. Intriguing links between animal behavior and anorexia nervosa. *Int J Eat Disord.* 1997;21(4):307–311

53. Hagan MM, Wauford PK, Chandler PC, Jarrett LA, Rybak RJ, Blackburn K. A new animal model of binge eating: key synergistic role of past caloric restriction and stress. *Physiol Behav.* 2002;77(1):45–54

54. Ackard DM, Fulkerson JA, Neumark-Sztainer D. Prevalence and utility of DSM-IV eating disorder criteria among youth. *Int J Eat Disord.* 2007;40(5):409–417

55. Hagan JF, Shaw JS, Duncan PM, eds. *Bright*

Futures: Guidelines for Health Supervision of Infants, Children, and Adolescents. 3rd ed. Elk Grove Village, IL: American Academy of Pediatrics; 2008

56. Morgan JF, Reid F. The SCOFF questionnaire: assessment of a new screening tool for eating disorders. *BMJ.* 1999;319(7223):1467–1468

57. Lask B, Bryant-Waugh R, Wright F, Campbell M, Willoughby K, Waller G. Family physician consultation patterns indicate high risk for early onset anorexia nervosa. *Int J Eat Disord.* 2005;38(3):269–272

58. Nicholls D, Chater R, Lask B. Children into DSM don't go: a comparison of classification systems for eating disorders in childhood and adolescence. *Int J Eat Disord.* 2000;28(3):317–324

59. Rosen DS. Eating disorders in children and young adolescents: etiology, classification, clinical features, and treatment. *Adolesc Med.* 2003;14(1):49–59

60. Wonderlich SA, Joiner TE, Keel PK, Williamson DA, Crosby RD. Eating disorder diagnoses: empirical approaches to classification. *Am Psychol.* 2007;62(3):167–180

61. Bravender T, Bryant-Waugh R, Herzog D, et al; Workgroup for Classification of Eating Disorders in Children and Adolescents. Classification of child and adolescent eating disturbances. *Int J Eat Disord.* 2007; 40(suppl):S117–S122

62. Nicholls D, Bryant-Waugh R. Eating disorders of infancy and childhood: definition, symptomatology, epidemiology, and comorbidity. *Child Adolesc Psychiatr Clin N Am.* 2009;18(1):17–30

63. Bunnell DW, Shenker IR, Nussbaum MP, et al. Subclinical versus formal eating disorders: differentiating psychological features. *Int J Eat Disord.* 1990;9(3): 357–362

64. Peebles R, Wilson JL, Lock JD. How do children with eating disorders differ from adolescents with eating disorders at initial evaluation. *J Adolesc Health.* 2006;39(6): 800–805

65. Godart NT, Flament MF, Curt F, et al. Anxiety disorders in subjects seeking treatment for eating disorders: a DSM-IV controlled study. *Psychiatry Res.* 2003;117(3): 245–258

66. Keel PK, Dorer DJ, Eddy KT, Franko D, Charatan DL, Herzog DB. Predictors of mortality in eating disorders. *Arch Gen Psychiatry.* 2003;60(2):179–183

67. Palla B, Litt IF. Medical complications of eating disorders in adolescents. *Pediatrics.* 1988;81(5):613–623

68. Fisher M. Medical complications of an-

orexia and bulimia nervosa. *Adolesc Med.* 1992;3(3):487–502

69. Nicholls D, Stanhope R. Medical complications of anorexia nervosa in children and young adolescents. *Eur Eat Disord Rev.* 2000;8(2):170–180

70. Brambilla F, Monteleone P. Physical complications and physiological aberrations in eating disorders: a review. In: Maj M, Halmi K, Lopez-Ibor JJ, Sartorius N, eds. *Eating Disorders.* Chichester, England: John Wiley and Sons; 2003:139–192

71. Rome ES, Ammerman S. Medical complications of eating disorders: an update. *J Adolesc Health.* 2003;33(6):418–426

72. Katzman, DK. Medical complications in adolescents with anorexia nervosa: a review of the literature. *Int J Eat Disord.* 2005; 37(suppl):S52–S59

73. Mitchell JE, Crow S. Medical complications of anorexia nervosa and bulimia nervosa. *Curr Opin Psychiatry.* 2006;19(4):438–443

74. Mehler PS, Anderson AE. *Guide to the Medical Care and Complications of Eating Disorders.* Baltimore, MD: Johns Hopkins University Press; 1999

75. Misra M, Aggarwal A, Miller KK, et al. Effects of anorexia nervosa on clinical, hematologic, biochemical, and bone density parameters in community-dwelling adolescent girls. *Pediatrics.* 2004;114(6): 1574–1583

76. Konrad KK, Careis RA, Garner DM. Metabolic and psychological changes during refeeding in anorexia nervosa. *Eat Weight Disord.* 2007;12(1):20–26

77. Panagiotopoulos C, McKrindle BW, Hick K, Katzman DK. Electrocardiographic findings in adolescents with eating disorders. *Pediatrics.* 2000;105(5):1100–1105

78. Casiero D, Frishman WH. Cardiovascular complications of eating disorders. *Cardiol Rev.* 2006;14(5):227–231

79. Lo Sauro C, Ravaldi C, Cabras PL, Faravelli C. Stress, hypothalamic-pituitary-adrenal axis and eating disorders. *Neuropsychobiology.* 2008;57(3):95–115

80. Wong JCH, Lewindon P, Mortimer R, Shepherd R. Bone mineral density in adolescent females with recently diagnosed anorexia nervosa. *Int J Eat Disord.* 2001;29(1):11–16

81. Grinspoon S, Thomas E, Pitts S, et al. Prevalence and predictive factors for regional osteopenia in women with anorexia nervosa. *Ann Intern Med.* 2000;133(10): 790–794

82. Castro J, Lazaro L, Pons F, Halperin I, Toro J. Predictors of bone mineral density reduction in adolescents with anorexia nervosa. *J Am Acad Child Adolesc Psychiatry.* 2000;39(11):1365–1370

83. Golden NH, Shenker IR. Amenorrhea in anorexia nervosa: etiology and implications. *Adolesc Med.* 1992;3(3):503–518

84. Chui HT, Christensen BK, Zipursky RB, et al. Cognitive function and brain structure in females with a history of adolescent-onset anorexia nervosa. *Pediatrics.* 2008;122(2). Available at: www.pediatrics.org/cgi/content/full/122/2/e426

85. Theander S. Anorexia nervosa with an early onset: selection, gender, outcome, and results of a long-term follow-up study. *J Youth Adolesc.* 1996;25(4):419–429

86. Swenne I. Weight requirements for catch-up growth in girls with eating disorders and onset of weight loss before puberty. *Int J Eat Disord.* 2005;38(4):340–345

87. Katzman DK, Zipursky RB. Adolescents and anorexia nervosa: impact of the disorder on bones and brains. *Ann N Y Acad Sci.* 1997;817:127–137

88. Misra M, Klibanski A. Anorexia nervosa and osteoporosis. *Rev Endocr Metab Disord.* 2006;7(1–2):91–99

89. Katzman DK, Zipursky RB, Lambe EK, Mikulis DJ. Longitudinal magnetic resonance imaging study of the brain changes in adolescents with anorexia nervosa. *Arch Pediatr Adolesc Med.* 1997;151(8):793–797

90. Van den Eynde F, Treasure J. Neuroimaging in eating disorders and obesity: implications for research. *Child Adolesc Psychiatr Clin N Am.* 2009;18(1):95–115

91. Golden NH, Katzman DK, Kreipe RE, et al; Society For Adolescent Medicine. Eating disorders in adolescents: a position paper of the Society for Adolescent Medicine. *J Adolesc Health.* 2003;33(6):496–503

92. Rock CL, Curran-Celentano J. Nutritional disorder of anorexia nervosa: a review. *Int J Eat Disord.* 1994;15(2):187–203

93. Rock CL, Curran-Celentano J. Nutritional management of eating disorders. *Psychiatr Clin North Am.* 1996;19(4):701–713

94. Rome ES, Vazquez IM, Emans SJ. Nutritional problems in adolescence: anorexia nervosa/bulimia nervosa for young athletes. In: Walker WA, Watkins JB, eds. *Nutrition in Pediatrics: Basic Science and Clinical Applications.* 2nd ed. Hamilton, Ontario, Canada: BC Decker Inc; 1997: 691–704

95. American Dietetic Association. Position of the American Dietetic Association: nutrition intervention in the treatment of anorexia nervosa, bulimia nervosa, and other eating disorders. *J Am Diet Assoc.* 2006;106(12):2073–2082

96. Kreipe R, Uphoff M. Treatment and outcome of adolescents with anorexia nervosa. *Adolesc Med.* 1992;3(3):519–540

97. Yager J. Psychosocial treatments for eating disorders. *Psychiatry.* 1994;57(2): 153–164

98. Powers PS. Initial assessment and early treatment options for anorexia nervosa and bulimia nervosa. *Psychiatr Clin North Am.* 1996;19(4):639–655

99. Robin AL, Gilroy M, Dennis AB. Treatment of eating disorders in children and adolescents. *Clin Psychol Rev.* 1998;18(4): 421–446

100. Golden NH, Jacobson MS, Schebendach J, Solanto MV, Hertz SM, Shenker IR. Resumption of menses in anorexia nervosa. *Arch Pediatr Adolesc Med.* 1997;151(1):16–21

101. Golden NH, Jacobson MS, Meyer-Sterling W, Hertz S. Treatment goal weight in adolescents with anorexia nervosa: use of BMI percentiles. *Int J Eat Disord.* 2008;41(4): 301–306

102. le Grange D, Eisler I. Family interventions in adolescent anorexia nervosa. *Child Adolesc Psychiatr Clin N Am.* 2009;18(1): 159–173

103. Lock J, Couturier J, Agras WS. Comparison of long-term outcomes in adolescents with anorexia nervosa treated with family therapy. *J Am Acad Child Adolesc Psychiatry.* 2006;45(6):666–672

104. Eisler I, Simic M, Russell GFM, Dare C. A randomized controlled treatment trial of two forms of family therapy in adolescent anorexia nervosa: a five year follow-up. *J Child Psychol Psychiatry.* 2007;48(6): 552–560

105. Findlay S, Pinzon J, Taddeo D, Katzman D; Canadian Paediatric Society, Adolescent Health Committee. Family-based treatment of children and adolescents with anorexia nervosa: guidelines for the community physician. *Paediatr Child Health.* 2010; 15(1):31–35

106. Lock J, le Grange D, Agras WS, Dare C. *Treatment Manual for Anorexia Nervosa: A Family-Based Approach.* New York, NY: Guilford Press; 2001

107. Lock J, le Grange D. *Help Your Teenager Beat an Eating Disorder.* New York, NY: Guilford Press; 2004

108. Schmidt U, Lee S, Beecham J, et al. A randomized controlled trial of family therapy and cognitive behavior therapy guided self-care for adolescents with bulimia nervosa and related disorders. *Am J Psychiatry.* 2007;164(4):591–598

109. Zipfel S, Reas DL, Thornton C, et al. Day hospitalization programs for eating

disorders: a systematic review of the literature. *Int J Eat Disord.* 2002;31(2):105–117

110. Kaplan AS, Olmstead MP. Partial hospitalization. In: Garner DM, Garfinkel PE, eds. *Handbook of Treatment for Eating Disorders.* 2nd ed. New York, NY: Guilford Press; 1997:354–360

111. Kaplan AS, Olmstead MP, Molleken L. Day treatment of eating disorders. In: Jimerson D, Kaye WH, eds. *Bailliere's Clinical Psychiatry, Eating Disorders.* Philadelphia, PA: Bailliere Tindall; 1997:275–289

112. Howard WT, Evans KK, Quintero-Howard CV, Bowers WA, Andersen AE. Predictors of success or failure of transition to day hospital treatment for inpatients with anorexia nervosa. *Am J Psychiatry.* 1999; 156(11):1697–1702

113. Fittig E, Jacobi C, Backmund H, et al. Effectiveness of day hospital treatment for anorexia and bulimia nervosa. *Eur Eat Disord Rev.* 2008;16(5):341–351

114. Dancyger I, Fornari V, Schneider M, et al. Adolescents and eating disorders: an examination of a day treatment program. *Eat Weight Disord.* 2003;8(3):242–248

115. National Institute for Clinical Excellence. *Eating Disorders: Core Interventions in the Treatment and Management of Anorexia Nervosa, Bulimia Nervosa, and Related Eating Disorders.* London, England: National Institute for Clinical Excellence; 2004

116. Silber TJ. Eating disorders and health insurance. *Arch Pediatr Adolesc Med.* 1994; 148(8):785–788

117. Sigman G. How has the care of eating disorder patients been altered and upset by payment and insurance issues? Let me count the ways. *J Adolesc Health.* 1996; 19(5):317–318

118. Baran SA, Weltzin TE, Kaye WH. Low discharge weight and outcome in anorexia nervosa. *Am J Psychiatry.* 1995;152(7): 1070–1072

119. Silber TJ, Robb AS, Orrell-Valente JK, Ellis N, Valadez-Meltzer A, Dadson MJ. Nocturnal nasogastric refeeding for hospitalized adolescent boys with anorexia nervosa. *J Dev Behav Pediatr.* 2004;25(6):415–418

120. Solomon SM, Kirby DF. The refeeding syndrome: a review. *JPEN J Parenter Enteral Nutr.* 1990;14(1):90–97

121. Birmingham CL, Alothman AF, Goldner EM. Anorexia nervosa: refeeding and hy-

pophosphatemia. *Int J Eat Disord.* 1996;20(2):211–213

122. Kohn MR, Golden NH, Shenker IR. Cardiac arrest and delirium: presentations of the refeeding syndrome in severely malnourished adolescents with anorexia nervosa. *J Adolesc Health.* 1998;22(3):239–243

123. Fisher M, Simpser E, Schneider M. Hypophosphatemia secondary to oral refeeding in anorexia nervosa. *Int J Eat Disord.* 2000;28(2):181–187

124. Powers PS, Bruty H. Pharmacotherapy for eating disorders and obesity. *Child Adolesc Psychiatr Clin N Am.* 2009;18(1): 175–187

125. Kaye W, Nagata T, Weltzin TE, et al. Double blind placebo controlled administration of fluoxetine in restricting type anorexia nervosa. *Biol Psychiatry.* 2001;49(7):644–652

126. Brambilla F, Garcia CS, Fassino S, et al. Olanzapine therapy in anorexia nervosa: psychobiological effects. *Int Clin Psychopharmacol.* 2007;22(4):197–204

127. Bissada H, Tasca GA, Barber AM, Bradwejn J. Olanzapine in the treatment of low body weight and obsessive thinking in women with anorexia nervosa: a randomized double-blind placebo-controlled trial. *Am J Psychiatry.* 2008;165(10):1281–1288

128. Fluoxetine Bulimia Nervosa Collaborative Study Group. Fluoxetine in the treatment of bulimia nervosa: a multi-center placebo-controlled double-blind trial. *Arch Gen Psychiatry.* 1992;49(2):139–147

129. McElroy SL, Arnold LM, Shapira NA, et al. Topirimate in the treatment of binge eating disorder associated with obesity: a randomized placebo-controlled trial [published correction appears in *Am J Psychiatry.* 2003;160(3):612]. *Am J Psychiatry.* 2003;160(2):255–261

130. Steffen KJ, Roerig JL, Mitchell JE, Uppala S. Emerging drugs for eating disorder treatment. *Expert Opin Emerg Drugs.* 2006; 11(2):315–336

131. Fisher M. Course and outcome of eating disorders in adults and adolescents: a review. *Adolesc Med.* 2003;14(1):149–158

132. Strober M, Freeman R, Morrell W. The long-term course of severe anorexia nervosa in adolescents: survival analysis of recovery, relapse, and outcome predictors over 10–15 years in a prospective study. *Int J Eat Disord.* 1997;22(4):339–360

133. Steinhausen HC. Outcome of anorexia ner-

vosa in the 20th century. *Am J Psychiatry.* 2002;159(8):1284–1293

134. Steinhausen HC. Outcome of eating disorders. *Child Adolesc Psychiatr Clin N Am.* 2009;18(1):225–242

135. Herpertz-Dahlmann B, Muller B, Herpertz S, Heussen N. Prospective 10-year follow-up in adolescent anorexia nervosa: course, outcome, psychiatric comorbidity, and psychosocial adaptation. *J Child Psychol Psychiatry.* 2001;42(5):603–612

136. Johnson JG, Cohen P, Kasen S, Brook JS. Eating disorders during adolescence and the risk of physical and mental disorders during early adulthood. *Arch Gen Psychiatry.* 2002;59(6):545–552

137. Silberg JL, Bulik CM. The developmental association between eating disorders symptoms and symptoms of depression and anxiety in juvenile twin girls. *J Child Psychol Psychiatry.* 2005;46(12):1317–1326

138. Adolescent Health Committee, Canadian Paediatric Society. Dieting in adolescence. *Paediatr Child Health.* 2004;9(7): 487–491

139. Shaw H, Stice E, Becker CB. Preventing eating disorders. *Child Adolesc Psychiatr Clin N Am.* 2009;18(1):199–207

140. Stice E, Shaw H. Eating disorder prevention programs: a meta-analytic review. *Psychol Bull.* 2004;130(2):206–227

141. Killen JD, Taylor CB, Hammer LD, et al. An attempt to modify unhealthful eating attitudes and weight regulation practices of young adolescent girls. *Int J Eat Disord.* 1993;13(4):369–384

142. Neumark-Sztainer D, Butler R, Palti H. Eating disturbances among adolescent girls: evaluation of a school-based primary prevention program. *J Nutr Educ.* 1995;27(1): 24–31

143. Neumark-Sztainer D. School-based programs for preventing eating disturbances. *J Sch Health.* 1996;66(2):64–71

144. Carter JC, Stewart DA, Dunn VJ, Fairburn CG. Primary prevention of eating disorders: might it do more harm than good? *Int J Eat Disord.* 1997;22(2):167–172

145. Martz DM, Bazzini DG. Eating disorder prevention programs may be failing: evaluation of 2 one-shot programs. *J Coll Stud Dev.* 1999;40(1):32–42

146. Hartley P. Does health education promote eating disorders? *Eur Eat Disord Rev.* 1996; 4(1):3–11

American Academy
of Pediatrics
DEDICATED TO THE HEALTH OF ALL CHILDREN™

Organizational Principles to Guide and Define the Child
Health Care System and/or Improve the Health of all Children

CLINICAL PRACTICE GUIDELINE

Management of Newly Diagnosed Type 2 Diabetes Mellitus (T2DM) in Children and Adolescents

abstract

Over the past 3 decades, the prevalence of childhood obesity has increased dramatically in North America, ushering in a variety of health problems, including type 2 diabetes mellitus (T2DM), which previously was not typically seen until much later in life. The rapid emergence of childhood T2DM poses challenges to many physicians who find themselves generally ill-equipped to treat adult diseases encountered in children. This clinical practice guideline was developed to provide evidence-based recommendations on managing 10- to 18-year-old patients in whom T2DM has been diagnosed. The American Academy of Pediatrics (AAP) convened a Subcommittee on Management of T2DM in Children and Adolescents with the support of the American Diabetes Association, the Pediatric Endocrine Society, the American Academy of Family Physicians, and the Academy of Nutrition and Dietetics (formerly the American Dietetic Association). These groups collaborated to develop an evidence report that served as a major source of information for these practice guideline recommendations. The guideline emphasizes the use of management modalities that have been shown to affect clinical outcomes in this pediatric population. Recommendations are made for situations in which either insulin or metformin is the preferred first-line treatment of children and adolescents with T2DM. The recommendations suggest integrating lifestyle modifications (ie, diet and exercise) in concert with medication rather than as an isolated initial treatment approach. Guidelines for frequency of monitoring hemoglobin A1c (HbA1c) and finger-stick blood glucose (BG) concentrations are presented. Decisions were made on the basis of a systematic grading of the quality of evidence and strength of recommendation. The clinical practice guideline underwent peer review before it was approved by the AAP. This clinical practice guideline is not intended to replace clinical judgment or establish a protocol for the care of all children with T2DM, and its recommendations may not provide the only appropriate approach to the management of children with T2DM. Providers should consult experts trained in the care of children and adolescents with T2DM when treatment goals are not met or when therapy with insulin is initiated. The AAP acknowledges that some primary care clinicians may not be confident of their ability to successfully treat T2DM in a child because of the child's age, coexisting conditions, and/or other concerns. At any point at which a clinician feels he or she is not adequately trained or is uncertain about treatment, a referral to a pediatric medical subspecialist should be made. If a diagnosis of T2DM is made by a pediatric medical subspecialist, the primary care clinician should develop a comanagement strategy with the subspecialist to ensure that the child continues to receive appropriate care consistent with a medical home model in which the pediatrician partners with parents to ensure that all health needs are met. *Pediatrics* 2013;131:364–382

Kenneth C. Copeland, MD, Janet Silverstein, MD, Kelly R. Moore, MD, Greg E. Prazar, MD, Terry Raymer, MD, CDE, Richard N. Shiffman, MD, Shelley C. Springer, MD, MBA, Vidhu V. Thaker, MD, Meaghan Anderson, MS, RD, LD, CDE, Stephen J. Spann, MD, MBA, and Susan K. Flinn, MA

KEY WORDS
diabetes, type 2 diabetes mellitus, childhood, youth, clinical practice guidelines, comanagement, management, treatment

ABBREVIATIONS
AAP—American Academy of Pediatrics
AAFP—American Academy of Family Physicians
BG—blood glucose
FDA—US Food and Drug Administration
HbA1c—hemoglobin A1c
PES—Pediatric Endocrine Society
T1DM—type 1 diabetes mellitus
T2DM—type 2 diabetes mellitus
TODAY—Treatment Options for type 2 Diabetes in Adolescents and Youth

This document is copyrighted and is property of the American Academy of Pediatrics and its Board of Directors. All authors have filed conflict of interest statements with the American Academy of Pediatrics. Any conflicts have been resolved through a process approved by the Board of Directors. The American Academy of Pediatrics has neither solicited nor accepted any commercial involvement in the development of the content of this publication.

The recommendations in this report do not indicate an exclusive course of treatment or serve as a standard of medical care. Variations, taking into account individual circumstances, may be appropriate.

All clinical practice guidelines from the American Academy of Pediatrics automatically expire 5 years after publication unless reaffirmed, revised, or retired at or before that time.

www.pediatrics.org/cgi/doi/10.1542/peds.2012-3494

doi:10.1542/peds.2012-3494

PEDIATRICS (ISSN Numbers: Print, 0031-4005; Online, 1098-4275).

Key action statements are as follows:

1. Clinicians must ensure that insulin therapy is initiated for children and adolescents with T2DM who are ketotic or in diabetic ketoacidosis and in whom the distinction between types 1 and 2 diabetes mellitus is unclear and, in usual cases, should initiate insulin therapy for patients

    a. who have random venous or plasma BG concentrations ≥250 mg/dL; or

    b. whose HbA1c is >9%.

2. In all other instances, clinicians should initiate a lifestyle modification program, including nutrition and physical activity, and start metformin as first-line therapy for children and adolescents at the time of diagnosis of T2DM.

3. The committee suggests that clinicians monitor HbA1c concentrations every 3 months and intensify treatment if treatment goals for finger-stick BG and HbA1c concentrations are not being met (intensification is defined in the Definitions box).

4. The committee suggests that clinicians advise patients to monitor finger-stick BG (see Key Action Statement 4 in the guideline for further details) concentrations in patients who

    a. are taking insulin or other medications with a risk of hypoglycemia; or

    b. are initiating or changing their diabetes treatment regimen; or

    c. have not met treatment goals; or

    d. have intercurrent illnesses.

5. The committee suggests that clinicians incorporate the Academy of Nutrition and Dietetics' *Pediatric Weight Management Evidence-Based Nutrition Practice Guidelines* in their dietary or nutrition counseling of patients with T2DM at the time of diagnosis and as part of ongoing management.

6. The committee suggests that clinicians encourage children and adolescents with T2DM to engage in moderate-to-vigorous exercise for at least 60 minutes daily and to limit nonacademic "screen time" to less than 2 hours a day.

Definitions

Adolescent: an individual in various stages of maturity, generally considered to be between 12 and 18 years of age.

Childhood T2DM: disease in the child who typically

- is overweight or obese (BMI ≥85th–94th and >95th percentile for age and gender, respectively);

- has a strong family history of T2DM;

- has substantial residual insulin secretory capacity at diagnosis (reflected by normal or elevated insulin and C-peptide concentrations);

- has insidious onset of disease;

- demonstrates insulin resistance (including clinical evidence of polycystic ovarian syndrome or acanthosis nigricans);

- lacks evidence for diabetic autoimmunity (negative for autoantibodies typically associated with T1DM). These patients are more likely to have hypertension and dyslipidemia than are those with T1DM.

Clinician: any provider within his or her scope of practice; includes medical practitioners (including physicians and physician extenders), dietitians, psychologists, and nurses.

Diabetes: according to the American Diabetes Association criteria, defined as

1. HbA1c ≥6.5% (test performed in an appropriately certified laboratory); or

2. fasting (defined as no caloric intake for at least 8 hours) plasma glucose ≥126 mg/dL (7.0 mmol/L); or

3. 2-hour plasma glucose ≥200 mg/dL (11.1 mmol/L) during an oral glucose tolerance test performed as described by the World Health Organization by using a glucose load containing the equivalent of 75 g anhydrous glucose dissolved in water; or

4. a random plasma glucose ≥200 mg/dL (11.1 mmol/L) with symptoms of hyperglycemia.

(In the absence of unequivocal hyperglycemia, criteria 1–3 should be confirmed by repeat testing.)

Diabetic ketoacidosis: acidosis resulting from an absolute or relative insulin deficiency, causing fat breakdown and formation of β hydroxybutyrate. Symptoms include nausea, vomiting, dehydration, Kussmaul respirations, and altered mental status.

Fasting blood glucose: blood glucose obtained before the first meal of the day and after a fast of at least 8 hours.

Glucose toxicity: The effect of high blood glucose causing both insulin resistance and impaired β-cell production of insulin.

Intensification: Increase frequency of blood glucose monitoring and adjustment of the dose and type of medication in an attempt to normalize blood glucose concentrations.

Intercurrent illnesses: Febrile illnesses or associated symptoms severe enough to cause the patient to stay home from school and/or seek medical care.

Microalbuminuria: Albumin:creatinine ratio ≥30 mg/g creatinine but <300 mg/g creatinine.

Moderate hyperglycemia: blood glucose = 180–250 mg/dL.

Moderate-to-vigorous exercise: exercise that makes the individual breathe hard and perspire and that raises his or her heart rate. An easy way to define exercise intensity for patients is the "talk test": during moderate physical activity a person can talk, but not sing. During vigorous activity, a person cannot talk without pausing to catch a breath.

Obese: BMI ≥95th percentile for age and gender.

Overweight: BMI between the 85th and 94th percentile for age and gender.

Prediabetes: Fasting plasma glucose ≥100–125 mg/dL or 2-hour glucose concentration during an oral glucose tolerance test ≥126 but <200 mg/dL or an HbA1c of 5.7% to 6.4%.

Severe hyperglycemia: blood glucose >250 mg/dL.

Thiazolidinediones (TZDs): Oral hypoglycemic agents that exert their effect at least in part by activation of the peroxisome proliferator-activated receptor γ.

Type 1 diabetes mellitus (T1DM): Diabetes secondary to autoimmune destruction of β cells resulting in absolute (complete or near complete) insulin deficiency and requiring insulin injections for management.

Type 2 diabetes mellitus (T2DM): The investigators' designation of the diagnosis was used for the purposes of the literature review. The committee acknowledges the distinction between T1DM and T2DM in this population is not always clear cut, and clinical judgment plays an important role. Typically, this diagnosis is made when hyperglycemia is secondary to insulin resistance accompanied by impaired β-cell function resulting in inadequate insulin production to compensate for the degree of insulin resistance.

Youth: used interchangeably with "adolescent" in this document.

INTRODUCTION

Over the past 3 decades, the prevalence of childhood obesity has increased dramatically in North America,[1–5] ushering in a variety of health problems, including type 2 diabetes mellitus (T2DM), which previously was not typically seen until much later in life. Currently, in the United States, up to 1 in 3 new cases of diabetes mellitus diagnosed in youth younger than 18 years is T2DM (depending on the ethnic composition of the patient population),[6,7] with a disproportionate representation in ethnic minorities[8,9] and occurring most commonly among youth between 10 and 19 years of age.[5,10] This trend is not limited to the United States but is occurring internationally[11]; it is projected that by the year 2030, an estimated 366 million people worldwide will have diabetes mellitus.[12]

The rapid emergence of childhood T2DM poses challenges to many physicians who find themselves generally ill-equipped to treat adult diseases encountered in children. Most diabetes education materials designed for pediatric patients are directed primarily to families of children with type 1 diabetes mellitus (T1DM) and emphasize insulin treatment and glucose monitoring, which may or may not be appropriate for children with

T2DM.[13,14] The National Diabetes Education Program TIP sheets (which can be ordered or downloaded from www.yourdiabetesinfo.org or ndep.nih.gov) provide guidance on healthy eating, physical activity, and dealing with T2DM in children and adolescents, but few other resources are available that are directly targeted at youth with this disease.[15] Most medications used for T2DM have been tested for safety and efficacy only in people older than 18 years, and there is scant scientific evidence for optimal management of children with T2DM.[16,17] Recognizing the scarcity of evidence-based data, this report provides a set of guidelines for the management and treatment of children with T2DM that is based on a review of current medical literature covering a period from January 1, 1990, to July 1, 2008.

Despite these limitations, the practicing physician is likely to be faced with the need to provide care for children with T2DM. Thus, the American Academy of Pediatrics (AAP), the Pediatric Endocrine Society (PES), the American Academy of Family Physicians (AAFP), American Diabetes Association, and the Academy of Nutrition and Dietetics (formerly the American Dietetic Association) partnered to develop a set of guidelines that might benefit endocrinologists and generalists, including pediatricians and family physicians alike. This clinical practice guideline may not provide the only appropriate approach to the management of children with T2DM. It is not expected to serve as a sole source of guidance in the management of children and adolescents with T2DM, nor is it intended to replace clinical judgment or establish a protocol for the care of all children with this condition. Rather, it is intended to assist clinicians in decision-making.

Primary care providers should endeavor to obtain the requisite skills to care for children and adolescents with T2DM, and should communicate and work closely with a diabetes team of subspecialists when such consultation is available, practical, and appropriate. The frequency of such consultations will vary, but should usually be obtained at diagnosis and then at least annually if possible. When treatment goals are not met, the committee encourages clinicians to consult with an expert trained in the care of children and adolescents with T2DM.[18,19] When first-line therapy (eg, metformin) fails, recommendations for intensifying therapy should be generally the same for pediatric and adult populations. The picture is constantly changing, however, as new drugs are introduced, and some drugs that initially appeared to be safe demonstrate adverse effects with wider use. Clinicians should, therefore, remain alert to new developments with regard to treatment of T2DM. Seeking the advice of an expert can help ensure that the treatment goals are appropriately set and that clinicians benefit from cutting-edge treatment information in this rapidly changing area.

The Importance of Family-Centered Diabetes Care

Family structure, support, and education help inform clinical decision-making and negotiations with the patient and family about medical preferences that affect medical decisions, independent of existing clinical recommendations. Because adherence is a major issue in any lifestyle intervention, engaging the family is critical not only to maintain needed changes in lifestyle but also to foster medication adherence.[20–22] The family's ideal role in lifestyle interventions varies, however, depending on the child's age. Behavioral interventions in younger children have shown a favorable effect. With adolescents, however, interventions based on target-age behaviors (eg, including phone or Internet-based interventions as well as face-to-face or peer-enhanced activities) appear to foster better results, at least for weight management.[23]

Success in making lifestyle changes to attain therapeutic goals requires the initial and ongoing education of the patient and the entire family about healthy nutrition and exercise. Any behavior change recommendations must establish realistic goals and take into account the families' health beliefs and behaviors. Understanding the patient and family's perception of the disease (and overweight status) before establishing a management plan is important to dispel misconceptions and promote adherence.[24] Because T2DM disproportionately affects minority populations, there is a need to ensure culturally appropriate, family-centered care along with ongoing education.[25–28] Several observational studies cite the importance of addressing cultural issues within the family.[20–22]

Restrictions in Creating This Document

In developing these guidelines, the following restrictions governed the committee's work:

- Although the importance of diabetes detection and screening of at-risk populations is acknowledged and referenced, the guidelines are restricted to patients meeting the diagnostic criteria for diabetes (eg, this document focuses on treatment postdiagnosis). Specifically, this document and its recommendations do not pertain to patients with impaired fasting plasma glucose (100–125 mg/dL) or impaired glucose tolerance (2-hour oral glucose tolerance test plasma glucose: 140–200 mg/dL) or isolated insulin resistance.

- Although it is noted that the distinction between types 1 and 2 diabetes mellitus in children may be difficult,[29,30] these recommendations pertain specifically to patients 10 to less than 18 years of age with T2DM (as defined above).

- Although the importance of high-risk care and glycemic control in pregnancy, including pregravid glycemia, is affirmed, the evidence considered and recommendations contained in this document do not pertain to diabetes in pregnancy, including diabetes in pregnant adolescents.

- Recommended screening schedules and management tools for select comorbid conditions (hypertension, dyslipidemia, nephropathy, microalbuminuria, and depression) are provided as resources in the accompanying technical report.[31] These therapeutic recommendations were adapted from other recommended guideline documents with references, without an independent assessment of their supporting evidence.

METHODS

A systematic review was performed and is described in detail in the accompanying technical report.[31] To develop the clinical practice guideline on the management of T2DM in children and adolescents, the AAP convened the Subcommittee on Management of T2DM in Children and Adolescents with the support of the American Diabetes Association, the PES, the AAFP, and the Academy of Nutrition and Dietetics. The subcommittee was co-chaired by 2 pediatric endocrinologists preeminent in their field and included experts in general pediatrics, family medicine, nutrition, Native American health, epidemiology, and medical informatics/guideline methodology. All panel members reviewed the AAP policy on Conflict of Interest and Voluntary Disclosure and declared all potential conflicts (see conflicts statements in the Task Force member list).

These groups partnered to develop an evidence report that served as a major source of information for these practice guideline recommendations.[31] Specific clinical questions addressed in the evidence review were as follows: (1) the effectiveness of treatment modalities for T2DM in children and adolescents, (2) the efficacy of pharmaceutical therapies for treatment of children and adolescents with T2DM, (3) appropriate recommendations for screening for comorbidities typically associated with T2DM in children and adolescents, and (4) treatment recommendations for comorbidities of T2DM in children and adolescents. The accompanying technical report contains more information on comorbidities.[31]

Epidemiologic project staff searched Medline, the Cochrane Collaboration, and Embase. MESH terms used in various combinations in the search included diabetes, mellitus, type 2, type 1, treatment, prevention, diet, pediatric, T2DM, T1DM, NIDDM, metformin, lifestyle, RCT, meta-analysis, child, adolescent, therapeutics, control, adult, obese, gestational, polycystic ovary syndrome, metabolic syndrome, cardiovascular, dyslipidemia, men, and women. In addition, the Boolean

operators NOT, AND, OR were included in various combinations. Articles addressing treatment of diabetes mellitus were prospectively limited to those that were published in English between January 1990 and June 2008, included abstracts, and addressed children between the ages of 120 and 215 months with an established diagnosis of T2DM. Studies in adults were considered for inclusion if >10% of the study population was 45 years of age or younger. The Medline search limits included the following: clinical trial; meta-analysis; randomized controlled trial; review; child: 6–12 years; and adolescent: 13–18 years. Additional articles were identified by review of reference lists of relevant articles and ongoing studies recommended by a technical expert advisory group. All articles were reviewed for compliance with the search limitations and appropriateness for inclusion in this document.

Initially, 199 abstracts were identified for possible inclusion, of which 52 were retained for systematic review. Results of the literature review were presented in evidence tables and published in the final evidence report. An additional literature search of Medline and the Cochrane Database of

FIGURE 1
Evidence quality. Integrating evidence quality appraisal with an assessment of the anticipated balance between benefits and harms if a policy is carried out leads to designation of a policy as a strong recommendation, recommendation, option, or no recommendation.[32] RCT, randomized controlled trial; Rec, recommendation.

TABLE 1 Definitions and Recommendation Implications

Statement	Definition	Implication
Strong recommendation	A *strong recommendation* in favor of a particular action is made when the anticipated benefits of the recommended intervention clearly exceed the harms (as a strong recommendation against an action is made when the anticipated harms clearly exceed the benefits) and the quality of the supporting evidence is excellent. In some clearly identified circumstances, strong recommendations may be made when high-quality evidence is impossible to obtain and the anticipated benefits strongly outweigh the harms.	Clinicians should follow a strong recommendation unless a clear and compelling rationale for an alternative approach is present.
Recommendation	A *recommendation* in favor of a particular action is made when the anticipated benefits exceed the harms but the quality of evidence is not as strong. Again, in some clearly identified circumstances, recommendations may be made when high-quality evidence is impossible to obtain but the anticipated benefits outweigh the harms.	Clinicians would be prudent to follow a recommendation but should remain alert to new information and sensitive to patient preferences.
Option	*Options* define courses that may be taken when either the quality of evidence is suspect or carefully performed studies have shown little clear advantage to 1 approach over another.	Clinicians should consider the option in their decision-making, and patient preference may have a substantial role.
No recommendation	*No recommendation* indicates that there is a lack of pertinent published evidence and that the anticipated balance of benefits and harms is presently unclear.	Clinicians should be alert to new published evidence that clarifies the balance of benefit versus harm.

It should be noted that, because childhood T2DM is a relatively recent medical phenomenon, there is a paucity of evidence for many or most of the recommendations provided. In some cases, supporting references for a specific recommendation are provided that do not deal specifically with childhood T2DM, such as T1DM, childhood obesity, or childhood "prediabetes," or that were not included in the original comprehensive search. Committee members have made every effort to identify those references that did not affect or alter the level of evidence for specific recommendations.

Systematic Reviews was performed in July 2009 for articles discussing recommendations for screening and treatment of 5 recognized comorbidities of T2DM: cardiovascular disease, dyslipidemia, retinopathy, nephropathy, and peripheral vascular disease. Search criteria were the same as for the search on treatment of T2DM, with the inclusion of the term "type 1 diabetes mellitus." Search terms included, in various combinations, the following: diabetes, mellitus, type 2, type 1, pediatric, T2DM, T1DM, NIDDM, hyperlipidemia, retinopathy, microalbuminuria, comorbidities, screening, RCT, meta-analysis, child, and adolescent. Boolean operators and search limits mirrored those of the primary search.

An additional 336 abstracts were identified for possible inclusion, of which 26 were retained for systematic review. Results of this subsequent literature review were also presented in evidence tables and published in

the final evidence report. An epidemiologist appraised the methodologic quality of the research before it was considered by the committee members.

The evidence-based approach to guideline development requires that the evidence in support of each key action statement be identified, appraised, and summarized and that an explicit link between evidence and recommendations be defined. Evidence-based recommendations reflect the quality of evidence and the balance of benefit and harm that is anticipated when the recommendation is followed. The AAP policy statement, "Classifying Recommendations for Clinical Practice Guidelines,"[32] was followed in designating levels of recommendation (see Fig 1 and Table 1).

To ensure that these recommendations can be effectively implemented, the Guidelines Review Group at Yale Center for Medical Informatics provided feedback

on a late draft of these recommendations, using the GuideLine Implementability Appraisal.[33] Several potential obstacles to successful implementation were identified and resolved in the final guideline. Evidence was incorporated systematically into 6 key action statements about appropriate management facilitated by BRIDGE-Wiz software (Building Recommendations in a Developer's Guideline Editor; Yale Center for Medical Informatics).

A draft version of this clinical practice guideline underwent extensive peer review by 8 groups within the AAP, the American Diabetes Association, PES, AAFP, and the Academy of Nutrition and Dietetics. Members of the subcommittee were invited to distribute the draft to other representatives and committees within their specialty organizations. The resulting comments were reviewed by the subcommittee and incorporated into the guideline, as appropriate. All AAP guidelines are reviewed every 5 years.

KEY ACTION STATEMENTS

Key Action Statement 1

Clinicians must ensure that insulin therapy is initiated for children and adolescents with T2DM who are ketotic or in diabetic ketoacidosis and in whom the distinction between T1DM and T2DM is unclear; and, in usual cases, should initiate insulin therapy for patients:

a. who have random venous or plasma BG concentrations ≥250 mg/dL; or

b. whose HbA1c is >9%.

(Strong Recommendation: evidence quality X, validating studies cannot be performed, and C, observational studies and expert opinion; preponderance of benefit over harm.)

Action Statement Profile KAS 1

Aggregate evidence quality	X (validating studies cannot be performed)
Benefits	Avoidance of progression of diabetic ketoacidosis (DKA) and worsening metabolic acidosis; resolution of acidosis and hyperglycemia; avoidance of coma and/or death. Quicker restoration of glycemic control, potentially allowing islet β cells to "rest and recover," increasing long-term adherence to treatment; avoiding progression to DKA if T1DM. Avoiding hospitalization. Avoidance of potential risks associated with the use of other agents (eg, abdominal discomfort, bloating, loose stools with metformin; possible cardiovascular risks with sulfonylureas).
Harms/risks/cost	Potential for hypoglycemia, insulin-induced weight gain, cost, patient discomfort from injection, necessity for BG testing, more time required by the health care team for patient training.
Benefits-harms assessment	Preponderance of benefit over harm.
Value judgments	Extensive clinical experience of the expert panel was relied on in making this recommendation.
Role of patient preferences	Minimal.
Exclusions	None.
Intentional vagueness	None.
Strength	Strong recommendation.

The presentation of T2DM in children and adolescents varies according to the disease stage. Early in the disease, before diabetes diagnostic criteria are met, insulin resistance predominates with compensatory high insulin secretion, resulting in normoglycemia. Over time, β cells lose their ability to secrete adequate amounts of insulin to overcome insulin resistance, and hyperglycemia results. Early in this process, blood glucose (BG) concentrations may be normal much of the time and the patient likely will be asymptomatic. At this stage, the disease may only be detected by abnormal BG concentrations identified during screening. As insulin secretion declines further, the patient is likely to develop symptoms of hyperglycemia, occasionally with ketosis or frank ketoacidosis. High glucose concentrations can cause a reversible toxicity to islet β cells that contributes further to insulin deficiency. Of adolescents in whom T2DM is subsequently diagnosed, 5% to 25% present with ketoacidosis.[34]

Diabetic ketoacidosis must be treated with insulin and fluid and electrolyte replacement to prevent worsening metabolic acidosis, coma, and death. Children and adolescents with symptoms of hyperglycemia (polyuria, polydipsia, and polyphagia) who are diagnosed with diabetes mellitus should be evaluated for ketosis (serum or urine ketones) and, if positive, for ketoacidosis (venous pH), even if their phenotype and risk factor status (obesity, acanthosis nigricans, positive family history of T2DM) suggests T2DM. Patients in whom ketoacidosis is diagnosed require immediate treatment with insulin and fluid replacement in an inpatient setting under the supervision of a physician who is experienced in treating this complication.

Youth and adolescents who present with T2DM with poor glycemic control (BG concentrations ≥250 mg/dL or HbA1c >9%) but who lack evidence of ketosis or ketoacidosis may also benefit from initial treatment with insulin, at least on a short-term basis.[34] This allows for quicker restoration of glycemic control and, theoretically, may allow islet β cells to "rest and recover."[35,36] Furthermore, it has been noted that initiation of insulin may increase long-term adherence to treatment in children and adolescents with T2DM by enhancing the patient's perception of the seriousness of the disease.[7,37–40] Many patients with T2DM can be weaned gradually from insulin therapy and subsequently managed with metformin and lifestyle modification.[34]

As noted previously, in some children and adolescents with newly diagnosed diabetes mellitus, it may be difficult to distinguish between type 1 and type 2 disease (eg, an obese child presenting with ketosis).[39,41] These patients are best managed initially with insulin therapy while appropriate tests are performed to differentiate between T1DM and T2DM. The care of children and adolescents who have either newly diagnosed T2DM or undifferentiated-type diabetes and who require initial insulin treatment should be supervised by a physician experienced in treating diabetic patients with insulin.

Key Action Statement 2

In all other instances, clinicians should initiate a lifestyle modification program, including nutrition

and physical activity, and start metformin as first-line therapy for children and adolescents at the time of diagnosis of T2DM. (Strong recommendation: evidence quality B; 1 RCT showing improved outcomes with metformin versus lifestyle; preponderance of benefits over harms.)

committee recommends starting the drug at a low dose of 500 mg daily, increasing by 500 mg every 1 to 2 weeks, up to an ideal and maximum dose of 2000 mg daily in divided doses.[41] It should be noted that the main gastrointestinal adverse effects (abdominal pain, bloating, loose stools) present at initiation of metformin often are transient and often

credible RCTs in adolescents with T2DM. The evidence to recommend initiating metformin at diagnosis along with lifestyle changes comes from 1 RCT, several observational studies, and consensus recommendations.

Lifestyle modifications (including nutrition interventions and increased physical activity) have long been the cornerstone of therapy for T2DM. Yet, medical practitioners recognize that effecting these changes is both challenging and often accompanied by regression over time to behaviors not conducive to maintaining the target range of BG concentrations. In pediatric patients, lifestyle change is most likely to be successful when a multidisciplinary approach is used and the entire family is involved. (Encouragement of healthy eating and physical exercise are discussed in Key Action Statements 5 and 6.) Unfortunately, efforts at lifestyle change often fail for a variety of reasons, including high rates of loss to follow-up; a high rate of depression in teenagers, which affects adherence; and peer pressure to participate in activities that often center on unhealthy eating.

Expert consensus is that fewer than 10% of pediatric T2DM patients will attain their BG goals through lifestyle interventions alone.[6,35,44] It is possible that the poor long-term success rates observed from lifestyle interventions stem from patients' perception that the intervention is not important because medications are not being prescribed. One might speculate that prescribing medications, particularly insulin therapy, may convey a greater degree of concern for the patient's health and the seriousness of the diagnosis, relative to that conveyed when medications are not needed, and that improved treatment adherence and follow-up may result from the use of medication. Indeed, 2 prospective observational studies revealed that treatment with

Action Statement Profile KAS 2

Aggregate evidence quality	B (1 randomized controlled trial showing improved outcomes with metformin versus lifestyle combined with expert opinion).
Benefit	Lower HbA1c, target HbA1c sustained longer, less early deterioration of BG, less chance of weight gain, improved insulin sensitivity, improved lipid profile.
Harm (of using metformin)	Gastrointestinal adverse effects or potential for lactic acidosis and vitamin B_{12} deficiency, cost of medications, cost to administer, need for additional instruction about medication, self-monitoring blood glucose (SMBG), perceived difficulty of insulin use, possible metabolic deterioration if T1DM is misdiagnosed and treated as T2DM, potential risk of lactic acidosis in the setting of ketosis or significant dehydration. It should be noted that there have been no cases reported of vitamin B_{12} deficiency or lactic acidosis with the use of metformin in children.
Benefits-harms assessment	Preponderance of benefit over harm.
Value judgments	Committee members valued faster achievement of BG control over not medicating children.
Role of patient preferences	Moderate; precise implementation recommendations likely will be dictated by patient preferences regarding healthy nutrition, potential medication adverse reaction, exercise, and physical activity.
Exclusions	Although the recommendation to start metformin applies to all, certain children and adolescents with T2DM will not be able to tolerate metformin. In addition, certain older or more debilitated patients with T2DM may be restricted in the amount of moderate-to-vigorous exercise they can perform safely. Nevertheless, this recommendation applies to the vast majority of children and adolescents with T2DM.
Intentional vagueness	None.
Policy level	Strong recommendation.

Metformin as First-Line Therapy

Because of the low success rate with diet and exercise alone in pediatric patients diagnosed with T2DM, metformin should be initiated along with the promotion of lifestyle changes, unless insulin is needed to reverse glucose toxicity in the case of significant hyperglycemia or ketoacidosis (see Key Action Statement 1). Because gastrointestinal adverse effects are common with metformin therapy, the

disappear completely if medication is continued. Generally, doses higher than 2000 mg daily do not provide additional therapeutic benefit.[34,42,43] In addition, the use of extended-release metformin, especially with evening dosing, may be considered, although data regarding the frequency of adverse effects with this preparation are scarce. Metformin is generally better tolerated when taken with food. It is important to recognize the paucity of lifestyle modification alone is associated with a higher rate of loss to follow-up than that found in patients who receive medication.[45]

Before initiating treatment with metformin, a number of important considerations must be taken into account. First, it is important to determine whether the child with a new diagnosis has T1DM or T2DM, and it is critical to err on the side of caution if there is any uncertainty. The 2009 *Clinical Practice Consensus Guidelines on Type 2 Diabetes in Children and Adolescents* from the International Society for Pediatric and Adolescent Diabetes provides more information on the classification of diabetes in children and adolescents with new diagnoses.[46] If the diagnosis is unclear (as may be the case when an obese child with diabetes presents also with ketosis), the adolescent must be treated with insulin until the T2DM diagnosis is confirmed.[47] Although it is recognized that some children with newly diagnosed T2DM may respond to metformin alone, the committee believes that the presence of either ketosis or ketoacidosis dictates an absolute initial requirement for insulin replacement. (This is addressed in Key Action Statement 1.)

Although there is little debate that a child presenting with significant hyperglycemia and/or ketosis requires insulin, children presenting with more modest levels of hyperglycemia (eg, random BG of 200–249 mg/dL) or asymptomatic T2DM present additional therapeutic challenges to the clinician. In such cases, metformin alone, insulin alone, or metformin with insulin all represent reasonable options. Additional agents are likely to become reasonable options for initial pharmacologic management in the near future. Although metformin and insulin are the only antidiabetic agents currently approved by the US Food and Drug Administration (FDA) for use in children, both thiazolidinediones and incretins are occasionally used in adolescents younger than 18 years.[48]

Metformin is recommended as the initial pharmacologic agent in adolescents presenting with mild hyperglycemia and without ketonuria or severe hyperglycemia. In addition to improving hepatic insulin sensitivity, metformin has a number of practical advantages over insulin:

- Potential weight loss or weight neutrality.[37,48]

- Because of a lower risk of hypoglycemia, less frequent finger-stick BG measurements are required with metformin, compared with insulin therapy or sulfonylureas.[37,42,49–51]

- Improves insulin sensitivity and may normalize menstrual cycles in females with polycystic ovary syndrome. (Because metformin may also improve fertility in patients with polycystic ovary syndrome, contraception is indicated for sexually active patients who wish to avoid pregnancy.)

- Taking pills does not have the discomfort associated with injections.

- Less instruction time is required to start oral medication, making it is easier for busy practitioners to prescribe.

- Adolescents do not always accept injections, so oral medication might enhance adherence.[52]

Potential advantages of insulin over metformin for treatment at diabetes onset include the following:

- Metabolic control may be achieved more rapidly with insulin compared with metformin therapy.[37]

- With appropriate education and targeting the regimen to the individual, adolescents are able to accept and use insulin therapy with improved metabolic outcomes.[53]

- Insulin offers theoretical benefits of improved metabolic control while preserving β-cell function or even reversing β-cell damage.[34,35]

- Initial use of insulin therapy may convey to the patient a sense of seriousness of the disease.[7,53]

Throughout the writing of these guidelines, the authors have been following the progress of the National Institute of Diabetes and Digestive and Kidney Diseases–supported Treatment Options for type 2 Diabetes in Adolescents and Youth (TODAY) trial,[54] designed to compare standard (metformin alone) therapy versus more aggressive therapy as the initial treatment of youth with recent-onset T2DM. Since the completion of these guidelines, results of the TODAY trial have become available and reveal that metformin alone is inadequate in effecting sustained glycemic control in the majority of youth with diabetes. The study also revealed that the addition of rosiglitazone to metformin is superior to metformin alone in preserving glycemic control. Direct application of these findings to clinical practice is problematic, however, because rosiglitazone is not FDA-approved for use in children, and its use, even in adults, is now severely restricted by the FDA because of serious adverse effects reported in adults. Thus, the results suggest that therapy that is more aggressive than metformin monotherapy may be required in these adolescents to prevent loss of glycemic control, but they do not provide specific guidance because it is not known whether the effect of the additional agent was specific to rosiglitazone or would be seen with the addition of other agents. Unfortunately, there are limited data for the use of other currently available oral or injected hypoglycemic agents in this age range, except for insulin. Therefore, the writing group for these guidelines continues to recommend metformin as first-line therapy in this age group but with close monitoring for glycemic deterioration and the early addition of insulin or another pharmacologic agent if needed.

Lifestyle Modification, Including Nutrition and Physical Activity

Although lifestyle changes are considered indispensable to reaching treatment goals in diabetes, no significant data from RCTs provide information on success rates with such an approach alone.

A potential downside for initiating lifestyle changes alone at T2DM onset is potential loss of patients to follow-up and worse health outcomes. The value of lifestyle modification in the management of adolescents with T2DM is likely forthcoming after a more detailed analysis of the lifestyle intervention arm of the multicenter TODAY trial becomes available.[54] As noted previously, although it was published after

plus-rosiglitazone intervention in maintaining glycemic control over time.[54]

Summary

As noted previously, metformin is a safe and effective agent for use at the time of diagnosis in conjunction with lifestyle changes. Although observational studies and expert opinion strongly support lifestyle changes as a key component of the regimen in addition to metformin, randomized trials are needed to delineate whether using lifestyle options alone is a reasonable first step in treating any select subgroups of children with T2DM.

Key Action Statement 3

The committee suggests that clinicians monitor HbA1c concentrations every 3 months and intensify treatment if treatment goals for BG and HbA1c concentrations are not being met. (Option: evidence quality D; expert opinion and studies in children with T1DM and in adults with T2DM; preponderance of benefits over harms.)

evaluated the relationship between glycemic control and the risk of developing microvascular and/or macrovascular complications in children and adolescents with T2DM. A number of studies of children with T1DM[55–57] and adults with T2DM have, however, shown a significant relationship between glycemic control (as measured by HbA1c concentration) and the risk of microvascular complications (eg, retinopathy, nephropathy, and neuropathy).[58,59] The relationship between HbA1c concentration and risk of microvascular complications appears to be curvilinear; the lower the HbA1c concentration, the lower the downstream risk of microvascular complications, with the greatest risk reduction seen at the highest HbA1c concentrations.[57]

It is generally recommended that HbA1c concentrations be measured every 3 months.[60] For adults with T1DM, the American Diabetes Association recommends target HbA1c concentrations of less than 7%; the American Association of Clinical Endocrinologists recommends target concentrations of less than 6.5%. Although HbA1c target concentrations for children and adolescents with T1DM are higher,[13] several review articles suggest target HbA1c concentrations of less than 7% for children and adolescents with T2DM.[40,61–63] The committee concurs that, ideally, target HbA1c concentration should be less than 7% but notes that specific goals must be achievable for the individual patient and that this concentration may not be applicable for all patients. For patients in whom a target concentration of less than 7% seems unattainable, individualized goals should be set, with the ultimate goal of reaching guideline target concentrations. In addition, in the absence of hypoglycemia, even lower HbA1c target concentrations can be considered on the basis of an absence of hypoglycemic events and other individual considerations.

Action Statement Profile KAS 3

Aggregate evidence quality	D (expert opinion and studies in children with T1DM and in adults with T2DM; no studies have been performed in children and adolescents with T2DM).
Benefit	Diminishing the risk of progression of disease and deterioration resulting in hospitalization; prevention of microvascular complications of T2DM.
Harm	Potential for hypoglycemia from overintensifying treatment to reach HbA1c target goals; cost of frequent testing and medical consultation; possible patient discomfort.
Benefits-harms assessment	Preponderance of benefits over harms.
Value judgments	Recommendation dictated by widely accepted standards of diabetic care.
Role of patient preferences	Minimal; recommendation dictated by widely accepted standards of diabetic care.
Exclusions	None.
Intentional vagueness	Intentional vagueness in the recommendation as far as setting goals and intensifying treatment attributable to limited evidence.
Policy level	Option.

this guideline was developed, the TODAY trial indicated that results from the metformin-plus-lifestyle intervention were not significantly different from either metformin alone or the metformin-

HbA1c provides a measure of glycemic control in patients with diabetes mellitus and allows an estimation of the individual's average BG over the previous 8 to 12 weeks. No RCTs have

When concentrations are found to be above the target, therapy should be intensified whenever possible, with the goal of bringing the concentration to target. Intensification activities may include, but are not limited to, increasing the frequency of clinic visits, engaging in more frequent BG monitoring, adding 1 or more antidiabetic agents, meeting with a registered dietitian and/or diabetes educator, and increasing attention to diet and exercise regimens. Patients whose HbA1c concentrations remain relatively stable may only need to be tested every 6 months. Ideally, real-time HbA1c concentrations should be available at the time of the patient's visit with the clinician to allow the physician and patient and/or parent to discuss intensification of therapy during the visit, if needed.

Key Action Statement 4

The committee suggests that clinicians advise patients to monitor finger-stick BG concentrations in those who

a. are taking insulin or other medications with a risk of hypoglycemia; or

b. are initiating or changing their diabetes treatment regimen; or

c. have not met treatment goals; or

d. have intercurrent illnesses.

(Option: evidence quality D; expert consensus. Preponderance of benefits over harms.)

Action Statement Profile KAS 4

Aggregate evidence quality	D (expert consensus).
Benefit	Potential for improved metabolic control, improved potential for prevention of hypoglycemia, decreased long-term complications.
Harm	Patient discomfort, cost of materials.
Benefits-harms assessment	Benefit over harm.
Value judgments	Despite lack of evidence, there were general committee perceptions that patient safety concerns related to insulin use or clinical status outweighed any risks from monitoring.
Role of patient preferences	Moderate to low; recommendation driven primarily by safety concerns.
Exclusions	None.
Intentional vagueness	Intentional vagueness in the recommendation about specific approaches attributable to lack of evidence and the need to individualize treatment.
Policy level	Option.

Glycemic control correlates closely with the frequency of BG monitoring in adolescents with T1DM.[64,65] Although studies evaluating the efficacy of frequent BG monitoring have not been conducted in children and adolescents with T2DM, benefits have been described in insulin-treated adults with T2DM who tested their BG 4 times per day, compared with adults following a less frequent monitoring regimen.[66] These data support the value of BG monitoring in adults treated with insulin, and likely are relevant to youth with T2DM as well, especially those treated with insulin, at the onset of the disease, when treatment goals are not met, and when the treatment regimen is changed. The committee believes that current (2011) ADA recommendations for finger-stick BG monitoring apply to most youth with T2DM[67]:

- Finger-stick BG monitoring should be performed 3 or more times daily for patients using multiple insulin injections or insulin pump therapy.

- For patients using less-frequent insulin injections, noninsulin therapies, or medical nutrition therapy alone, finger-stick BG monitoring may be useful as a guide to the success of therapy.

- To achieve postprandial glucose targets, postprandial finger-stick BG monitoring may be appropriate.

Recognizing that current practices may not always reflect optimal care, a 2004 survey of practices among members of the PES revealed that 36% of pediatric endocrinologists asked their pediatric patients with T2DM to monitor BG concentrations twice daily; 12% asked patients to do so once daily; 13% asked patients to do so 3 times per day; and 12% asked patients to do so 4 times daily.[61] The questionnaire provided to the pediatric endocrinologists did not ask about the frequency of BG monitoring in relationship to the diabetes regimen, however.

Although normoglycemia may be difficult to achieve in adolescents with T2DM, a fasting BG concentration of 70 to 130 mg/dL is a reasonable target for most. In addition, because postprandial hyperglycemia has been associated with increased risk of cardiovascular events in adults, postprandial BG testing may be valuable in select patients. BG concentrations obtained 2 hours after meals (and paired with pre-meal concentrations) provide an index of glycemic excursion, and may be useful in improving glycemic control, particularly for the patient whose fasting plasma glucose is normal but whose HbA1c is not at target.[68] Recognizing the limited evidence for benefit of FSBG testing in this population, the committee provides suggested guidance for testing frequency, tailored to the medication regimen, as follows:

BG Testing Frequency for Patients With Newly Diagnosed T2DM: Fasting, Premeal, and Bedtime Testing

The committee suggests that all patients with newly diagnosed T2DM, regardless of prescribed treatment plan, should perform finger-stick BG monitoring before meals (including a morning fasting concentration) and at bedtime until reasonable metabolic control is achieved.[69] Once BG concentrations are at target levels, the frequency of monitoring can be modified depending on the medication used, the regimen's intensity, and the patient's metabolic control. Patients who are prone to marked hyperglycemia or hypoglycemia or who are on a therapeutic regimen associated with increased risk of hypoglycemia will require continued frequent BG testing. Expectations for frequency and timing of BG monitoring should be clearly defined through shared goal-setting between the patient and clinician. The adolescent and family members should be given a written action plan stating the medication regimen, frequency and timing of expected BG monitoring, as well as follow-up instructions.

BG Testing Frequency for Patients on Single Insulin Daily Injections and Oral Agents

Single bedtime long-acting insulin: The simplest insulin regimen consists of a single injection of long-acting insulin at bedtime (basal insulin only). The appropriateness of the insulin dose for patients using this regimen is best defined by the fasting/prebreakfast BG test. For patients on this insulin regimen, the committee suggests daily fasting BG measurements. This regimen is associated with some risk of hypoglycemia (especially overnight or fasting hypoglycemia) and may not provide adequate insulin coverage for mealtime ingestions throughout the day, as reflected by fasting BG concentrations in target, but daytime readings above target. In such cases, treatment with meglitinide (Prandin [Novo Nordisk Pharmaceuticals] or Starlix [Novartis Pharmaceuticals]) or a short-acting insulin before meals (see below) may be beneficial.

Oral agents: Once treatment goals are met, the frequency of monitoring can be decreased; however, the committee recommends some continued BG testing for all youth with T2DM, at a frequency determined within the clinical context (e.g. medication regimen, HbA1c, willingness of the patient, etc.). For example, an infrequent or intermittent monitoring schedule may be adequate when the patient is using exclusively an oral agent associated with a low risk of hypoglycemia and if HbA1c concentrations are in the ideal or non-diabetic range. A more frequent monitoring schedule should be advised during times of illness or if symptoms of hyperglycemia or hypoglycemia develop.

Oral agent plus a single injection of a long-acting insulin: Some youth with T2DM can be managed successfully with a single injection of long-acting insulin in conjunction with an oral agent. Twice a day BG monitoring (fasting plus a second BG concentration – ideally 2-hour post prandial) often is recommended, as long as HbA1c and BG concentrations remain at goal and the patient remains asymptomatic.

BG Testing Frequency for Patients Receiving Multiple Daily Insulin Injections (eg, Basal Bolus Regimens): Premeal and Bedtime Testing

Basal bolus regimens are commonly used in children and youth with T1DM and may be appropriate for some youth with T2DM as well. They are the most labor intensive, providing both basal insulin plus bolus doses of short-acting insulin at meals. Basal insulin is provided through either the use of long-acting, relatively peak-free insulin (by needle) or via an insulin pump. Bolus insulin doses are given at meal-time, using one of the rapid-acting insulin analogs. The bolus dose is calculated by using a correction algorithm for the premeal BG concentration as well as a "carb ratio," in which 1 unit of

a rapid-acting insulin analog is given for "X" grams of carbohydrates ingested (see box below). When using this method, the patient must be willing and able to count the number of grams of carbohydrates in the meal and divide by the assigned "carb ratio (X)" to know how many units of insulin should be taken. In addition, the patient must always check BG concentrations before the meal to determine how much additional insulin should be given as a correction dose using an algorithm assigned by the care team if the fasting BG is not in target. Insulin pumps are based on this concept of "basal-bolus" insulin administration and have the capability of calculating a suggested bolus dosage, based on inputted grams of carbohydrates and BG concentrations. Because the BG value determines the amount of insulin to be given at each meal, the recommended testing frequency for patients on this regimen is before every meal.

Box 1 Example of Basal Bolus Insulin Regimen

If an adolescent has a BG of 250 mg/dL, is to consume a meal containing 60 g of carbohydrates, with a carbohydrate ratio of 1:10 and an assigned correction dose of 1:25>125 (with 25 being the insulin sensitivity and 125 mg/dL the target blood glucose level), the mealtime bolus dose of insulin would be as follows:

60 g/10 "carb ratio" =

6 units rapid-acting insulin for meal

plus

(250–125)/25 = 125/25 =

5 units rapid-acting insulin for correction

Thus, total bolus insulin coverage at mealtime is: **11 U** (6 + 5) of rapid-acting insulin.

Key Action Statement 5

The committee suggests that clinicians incorporate the Academy of Nutrition and Dietetics' *Pediatric Weight Management Evidence-Based Nutrition Practice Guidelines* **in the nutrition counseling of patients with T2DM both at the time of diagnosis and as part of ongoing management. (Option; evidence quality D; expert opinion; preponderance of benefits over harms. Role of patient preference is dominant.)**

Action Statement Profile KAS 5

Aggregate evidence quality	D (expert opinion).
Benefit	Promotes weight loss; improves insulin sensitivity; contributes to glycemic control; prevents worsening of disease; facilitates a sense of well-being; and improves cardiovascular health.
Harm	Costs of nutrition counseling; inadequate reimbursement of clinicians' time; lost opportunity costs vis-a-vis time and resources spent in other counseling activities.
Benefits-harms assessment	Benefit over harm.
Value judgments	There is a broad societal agreement on the benefits of dietary recommendations.
Role of patient preference	Dominant. Patients may have different preferences for how they wish to receive assistance in managing their weight-loss goals. Some patients may prefer a referral to a nutritionist while others might prefer accessing online sources of help. Patient preference should play a significant role in determining an appropriate weight-loss strategy.
Exclusions	None.
Intentional vagueness	Intentional vagueness in the recommendation about specific approaches attributable to lack of evidence and the need to individualize treatment.
Policy level	Option.

Consuming more calories than one uses results in weight gain and is a major contributor to the increasing incidence of T2DM in children and adolescents. Current literature is inconclusive about a single best meal plan for patients with diabetes mellitus, however, and studies specifically addressing the diet of children and adolescents with T2DM are limited. Challenges to making recommendations stem from the small sample size of these studies, limited specificity for children and adolescents, and difficulties in generalizing the data from dietary research studies to the general population.

Although evidence is lacking in children with T2DM, numerous studies have been conducted in overweight children and adolescents, because the great majority of children with T2DM are obese or overweight at diagnosis.[26] The committee suggests that clinicians encourage children and adolescents with T2DM to follow the Academy of Nutrition and Dietetics' recommendations for maintaining healthy weight to promote health and reduce obesity in this population. The committee recommends that clinicians refer patients to a registered dietitian who has expertise in the nutritional needs of youth with T2DM. Clinicians should incorporate the Academy of Nutrition and Dietetics' *Pediatric Weight Management Evidence-Based Nutrition Practice Guidelines*, which describe effective, evidence-based treatment options for weight management, summarized below (A complete list of these recommendations is accessible to health care professionals at: http://www.andevidencelibrary.com/topic.cfm?cat=4102&auth=1.)

According to the Academy of Nutrition and Dietetics' guidelines, when incorporated with lifestyle changes, balanced macronutrient diets at 900 to 1200 kcal per day are associated with both short- and long-term (eg, ≥ 1 year) improvements in weight status and body composition in children 6 to 12 years of age.[70] These calorie recommendations are to be incorporated with lifestyle changes, including increased activity and possibly medication. Restrictions of no less than 1200 kcal per day in adolescents 13 to 18 years old result in improved weight status and body composition as well.[71] The Diabetes Prevention Program demonstrated that participants assigned to the intensive lifestyle-intervention arm had a reduction in daily energy intake of 450 kcal and a 58% reduction in progression to diabetes at the 2.8-year follow-up.[71] At the study's end, 50% of the lifestyle-arm participants had achieved the goal weight loss of at least 7% after the 24-week curriculum and 38% showed weight loss of at least 7% at the time of their most recent visit.[72] The Academy of Nutrition and Dietetics recommends that protein-sparing, modified-fast (ketogenic) diets be restricted to children who are >120% of their ideal body weight and who have a serious medical complication that would benefit from rapid weight loss.[71] Specific recommendations are for the intervention to be short-term (typically 10 weeks) and to be conducted under the supervision of a multidisciplinary team specializing in pediatric obesity.

Regardless of the meal plan prescribed, some degree of nutrition education must be provided to maximize adherence and positive results. This education should encourage patients to follow healthy eating patterns, such as consuming 3 meals with planned snacks per day, not eating while watching television or using computers, using smaller plates to make portions appear larger, and leaving small amounts of food on the plate.[73] Common dietary recommendations to reduce calorie intake and to promote weight loss in children include the following: (1) eating regular meals and snacks; (2) reducing portion sizes; (3) choosing calorie-free beverages, except for milk; (4) limiting juice to 1 cup per day; (5) increasing consumption of fruits and vegetables; (6) consuming 3 or 4 servings of low-fat dairy products per day; (7) limiting intake of high-fat foods; (8) limiting frequency and size of snacks; and (9) reducing calories consumed in fast-food meals.[74]

Key Action Statement 6

The committee suggests that clinicians encourage children and adolescents with T2DM to engage in moderate-to-vigorous exercise for at least 60 minutes daily and to limit nonacademic screen time to less than 2 hours per day. (Option: evidence quality D, expert opinion and evidence from studies of metabolic syndrome and obesity; preponderance of benefits over harms. Role of patient preference is dominant.)

Action Statement Profile KAS 6

Aggregate evidence quality	D (expert opinion and evidence from studies of metabolic syndrome and obesity).
Benefit	Promotes weight loss; contributes to glycemic control; prevents worsening of disease; facilitates the ability to perform exercise; improves the person's sense of well-being; and fosters cardiovascular health.
Harm	Cost for patient of counseling, food, and time; costs for clinician in taking away time that could be spent on other activities; inadequate reimbursement for clinician's time.
Benefits-harms assessment	Preponderance of benefit over harm.
Value judgments	Broad consensus.
Role of patient preference	Dominant. Patients may seek various forms of exercise. Patient preference should play a significant role in creating an exercise plan.
Exclusions	Although certain older or more debilitated patients with T2DM may be restricted in the amount of moderate-to-vigorous exercise they can perform safely, this recommendation applies to the vast majority of children and adolescents with T2DM.
Intentional vagueness	Intentional vagueness on the sequence of follow-up contact attributable to the lack of evidence and the need to individualize care.
Policy level	Option.

Recommendations From the Academy of Nutrition and Dietetics	
Pediatric Weight Management Evidence-Based Nutrition Practice Guidelines	
Recommendation	Strength
Interventions to reduce pediatric obesity should be multicomponent and include diet, physical activity, nutritional counseling, and parent or caregiver participation.	Strong
A nutrition prescription should be formulated as part of the dietary intervention in a multicomponent pediatric weight management program.	Strong
Dietary factors that may be associated with an increased risk of overweight are increased total dietary fat intake and increased intake of calorically sweetened beverages.	Strong
Dietary factors that may be associated with a decreased risk of overweight are increased fruit and vegetable intake.	Strong
A balanced macronutrient diet that contains no fewer than 900 kcal per day is recommended to improve weight status in children aged 6–12 y who are medically monitored.	Strong
A balanced macronutrient diet that contains no fewer than 1200 kcal per day is recommended to improve weight status in adolescents aged 13–18 y who are medically monitored.	Strong
Family diet behaviors that are associated with an increased risk of pediatric obesity are parental restriction of highly palatable foods, consumption of food away from home, increased meal portion size, and skipping breakfast.	Fair

Engaging in Physical Activity

Physical activity is an integral part of weight management for prevention and treatment of T2DM. Although there is a paucity of available data from children and adolescents with T2DM, several well-controlled studies performed in obese children and adolescents at risk of metabolic syndrome and T2DM provide guidelines for physical activity. (See the Resources section for tools on this subject.) A summary of the references supporting the evidence for this guideline can be found in the technical report.[31]

At present, moderate-to-vigorous exercise of at least 60 minutes daily is recommended for reduction of BMI and improved glycemic control in patients with T2DM.[75] "Moderate to vigorous exercise" is defined as exercise that makes the individual breathe hard and perspire and that raises his or her heart rate. An easy way to define exercise intensity for patients is the "talk test"; during moderate physical activity a person can talk but not sing. During vigorous activity, a person cannot talk without pausing to catch a breath.[76]

Adherence may be improved if clinicians provide the patient with a written prescription to engage in physical activity, including a "dose" describing ideal duration, intensity, and frequency.[75] When prescribing physical exercise, clinicians are encouraged to be sensitive to the needs of children, adolescents, and their families. Routine, organized exercise may be beyond the family's logistical and/or financial means, and some families may not be able to provide structured exercise programs for their children. It is most helpful to recommend an individualized approach that can be incorporated into the daily routine, is tailored to the patients' physical abilities and preferences, and recognizes the families' circumstances.[77] For example, clinicians might recommend only daily walking, which has been shown to improve weight loss and insulin sensitivity in adults with T2DM[78] and may constitute "moderate to vigorous activity" for some children with T2DM. It is also important to recognize that the recommended 60 minutes of exercise do not have to be accomplished in 1 session but can be completed through several, shorter increments (eg, 10–15 minutes). Patients should be encouraged to identify a variety of forms of activity that can be performed both easily and frequently.[77] In addition, providers should be cognizant of the potential need to adjust the medication dosage, especially if the patient is receiving insulin, when initiating an aggressive physical activity program.

Reducing Screen Time

Screen time contributes to a sedentary lifestyle, especially when the child or adolescent eats while watching television or playing computer games. The US Department of Health and Human Services recommends that individuals limit "screen time" spent watching television and/or using computers and handheld devices to less than 2 hours per day unless the use is related to work or homework.[79] Physical activity may be gained either through structured games and sports or through everyday activities, such as walking, ideally with involvement of the parents as good role models.

Increased screen time and food intake and reduced physical activity are associated with obesity. There is good evidence that modifying these factors can help prevent T2DM by reducing the individual's rate of weight gain. The evidence profile in pediatric patients with T2DM is inadequate at this time, however. Pending new data, the committee suggests that clinicians follow the AAP Committee on Nutrition's guideline, *Prevention of Pediatric Overweight and Obesity.* The guideline recommends restricting nonacademic screen time to a maximum of 2 hours per day and discouraging the presence of video screens and television sets in children's bedrooms.[80–82] The American Medical Association's Expert Panel on Childhood Obesity has endorsed this guideline.

Valuable recommendations for enhancing patient health include the following:

- With patients and their families, jointly determining an individualized plan that includes specific goals to reduce sedentary behaviors and increase physical activity.

- Providing a written prescription for engaging in 60-plus minutes of moderate-to-vigorous physical activities per day that includes

dose, timing, and duration. It is important for clinicians to be sensitive to the needs of children, adolescents, and their families in encouraging daily physical exercise. Graded duration of exercise is recommended for those youth who cannot initially be active for 60 minutes daily, and the exercise may be accomplished through several, shorter increments (eg, 10–15 minutes).

- Incorporating physical activities into children's and adolescents' daily routines. Physical activity may be gained either through structured games and sports or through everyday activities, such as walking.

- Restricting nonacademic screen time to a maximum of 2 hours per day.

- Discouraging the presence of video screens and television sets in children's bedrooms.

Conversations pertaining to the Key Action Statements should be clearly documented in the patient's medical record.

AREAS FOR FUTURE RESEARCH

As noted previously, evidence for medical interventions in children in general is scant and is especially lacking for interventions directed toward children who have developed diseases not previously seen commonly in youth, such as childhood T2DM. Recent studies such as the Search for Diabetes in Youth Study (SEARCH)—an observational multicenter study in 2096 youth with T2DM funded by the Centers for Disease Control and Prevention and the National Institute of Diabetes and Digestive and Kidney Diseases—now provide a detailed description of childhood diabetes. Subsequent trials will describe the short-term and enduring effects of specific interventions on the progression of the disease with time.

Although it is likely that children and adolescents with T2DM have an aggressive form of diabetes, as reflected by the age of onset, future research should determine whether the associated comorbidities and complications of diabetes also are more aggressive in pediatric populations than in adults and if they are more or less responsive to therapeutic interventions. Additional research should explore whether early introduction of insulin or the use of particular oral agents will preserve β-cell function in these children, and whether recent technologic advances (such as continuous glucose monitoring and insulin pumps) will benefit this population. Additional issues that require further study include the following:

- To delineate whether using lifestyle options without medication is a reliable first step in treating selected children with T2DM.

- To determine whether BG monitoring should be recommended to all children and youth with T2DM, regardless of therapy used; what the optimal frequency of BG monitoring is for pediatric patients on the basis of treatment regimen; and which subgroups will be able to successfully maintain glycemic goals with less frequent monitoring.

- To explore the efficacy of school- and clinic-based diet and physical activity interventions to prevent and manage pediatric T2DM.

- To explore the association between increased "screen time" and reduced physical activity with respect to T2DM's risk factors.

RESOURCES

Several tools are available online to assist providers in improving patient adherence to lifestyle modifications, including examples of activities to be recommended for patients:

- The American Academy of Pediatrics:

  - www.healthychildren.org

  - www.letsmove.gov

  - Technical Report: Management of Type 2 Diabetes Mellitus in Children and Adolescents.[31]
    - Includes an overview and screening tools for a variety of comorbidities.

  - Gahagan S, Silverstein J; Committee on Native American Child Health and Section on Endocrinology. Clinical report: prevention and treatment of type 2 diabetes mellitus in children, with special emphasis on American Indian and Alaska Native Children. *Pediatrics*. 2003;112 (4):e328–e347. Available at: http://www.pediatrics.org/cgi/content/full/112/4/e328[63]
    - Fig 3 presents a screening tool for microalbumin.

  - Bright Futures: http://brightfutures.aap.org/

  - Daniels SR, Greer FR; Committee on Nutrition. Lipid screening and cardiovascular health in childhood. *Pediatrics*. 2008;122 (1):198–208. Available at:

- The American Diabetes Association: www.diabetes.org

  - Management of dyslipidemia in children and adolescents with diabetes. *Diabetes Care*. 2003;26(7):2194–2197. Available at: http://care.diabetesjournals.org/content/26/7/2194.full

- Academy of Nutrition and Dietetics:

  - http://www.eatright.org/childhoodobesity/

  - http://www.eatright.org/kids/

  - http://www.eatright.org/cps/rde/xchg/ada/hs.xsl/index.html

- Pediatric Weight Management Evidence-Based Nutrition Practice Guidelines: http://www.adaevidencelibrary.com/topic.cfm?cat=2721

- American Heart Association:

  - American Heart Association *Circulation*. 2006 Dec 12;114(24):2710-2738. Epub 2006 Nov 27. Review.

- Centers for Disease Control and Prevention:

  - http://www.cdc.gov/obesity/childhood/solutions.html

  - BMI and other growth charts can be downloaded and printed from the CDC Web site: http://www.cdc.gov/growth-charts.

  - Center for Epidemiologic Studies Depression Scale (CES-D): http://www.chcr.brown.edu/pcoc/cesdscale.pdf; see attachments

- *Diagnostic and Statistical Manual of Mental Disorders*. 4th ed. Washington, DC: American Psychiatric Association; 1994

- Let's Move Campaign: www.letsmove.gov

- The Reach Institute. *Guidelines for Adolescent Depression in Primary Care (GLAD-PC) Toolkit*, 2007. Contains a listing of the criteria for major depressive disorder as defined by the DSM-IV-TR. Available at: http://www.gladpc.org

- The National Heart, Lung, and Blood Institute (NHLBI) hypertension guidelines: http://www.nhlbi.nih.gov/guidelines/hypertension/child_tbl.htm

- The National Diabetes Education Program and TIP sheets (including tip sheets on youth transitioning to adulthood and adult providers, Staying Active, Eating Healthy, Ups and Downs of Diabetes, etc): www.ndep.nih.gov or www.yourdiabetesinfo.org

- National High Blood Pressure Education Program Working Group on High Blood Pressure in Children and Adolescents, The Fourth Report on the Diagnosis, Evaluation, and Treatment of High Blood Pressure in Children and Adolescents: *Pediatrics*. 2004;114:555–576. Available at: http://pediatrics.aappublications.org/content/114/Supplement_2/555.long
- National Initiative for Children's Healthcare Quality (NICHQ): childhood obesity section: http://www.nichq.org/childhood_obesity/index.html
- The National Institute of Child Health and Human Development (NICHD): www.NICHD.org
- President's Council on Physical Fitness and Sports: http://www.presidentchallenge.org/home_kids.aspx
- US Department of Agriculture's "My Pyramid" Web site:

- http://www.choosemyplate.gov/
- http://fnic.nal.usda.gov/life-cycle-nutrition/child-nutrition-and-health

SUBCOMMITTEE ON TYPE 2 DIABETES (OVERSIGHT BY THE STEERING COMMITTEE ON QUALITY IMPROVEMENT AND MANAGEMENT, 2008–2012)

Kenneth Claud Copeland, MD, FAAP: Co-chair—Endocrinology and Pediatric Endocrine Society Liaison (2009: Novo Nordisk, Genentech, Endo [National Advisory Groups]; 2010: Novo Nordisk [National Advisory Group]); published research related to type 2 diabetes

Janet Silverstein, MD, FAAP: Co-chair—Endocrinology and American Diabetes Association Liaison (small grants with Pfizer, Novo Nordisk, and Lilly; grant review committee for Genentech; was on an advisory committee for Sanofi Aventis, and Abbott Laboratories for a 1-time meeting); published research related to type 2 diabetes

Kelly Roberta Moore, MD, FAAP: General Pediatrics, Indian Health, AAP Committee on Native American Child Health Liaison (board member of the Merck Company Foundation Alliance to Reduce Disparities in Diabetes. Their national program office is the University of Michigan's Center for Managing Chronic Disease.)

Greg Edward Prazar, MD, FAAP: General Pediatrics (no conflicts)

Terry Raymer, MD, CDE: Family Medicine, Indian Health Service (no conflicts)

Richard N. Shiffman, MD, FAAP: Partnership for Policy Implementation Informatician, General Pediatrics (no conflicts)

Shelley C. Springer, MD, MBA, FAAP: Epidemiologist (no conflicts)

Meaghan Anderson, MS, RD, LD, CDE: Academy of Nutrition and Dietetics Liaison (formerly a Certified Pump Trainer for Animas)

Stephen J. Spann, MD, MBA, FAAFP: American Academy of Family Physicians Liaison (no conflicts)

Vidhu V. Thaker, MD, FAAP: QuIIN Liaison, General Pediatrics (no conflicts)

CONSULTANT

Susan K. Flinn, MA: Medical Writer (no conflicts)

STAFF

Caryn Davidson, MA

REFERENCES

1. Centers for Disease Control and Prevention. Data and Statistics. Obesity rates among children in the United States. Available at: www.cdc.gov/obesity/childhood/prevalence.html. Accessed August 13, 2012

2. Copeland KC, Chalmers LJ, Brown RD. Type 2 diabetes in children: oxymoron or medical metamorphosis? *Pediatr Ann*. 2005;34(9):686–697

3. Narayan KM, Boyle JP, Thompson TJ, Sorensen SW, Williamson DF. Lifetime risk for diabetes mellitus in the United States. *JAMA*. 2003;290(14):1884–1890

4. Chopra M, Galbraith S, Darnton-Hill I. A global response to a global problem: the epidemic of overnutrition. *Bull World Health Organ*. 2002;80(12):952–958

5. Liese AD, D'Agostino RB, Jr, Hamman RF, et al; SEARCH for Diabetes in Youth Study Group. The burden of diabetes mellitus among US youth: prevalence estimates from the SEARCH for Diabetes in Youth Study. *Pediatrics*. 2006;118(4):1510–1518

6. Silverstein JH, Rosenbloom AL. Type 2 diabetes in children. *Curr Diab Rep*. 2001;1(1):19–27

7. Pinhas-Hamiel O, Zeitler P. Clinical presentation and treatment of type 2 diabetes in children. *Pediatr Diabetes*. 2007;8(suppl 9):16–27

8. Dabelea D, Bell RA, D'Agostino RB Jr, et al; Writing Group for the SEARCH for Diabetes in Youth Study Group. Incidence of diabetes in youth in the United States. *JAMA*. 2007;297(24):2716–2724

9. Mayer-Davis EJ, Bell RA, Dabelea D, et al; SEARCH for Diabetes in Youth Study Group. The many faces of diabetes in American youth: type 1 and type 2 diabetes in five race and ethnic populations: the SEARCH for Diabetes in Youth Study. *Diabetes Care*. 2009;32(suppl 2):S99–S101

10. Copeland KC, Zeitler P, Geffner M, et al; TODAY Study Group. Characteristics of adolescents and youth with recent-onset type 2 diabetes: the TODAY cohort at baseline. *J Clin Endocrinol Metab*. 2011;96(1):159–167

11. Narayan KM, Williams R. Diabetes—a global problem needing global solutions. *Prim Care Diabetes*. 2009;3(1):3–4

12. Wild S, Roglic G, Green A, Sicree R, King H. Global prevalence of diabetes: estimates for the year 2000 and projections for 2030. *Diabetes Care*. 2004;27(5):1047–1053

13. Silverstein J, Klingensmith G, Copeland K, et al; American Diabetes Association. Care of children and adolescents with type 1 diabetes: a statement of the American Diabetes Association. *Diabetes Care*. 2005;28(1):186–212

14. Pinhas-Hamiel O, Zeitler P. Barriers to the treatment of adolescent type 2 diabetes—a survey of provider perceptions. *Pediatr Diabetes*. 2003;4(1):24–28

15. Moore KR, McGowan MK, Donato KA, Kollipara S, Roubideaux Y. Community resources for promoting youth nutrition and physical activity. *Am J Health Educ*. 2009;40(5):298–303

16. Zeitler P, Epstein L, Grey M, et al; The TODAY Study Group. Treatment Options for type 2 diabetes mellitus in Adolescents and Youth: a study of the comparative efficacy of metformin alone or in combination with rosiglitazone or lifestyle intervention in adolescents with type 2 diabetes mellitus. *Pediatr Diabetes*. 2007;8(2):74–87

17. Kane MP, Abu-Baker A, Busch RS. The utility of oral diabetes medications in type 2

diabetes of the young. *Curr Diabetes Rev.* 2005;1(1):83–92

18. De Berardis G, Pellegrini F, Franciosi M, et al. Quality of care and outcomes in type 2 diabetes patientes. *Diabetes Care.* 2004;27 (2):398–406

19. Ziemer DC, Miller CD, Rhee MK, et al. Clinical inertia contributes to poor diabetes control in a primary care setting. *Diabetes Educ.* 2005;31(4):564–571

20. Bradshaw B. The role of the family in managing therapy in minority children with type 2 diabetes mellitus. *J Pediatr Endocrinol Metab.* 2002;15(suppl 1):547–551

21. Pinhas-Hamiel O, Standiford D, Hamiel D, Dolan LM, Cohen R, Zeitler PS. The type 2 family: a setting for development and treatment of adolescent type 2 diabetes mellitus. *Arch Pediatr Adolesc Med.* 1999; 153(10):1063–1067

22. Mulvaney SA, Schlundt DG, Mudasiru E, et al. Parent perceptions of caring for adolescents with type 2 diabetes. *Diabetes Care.* 2006;29(5):993–997

23. Summerbell CD, Ashton V, Campbell KJ, Edmunds L, Kelly S, Waters E. Interventions for treating obesity in children. *Cochrane Database Syst Rev.* 2003;(3):CD001872

24. Skinner AC, Weinberger M, Mulvaney S, Schlundt D, Rothman RL. Accuracy of perceptions of overweight and relation to self-care behaviors among adolescents with type 2 diabetes and their parents. *Diabetes Care.* 2008;31(2):227–229

25. American Diabetes Association. Type 2 diabetes in children and adolescents. *Diabetes Care.* 2000;23(3):381–389

26. Pinhas-Hamiel O, Zeitler P. Type 2 diabetes in adolescents, no longer rare. *Pediatr Rev.* 1998;19(12):434–435

27. Fagot-Campagna A, Pettitt DJ, Engelgau MM, et al. Type 2 diabetes among North American children and adolescents: an epidemiologic review and a public health perspective. *J Pediatr.* 2000;136(5):664–672

28. Rothman RL, Mulvaney S, Elasy TA, et al. Self-management behaviors, racial disparities, and glycemic control among adolescents with type 2 diabetes. *Pediatrics.* 2008;121(4). Available at: www.pediatrics.org/cgi/content/full/121/4/e912

29. Scott CR, Smith JM, Cradock MM, Pihoker C. Characteristics of youth-onset noninsulin-dependent diabetes mellitus and insulin-dependent diabetes mellitus at diagnosis. *Pediatrics.* 1997;100(1):84–91

30. Libman IM, Pietropaolo M, Arslanian SA, LaPorte RE, Becker DJ. Changing prevalence of overweight children and adolescents at onset of insulin-treated diabetes. *Diabetes Care.* 2003;26(10):2871–2875

31. Springer SC, Copeland KC, Silverstein J, et al. Technical report: management of type 2 diabetes mellitus in children and adolescents. *Pediatrics.* 2012, In press

32. American Academy of Pediatrics Steering Committee on Quality Improvement and Management. Classifying recommendations for clinical practice guidelines. *Pediatrics.* 2004;114(3):874–877

33. Shiffman RN, Dixon J, Brandt C, et al. The GuideLine Implementability Appraisal (GLIA): development of an instrument to identify obstacles to guideline implementation. *BMC Med Inform Decis Mak.* 2005;5:23

34. Gungor N, Hannon T, Libman I, Bacha F, Arslanian S. Type 2 diabetes mellitus in youth: the complete picture to date. *Pediatr Clin North Am.* 2005;52(6):1579–1609

35. Daaboul JJ, Siverstein JH. The management of type 2 diabetes in children and adolescents. *Minerva Pediatr.* 2004;56(3):255–264

36. Kadmon PM, Grupposo PA. Glycemic control with metformin or insulin therapy in adolescents with type 2 diabetes mellitus. *J Pediatr Endocrinol.* 2004;17(9):1185–1193

37. Owada M, Nitadori Y, Kitagawa T. Treatment of NIDDM in youth. *Clin Pediatr (Phila).* 1998;37(2):117–121

38. Pinhas-Hamiel O, Zeitler P. Advances in epidemiology and treatment of type 2 diabetes in children. *Adv Pediatr.* 2005;52: 223–259

39. Jones KL, Haghi M. Type 2 diabetes mellitus in children and adolescence: a primer. *Endocrinologist.* 2000;10:389–396

40. Kawahara R, Amemiya T, Yoshino M, et al. Dropout of young non-insulin-dependent diabetics from diabetic care. *Diabetes Res Clin Pract.* 1994;24(3):181–185

41. Kaufman FR. Type 2 diabetes mellitus in children and youth: a new epidemic. *J Pediatr Endocrinol Metab.* 2002;15(suppl 2): 737–744

42. Garber AJ, Duncan TG, Goodman AM, Mills DJ, Rohlf JL. Efficacy of metformin in type II diabetes: results of a double-blind, placebo-controlled, dose-response trial. *Am J Med.* 1997;103(6):491–497

43. Dabelea D, Pettitt DJ, Jones KL, Arslanian SA. Type 2 diabetes mellitus in minority children and adolescents: an emerging problem. *Endocrinol Metabo Clin North Am.* 1999;28(4):709–729

44. Miller JL, Silverstein JH. The management of type 2 diabetes mellitus in children and adolescents. *J Pediatr Endocrinol Metab.* 2005;18(2):111–123

45. Reinehr T, Schober E, Roth CL, Wiegand S, Holl R; DPV-Wiss Study Group. Type 2 diabetes in children and adolescents in a 2-year

follow-up: insufficient adherence to diabetes centers. *Horm Res.* 2008;69(2):107–113

46. Rosenbloom AL, Silverstein JH, Amemiya S, Zeitler P, Klingensmith GJ. Type 2 diabetes in children and adolescents. *Pediatr Diabetes.* 2009;10(suppl 12):17–32

47. Zuhri-Yafi MI, Brosnan PG, Hardin DS. Treatment of type 2 diabetes mellitus in children and adolescents. *J Pediatr Endocrinol Metab.* 2002;15(suppl 1):541–546

48. Rapaport R, Silverstein JH, Garzarella L, Rosenbloom AL. Type 1 and type 2 diabetes mellitus in childhood in the United States: practice patterns by pediatric endocrinologists. *J Pediatr Endocrinol Metab.* 2004;17 (6):871–877

49. Glaser N, Jones KL. Non-insulin-dependent diabetes mellitus in children and adolescents. *Adv Pediatr.* 1996;43:359–396

50. Miller JL, Silverstein JH. The treatment of type 2 diabetes mellitus in youth: which therapies? *Treat Endocrinol.* 2006;5(4):201–210

51. Silverstein JH, Rosenbloom AL. Treatment of type 2 diabetes mellitus in children and adolescents. *J Pediatr Endocrinol Metab.* 2000;13(suppl 6):1403–1409

52. Dean H. Treatment of type 2 diabetes in youth: an argument for randomized controlled studies. *Paediatr Child Health (Oxford).* 1999;4(4):265–270

53. Sellers EAC, Dean HJ. Short-term insulin therapy in adolescents with type 2 diabetes mellitus. *J Pediatr Endocrinol Metab.* 2004; 17(11):1561–1564

54. Zeitler P, Hirst K, Pyle L, et al; TODAY Study Group. A clinical trial to maintain glycemic control in youth with type 2 diabetes. *N Engl J Med.* 2012;366(24):2247–2256

55. White NH, Cleary PA, Dahms W, Goldstein D, Malone J, Tamborlane WV; Diabetes Control and Complications Trial (DCCT)/Epidemiology of Diabetes Interventions and Complications (EDIC) Research Group. Beneficial effects of intensive therapy of diabetes during adolescence: outcomes after the conclusion of the Diabetes Control and Complications Trial (DCCT). *J Pediatr.* 2001;139(6):804–812

56. The Diabetes Control and Complications Trial Research Group. The effect of intensive treatment of diabetes on the development and progression of long-term complications in insulin-dependent diabetes mellitus. *N Engl J Med.* 1993;329(14):977–986

57. Orchard TJ, Olson JC, Erbey JR, et al. Insulin resistance-related factors, but not glycemia, predict coronary artery disease in type 1 diabetes: 10-year follow-up data from the Pittsburgh Epidemiology of Diabetes Complications Study. *Diabetes Care.* 2003;26(5):1374–1379

58. UK Prospective Diabetes Study Group. U.K. prospective diabetes study 16. Overview of 6 years' therapy of type II diabetes: a progressive disease. *Diabetes*. 1995;44(11): 1249–1258

59. Shichiri M, Kishikawa H, Ohkubo Y, Wake N. Long-term results of the Kumamoto Study on optimal diabetes control in type 2 diabetic patients. *Diabetes Care*. 2000;23 (suppl 2):B21–B29

60. Baynes JW, Bunn HF, Goldstein D, et al; National Diabetes Data Group. National Diabetes Data Group: report of the expert committee on glucosylated hemoglobin. *Diabetes Care*. 1984;7(6):602–606

61. Dabiri G, Jones K, Krebs J, et al. Benefits of rosiglitazone in children with type 2 diabetes mellitus [abstract]. *Diabetes*. 2005; A457

62. Ponder SW, Sullivan S, McBath G. Type 2 diabetes mellitus in teens. *Diabetes Spectrum*. 2000;13(2):95–119

63. Gahagan S, Silverstein J, and the American Academy of Pediatrics Committee on Native American Child Health. Prevention and treatment of type 2 diabetes mellitus in children, with special emphasis on American Indian and Alaska Native children. *Pediatrics*. 2003;112(4). Available at: www.pediatrics.org/cgi/content/full/112/4/e328

64. Levine BS, Anderson BJ, Butler DA, Antisdel JE, Brackett J, Laffel LM. Predictors of glycemic control and short-term adverse outcomes in youth with type 1 diabetes. *J Pediatr*. 2001;139(2):197–203

65. Haller MJ, Stalvey MS, Silverstein JH. Predictors of control of diabetes: monitoring may be the key. *J Pediatr*. 2004;144(5):660–661

66. Murata GH, Shah JH, Hoffman RM, et al; Diabetes Outcomes in Veterans Study (DOVES). Intensified blood glucose monitoring improves glycemic control in stable, insulin-treated veterans with type 2 diabetes: the Diabetes Outcomes in Veterans Study (DOVES). *Diabetes Care*. 2003;26(6): 1759–1763

67. American Diabetes Association. Standards of medical care in diabetes—2011. *Diabetes Care*. 2011;34(suppl 1):S11–S61

68. Hanefeld M, Fischer S, Julius U, et al. Risk factors for myocardial infarction and death in newly detected NIDDM: the Diabetes Intervention Study, 11-year follow-up. *Diabetologia*. 1996;39(12):1577–1583

69. Franciosi M, Pellegrini F, De Berardis G, et al; QuED Study Group. The impact of blood glucose self-monitoring on metabolic control and quality of life in type 2 diabetic patients: an urgent need for better educational strategies. *Diabetes Care*. 2001;24 (11):1870–1877

70. American Dietetic Association. Recommendations summary: pediatric weight management (PWM) using protein sparing modified fast diets for pediatric weight loss. Available at: www.adaevidencelibrary.com/template.cfm?template=guide_-summary&key=416. Accessed August 13, 2012

71. Knowler WC, Barrett-Connor E, Fowler SE, et al; Diabetes Prevention Program Research Group. Reduction in the incidence of type 2 diabetes with lifestyle intervention or metformin. *N Engl J Med*. 2002;346(6): 393–403

72. Willi SM, Martin K, Datko FM, Brant BP. Treatment of type 2 diabetes in childhood using a very-low-calorie diet. *Diabetes Care*. 2004;27(2):348–353

73. Berry D, Urban A, Grey M. Management of type 2 diabetes in youth (part 2). *J Pediatr Health Care*. 2006;20(2):88–97

74. Loghmani ES. Nutrition therapy for overweight children and adolescents with type 2 diabetes. *Curr Diab Rep*. 2005;5(5):385–390

75. McGavock J, Sellers E, Dean H. Physical activity for the prevention and management of youth-onset type 2 diabetes mellitus: focus on cardiovascular complications. *Diab Vasc Dis Res*. 2007;4(4):305–310

76. Centers for Disease Control and Prevention. Physical activity for everyone: how much physical activity do you need? Atlanta, GA: Centers for Disease Control and Prevention; 2008. Available at: www.cdc.gov/physicalactivity/everyone/guidelines/children.html. Accessed August 13, 2012

77. Pinhas-Hamiel O, Zeitler P. A weighty problem: diagnosis and treatment of type 2 diabetes in adolescents. *Diabetes Spectrum*. 1997;10(4):292–298

78. Yamanouchi K, Shinozaki T, Chikada K, et al. Daily walking combined with diet therapy is a useful means for obese NIDDM patients not only to reduce body weight but also to improve insulin sensitivity. *Diabetes Care*. 1995;18(6):775–778

79. National Heart, Lung, and Blood Institute, US Department of Health and Human Services, National Institutes of Health. Reduce screen time. Available at: www.nhlbi.nih.gov/health/public/heart/obesity/wecan/reduce-screen-time/index.htm. Accessed August 13, 2012

80. Krebs NF, Jacobson MS; American Academy of Pediatrics Committee on Nutrition. Prevention of pediatric overweight and obesity. *Pediatrics*. 2003;112(2):424–430

81. American Academy of Pediatrics Committee on Public Education. American Academy of Pediatrics: children, adolescents, and television. *Pediatrics*. 2001;107(2):423–426

82. American Medical Association. Appendix. Expert Committee recommendations on the assessment, prevention, and treatment of child and adolescent overweight and obesity. Chicago, IL: American Medical Association; January 25, 2007. Available at: www.ama-assn.org/ama1/pub/upload/mm/433/ped_obesity_recs.pdf. Accessed August 13, 2012

Copeland et al. Clinical Practice Guideline: Management of Newly Diagnosed Type 2 Diabetes Mellitus (T2DM) in Children and Adolescents. *Pediatrics.* 2013;131(2):364–382

Several inaccuracies occurred in the American Academy of Pediatrics "Clinical Practice Guideline: Management of Newly Diagnosed Type 2 Diabetes Mellitus (T2DM) in Children and Adolescents" published in the February 2013 issue of *Pediatrics* (2013;131[2]:364–382).

On page 366 in the table of definitions, "Prediabetes" should be defined as "Fasting plasma glucose ≥100–125 mg/dL or 2-hour glucose concentration during an oral glucose tolerance test of ≥140 but <200 mg/dL or an HbA1c of 5.7% to 6.4%."

On page 378, middle column, under "Reducing Screen Time," the second sentence should read as follows: "The US Department of Health and Human Services reflects the American Academy of Pediatrics policies by recommending that individuals limit "screen time" spent watching television and/or using computers and handheld devices to <2 hours per day unless the use is related to work or homework."[79–81,83]

Also on page 378, middle column, in the second paragraph under "Reducing Screen Time," the fourth sentence should read: "Pending new data, the committee suggests that clinicians follow the policy statement 'Children, Adolescents, and Television' from the AAP Council on Communications and Media (formerly the Committee on Public Education)." The references cited in the next sentence should be 80–83.

Reference 82 should be replaced with the following reference: Barlow SE; Expert Committee. Expert committee recommendations regarding the prevention, assessment, and treatment of child and adolescent overweight and obesity: summary report. *Pediatrics.* 2007;120(suppl 4):S164–S192

Finally, a new reference 83 should be added: American Academy of Pediatrics, Council on Communications and Media. Policy statement: children, adolescents, obesity, and the media. *Pediatrics.* 2011;128(1):201–208

doi:10.1542/peds.2013-0666

AMERICAN ACADEMY OF PEDIATRICS

POLICY STATEMENT
Organizational Principles to Guide and Define the Child Health Care System and/or Improve the Health of All Children

Committee on Nutrition

Prevention of Pediatric Overweight and Obesity

ABSTRACT. The dramatic increase in the prevalence of childhood overweight and its resultant comorbidities are associated with significant health and financial burdens, warranting strong and comprehensive prevention efforts. This statement proposes strategies for early identification of excessive weight gain by using body mass index, for dietary and physical activity interventions during health supervision encounters, and for advocacy and research.

ABBREVIATION. BMI, body mass index.

INTRODUCTION

Prevention is one of the hallmarks of pediatric practice and includes such diverse activities as newborn screenings, immunizations, and promotion of car safety seats and bicycle helmets. Documented trends in increasing prevalence of overweight and inactivity mean that pediatricians must focus preventive efforts on childhood obesity, with its associated comorbid conditions in childhood and likelihood of persistence into adulthood. These trends pose an unprecedented burden in terms of children's health as well as present and future health care costs. A number of statements have been published that address the scope of the problem and treatment strategies.[1-6]

The intent of this statement is to propose strategies to foster prevention and early identification of overweight and obesity in children. Evidence to support the recommendations for prevention is presented when available, but unfortunately, too few studies on prevention have been performed. The enormity of the epidemic, however, necessitates this call to action for pediatricians using the best information available.

DEFINITIONS AND DESCRIPTION OF THE PROBLEM

Body mass index (BMI) is the ratio of weight in kilograms to the square of height in meters. BMI is widely used to define overweight and obesity, because it correlates well with more accurate measures of body fatness and is derived from commonly available data—weight and height.[7] It has also been correlated with obesity-related comorbid conditions in

adults and children. Clinical judgment must be used in applying these criteria to a patient, because obesity refers to excess adiposity rather than excess weight, and BMI is a surrogate for adiposity. The pediatric growth charts for the US population now include BMI for age and gender, are readily available online (http://www.cdc.gov/growthcharts), and allow longitudinal tracking of BMI.[8]

BMI between 85th and 95th percentile for age and sex is considered at risk of overweight, and BMI at or above the 95th percentile is considered overweight or obese.[9,10] The prevalence of childhood overweight and obesity is increasing at an alarming rate in the United States as well as in other developed and developing countries. Prevalence among children and adolescents has doubled in the past 2 decades in the United States. Currently, 15.3% of 6- to 11-year-olds and 15.5% of 12- to 19-year-olds are at or above the 95th percentile for BMI on standard growth charts based on reference data from the 1970s, with even higher rates among subpopulations of minority and economically disadvantaged children.[10,11] Recent data from the Centers for Disease Control and Prevention also indicate that children younger than 5 years across all ethnic groups have had significant increases in the prevalence of overweight and obesity.[12,13] American children and adolescents today are less physically active as a group than were previous generations, and less active children are more likely to be overweight and to have higher blood pressure, insulin and cholesterol concentrations and more abnormal lipid profiles.[14,15]

Obesity is associated with significant health problems in the pediatric age group and is an important early risk factor for much of adult morbidity and mortality.[15,16] Medical problems are common in obese children and adolescents and can affect cardiovascular health (hypercholesterolemia and dyslipidemia, hypertension),[14,17-19] the endocrine system (hyperinsulinism, insulin resistance, impaired glucose tolerance, type 2 diabetes mellitus, menstrual irregularity),[20-22] and mental health (depression, low self-esteem).[23,24] Because of the increasing incidence of type 2 diabetes mellitus among obese adolescents and because diabetes-related morbidities may worsen if diagnosis is delayed, the clinician should be alert to the possibility of type 2 diabetes mellitus in all obese adolescents, especially those with a family history of early-onset (younger than 40 years) type 2 diabetes mellitus.[25] The psychologic stress of social stigmatization imposed on obese children may be just as damaging as the medical morbidities. The negative images of obesity are so strong that growth failure and pubertal delay have been reported in children practicing self-imposed caloric restriction because of fears of becoming obese.[26] Other important complications and associations include pulmonary (asthma, obstructive sleep apnea syndrome, pickwickian syndrome),[27–32] orthopedic (genu varum, slipped capital femoral epiphysis),[33,34] and gastrointestinal/hepatic (nonalcoholic steatohepatitis)[35] complications. All these disturbances are seen at an increased rate in obese individuals and have become more common in the pediatric population. The probability of childhood obesity persisting into adulthood is estimated to increase from approximately 20% at 4 years of age to approximately 80% by adolescence.[36] In addition, it is probable that comorbidities will persist into adulthood.[16,37] Thus, the potential future health care costs associated with pediatric obesity and its comorbidities are staggering, prompting the surgeon general to predict that preventable morbidity and mortality associated with obesity may exceed those associated with cigarette smoking.[10,38]

Although treatment approaches for pediatric obesity may be effective in the short term,[39–44] long-term outcome data for successful treatment approaches are limited.[45,46] The intractable nature of adult obesity is well known. Therefore, it is incumbent on the pediatric community to take a leadership role in prevention and early recognition of pediatric obesity.

RISK FACTORS

Development of effective prevention strategies mandates that physicians recognize populations and individuals at risk. Interactions between genetic, biological, psychologic, sociocultural, and environmental factors clearly are evident in childhood obesity. Elucidation of hormonal and neurochemical mechanisms that promote the energy imbalance that generates obesity has come from molecular genetics and neurochemistry. Knowledge of the genetic basis of differences in the complex of hormones and neurotransmitters (including growth hormone, leptin, ghrelin, neuropeptide Y, melanocortin, and others) that are responsible for regulating satiety, hunger, lipogenesis, and lipolysis as well as growth and reproductive development will eventually refine our understanding of risk of childhood overweight and obesity and may lead to more effective therapies.[47,48]

Genetic conditions known to be associated with propensity for obesity include Prader-Willi syndrome, Bardet-Biedl syndrome, and Cohen syndrome. In these conditions, early diagnosis allows collaboration with subspecialists, such as geneticists, endocrinologists, behavioralists, and nutritionists, to optimize growth and development while promoting healthy eating and activity patterns from a young age. For example, data suggest that growth hormone may improve some of the signs of Prader-Willi syndrome.[49–51]

It has long been recognized that obesity "runs in families"—high birth weight, maternal diabetes, and obesity in family members all are factors—but there are likely to be multiple genes and a strong interaction between genetics and environment that influence the degree of adiposity.[47,48,52,53] For young children, if 1 parent is obese, the odds ratio is approximately 3 for obesity in adulthood, but if both parents are obese, the odds ratio increases to more than 10. Before 3 years of age, parental obesity is a stronger predictor of obesity in adulthood than the child's weight status.[54] Such observations have important implications for recognition of risk and routine anticipatory guidance that is directed toward healthy eating and activity patterns in families.

There are critical periods of development for excessive weight gain. Extent and duration of breastfeeding have been found to be inversely associated with risk of obesity in later childhood, possibly mediated by physiologic factors in human milk as well as by the feeding and parenting patterns associated with nursing.[55–58] Investigations of dietary factors in infancy, such as high protein intake or the timing of introduction of complementary foods, have not consistently revealed effects on childhood obesity. It has been known for decades that adolescence is another critical period for development of obesity.[59] The normal tendency during early puberty for insulin resistance may be a natural cofactor for excessive weight gain as well as various comorbidities of obesity.[60] Early menarche is clearly associated with degree of overweight, with a twofold increase in rate of early menarche associated with BMI greater than the 85th percentile.[61] The risk of obesity persisting into adulthood is higher among obese adolescents than among younger children.[54] The roles of leptin, adiponectin, ghrelin, fat mass, and puberty on development of adolescent obesity are being actively investigated. Data suggest that adolescents who engage in high-risk behaviors, such as smoking, ethanol use, and early sexual experimentation also may be at greater risk of poor dietary and exercise habits.[62]

Environmental risk factors for overweight and obesity, including family and parental dynamics, are numerous and complicated. Although clinical interventions cannot change these factors directly, they can influence patients' adaptations to them, and the physician can advocate for change at the community level. Food insecurity may contribute to the inverse relation of obesity prevalence with socioeconomic status, but the relationship is a complex one.[63] Other barriers low-income families may face are lack of safe places for physical activity and lack of consistent access to healthful food choices, particularly fruits and vegetables. Low cognitive stimulation in the home, low socioeconomic status, and maternal obesity all predict development of obesity.[64] In research settings, there is accumulating evidence for the detrimental effects of overcontrolling parental behavior on children's ability to self-regulate energy intake. For example, maternal-child feeding practices, maternal perception of daughter's risk of overweight,[65] maternal restraint, verbal prompting to eat at mealtime, attentiveness to noneating behavior, and close parental monitoring[66] all may promote undesired consequences for children's eating behaviors. Parental food choices influence child food preferences,[67] and degree of parental adiposity is a marker for children's fat preferences.[68] Children and adolescents of lower socioeconomic status have been reported to be less likely to eat fruits and vegetables and to have a higher intake of total and saturated fat.[69–71] Absence of family meals is associated with lower fruit and vegetable consumption as well as consumption of more fried food and carbonated beverages. Although our understanding of the development of eating behaviors is improving, there are not yet good trials to demonstrate effective translation of this knowledge base into clinical practices to prevent obesity. At a minimum, however, pediatricians need to proactively discuss and promote healthy eating behaviors for children at an early age and empower parents to promote children's ability to self-regulate energy intake while providing appropriate structure and boundaries around eating.

Widespread and profound societal changes during the last several decades have affected child rearing, which in turn has affected childhood patterns of physical activity as well as diet. National survey data indicate that children are currently less active than they have been in previous surveys. Leisure activity is increasingly sedentary, with wide availability of entertainment such as television, videos, and computer games. In addition, with increasing urbanization, there has been a decrease in frequency and duration of physical activities of daily living for children, such as walking to school and doing household chores. Changes in availability and requirements of school physical education programs have also generally decreased children's routine physical activity, with the possible exception of children specifically enrolled in athletic programs. All these factors play a potential part in the epidemic of overweight.[72]

National survey data indicate that 20% of US children 8 to 16 years of age reported 2 or fewer bouts of vigorous physical activity per week, and more than 25% watched at least 4 hours of television per day.[73] Children who watched 4 or more hours of television per day had significantly greater BMI, compared with those watching fewer than 2 hours per day.[73] Furthermore, having a television in the bedroom has been reported to be a strong predictor of being overweight, even in preschool-aged children.[74] Some cross-sectional data have found significant correlation between obesity prevalence and television viewing,[75–77] but others have not.[78,79] The results of a randomized trial to decrease television viewing for school-aged children has provided the strongest evidence to support the role of limiting television in prevention of obesity. In this study, decreasing "media use" without specifically promoting more active behaviors in the intervention group resulted in a significantly lower increase in BMI at the 1-year follow-up, compared with the control group.[80] Additional support for the importance of decreasing television viewing comes from controlled investigations that demonstrated that obese children who were reinforced for decreasing sedentary activity (and following an energy-restricted diet) had significantly greater weight loss than those who were reinforced for increasing physical activity.[42] These findings have important implications for anticipatory guidance and provide additional support for recommendations to limit television exposure for young children.[2]

EARLY RECOGNITION

Routine assessments of eating and activity patterns in children and recognition of excessive weight gain relative to linear growth are essential throughout childhood. At any age, an excessive rate of weight gain relative to linear growth should be recognized, and underlying predisposing factors should be addressed with parents and other caregivers. The Centers for Disease Control and Prevention percentile grids for BMI are important tools for anticipatory guidance and discussion of longitudinal tracking of a child's BMI. Significant changes on growth patterns (eg, upward crossing of weight for age or BMI percentiles) can be recognized and addressed before children are severely overweight.[81] An increase in BMI percentiles should be discussed with parents, some of whom may be overly concerned and some of whom may not recognize or accept potential risk.[82]

Although data are extremely limited, it is likely that anticipatory guidance or treatment intervention before obesity has become severe will be more successful. Discussions to raise parental awareness should be conducted in a nonjudgmental, blame-free manner so that unintended negative impact on the child's self-concept is avoided.[24] Data from adult patient surveys indicate that those who were asked by their physician about diet were more likely to report positive changes.[83] Similarly, the efficacy of physicians discussing physical activity,[84] breastfeeding,[85] and smoking prevention[86] is well documented. Thus, pediatricians are strongly encouraged to incorporate assessment and anticipatory guidance about diet, weight, and physical activity into routine clinical practice, being careful to discuss habits rather than focusing on habitus to avoid stigmatizing the child, adolescent, or family.

ADVOCACY

Abundant opportunities exist for pediatricians to take a leadership role in this critical area of child health, including action in the following areas: opportunities for physical activity, the food supply, research, and third-party reimbursement. Change is desperately needed in opportunities for physical activity in child care centers, schools, after-school programs, and other community settings. As leaders in their communities, pediatricians can be effective advocates for health- and fitness-promoting programs and policies. Foods that are nutrient rich and palatable yet low in excess energy from added sugars and fat need to be readily available to parents, school and child care food services, and others responsible for feeding children. Potential affordable sources include community gardens and farmers' market projects. Advertising and promotion of energy-dense, nutrient-poor food products to children may need to be regulated or curtailed. The increase in

426   PREVENTION OF PEDIATRIC OVERWEIGHT AND OBESITY

carbonated beverage intake has been linked to obesity[87]; therefore, the sale of such beverages should not be promoted at school. Pediatricians are encouraged to work with school administrators and others in the community on ways to decrease the availability of foods and beverages with little nutritional value and to decrease the dependence on vending machines, snack bars, and school stores for school revenue. Regarding physical activity, advocacy is sorely needed for physical education programs that emphasize and model learning of daily activities for personal fitness (as opposed to physical education limited to a few team sports).

New initiatives for pilot projects to test prevention strategies have been funded by the National Institutes of Health and other organizations, but a long-term commitment of substantial funds from many sources and to many disciplines will be needed to attack this serious, widespread, and potentially intractable problem. Support for development and testing of primary prevention strategies for the primary care setting will be critical. Likewise, investment of substantial resources will be required for development of effective treatment approaches for normalizing or improving body weight and fitness and for determining long-term effects of weight loss on comorbidities of childhood obesity. Collaboration and coalitions with nutrition, behavioral health, physical therapy, and exercise physiology professionals will be needed. Working with communities and schools to develop needed counseling services, physical activity opportunities, and strategies to reinforce the gains made in clinical management is also important.

Pediatric referral centers will need to develop specialized programs for treatment of complex and difficult cases, and for research into etiology and new methods of prevention and treatment. Efforts are needed to ensure adequate health care coverage for preventive and treatment services. Even when serious comorbidities are documented, insurance reimbursement is limited.[88] Lack of reimbursement is a disincentive for physicians to develop prevention and treatment programs and presents a significant barrier to families seeking professional care.

SUMMARY/CONCLUSIONS

1. Prevalence of overweight and its significant comorbidities in pediatric populations has rapidly increased and reached epidemic proportions.
2. Prevention of overweight is critical, because long-term outcome data for successful treatment approaches are limited.
3. Genetic, environmental, or combinations of risk factors predisposing children to obesity can and should be identified.
4. Early recognition of excessive weight gain relative to linear growth should become routine in pediatric ambulatory care settings. BMI (kg/m^2 [see http://www.cdc.gov/growthcharts]) should be calculated and plotted periodically.
5. Families should be educated and empowered through anticipatory guidance to recognize the impact they have on their children's development

of lifelong habits of physical activity and nutritious eating.
6. Dietary practices should be fostered that encourage moderation rather than overconsumption, emphasizing healthful choices rather than restrictive eating patterns.
7. Regular physical activity should be consciously promoted, prioritized, and protected within families, schools, and communities.
8. Optimal approaches to prevention need to combine dietary and physical activity interventions.
9. Advocacy is needed in the areas of physical activity and food policy for children; research into pathophysiology, risk factors, and early recognition and management of overweight and obesity; and improved insurance coverage and third-party reimbursement for obesity care.

RECOMMENDATIONS

1. Health supervision
   a. Identify and track patients at risk by virtue of family history, birth weight, or socioeconomic, ethnic, cultural, or environmental factors.
   b. Calculate and plot BMI once a year in all children and adolescents.
   c. Use change in BMI to identify rate of excessive weight gain relative to linear growth.
   d. Encourage, support, and protect breastfeeding.
   e. Encourage parents and caregivers to promote healthy eating patterns by offering nutritious snacks, such as vegetables and fruits, low-fat dairy foods, and whole grains; encouraging children's autonomy in self-regulation of food intake and setting appropriate limits on choices; and modeling healthy food choices.
   f. Routinely promote physical activity, including unstructured play at home, in school, in child care settings, and throughout the community.
   g. Recommend limitation of television and video time to a maximum of 2 hours per day.
   h. Recognize and monitor changes in obesity-associated risk factors for adult chronic disease, such as hypertension, dyslipidemia, hyperinsulinemia, impaired glucose tolerance, and symptoms of obstructive sleep apnea syndrome.
2. Advocacy
   a. Help parents, teachers, coaches, and others who influence youth to discuss health habits, not body habitus, as part of their efforts to control overweight and obesity.
   b. Enlist policy makers from local, state, and national organizations and schools to support a healthful lifestyle for all children, including proper diet and adequate opportunity for regular physical activity.
   c. Encourage organizations that are responsible for health care and health care financing to provide coverage for effective obesity prevention and treatment strategies.
   d. Encourage public and private sources to direct funding toward research into effective strategies to prevent overweight and obesity and to maximize limited family and community re-

sources to achieve healthful outcomes for youth.

e. Support and advocate for social marketing intended to promote healthful food choices and increased physical activity.

COMMITTEE ON NUTRITION, 2002–2003
*Nancy F. Krebs, MD, Chairperson
Robert D. Baker, Jr, MD, PhD
Frank R. Greer, MD
Melvin B. Heyman, MD
Tom Jaksic, MD, PhD
Fima Lifshitz, MD

*Marc S. Jacobson, MD
   Past Committee Member

LIAISONS
Donna Blum-Kemelor, MS, RD
   US Department of Agriculture
Margaret P. Boland, MD
   Canadian Paediatric Society
William Dietz, MD, PhD
   Centers for Disease Control and Prevention
Van S. Hubbard, MD, PhD
   National Institute of Diabetes and Digestive and Kidney Diseases
Elizabeth Yetley, PhD
   US Food and Drug Administration

STAFF
Pamela Kanda, MPH

*Lead authors

REFERENCES

1. American Academy of Pediatrics, Committee on Sports Medicine and Fitness. Promotion of healthy weight-control practices in young athletes. *Pediatrics.* 1996;97:752–753
2. American Academy of Pediatrics, Committee on Public Education. Children, adolescents, and television. *Pediatrics.* 2001;107:423–426
3. American Dietetic Association. Position of the American Dietetic Association. Dietary guidance for healthy children aged 2 to 11 years. *J Am Diet Assoc.* 1999;99:93–101
4. Gidding SS, Leibel RL, Daniels S, Rosenbaum M, Van Horn L, Marx GR. Understanding obesity in youth. A statement for healthcare professionals from the Committee on Atherosclerosis and Hypertension in the Young of the Committee on Cardiovascular Disease in the Young and Nutrition Committee, American Heart Association. *Circulation.* 1996;94: 3383–3387
5. American Medical Association, Council on Scientific Affairs. *Obesity as a Major Public Health Problem.* Chicago, IL: American Medical Association; 1999. Available at: http://www.ama-assn.org/meetings/public/annual99/reports/csa/rtf/csa6.rtf. Accessed September 4, 2002
6. Barlow SE, Dietz WH. Obesity evaluation and treatment: expert committee recommendations. The Maternal and Child Health Bureau, Health Resources and Services Administration and the Department of Health and Human Services. *Pediatrics.* 1998;102(3). Available at: http://www.pediatrics.org/cgi/content/full/102/3/e29
7. Pietrobelli A, Faith MS, Allison DB, Gallagher D, Chiumello G, Heymsfield SB. Body mass index as a measure of adiposity among children and adolescents: a validation study. *J Pediatr.* 1998;132:204–210
8. Kuczmarski RJ, Ogden CL, Grummer-Strawn LM, et al. CDC growth charts: United States. *Adv Data.* 2000 Jun 8;(314):1–27
9. Himes JH, Dietz WH. Guidelines for overweight in adolescent preventive services: recommendations from an expert committee. *Am J Clin Nutr.* 1994;59:307–316
10. US Dept Health and Human Services. *The Surgeon General's Call to Action to Prevent and Decrease Overweight and Obesity.* Rockville, MD: US Department of Health and Human Services, Public Health Service, Office of the Surgeon General; 2001
11. Ogden CL, Flegal KM, Carroll MD, Johnson CL. Prevalence and trends in overweight among US children and adolescents, 1999–2000. *JAMA.* 2002;288:1728–1732
12. Mei Z, Scanlon KS, Grummer-Strawn LM, Freedman DS, Yip R, Trowbridge FL. Increasing prevalence of overweight among US low-income preschool children: The Centers for Disease Control and Prevention Pediatric Nutrition Surveillance, 1983 to 1995. *Pediatrics.* 1998;101(1). Available at: http://www.pediatrics.org/cgi/content/full/101/1/e12
13. Ogden CL, Troiano RP, Breifel RR, Kuczmarski RJ, Flegal KM, Johnson CL. Prevalence of overweight among preschool children in the United States, 1971 through 1994. *Pediatrics.* 1997;99(4). Available at: http://www.pediatrics.org/cgi/content/full/99/4/e1
14. Gidding SS, Bao W, Srinivasan SR, Berenson GW. Effects of secular trends in obesity on coronary risk factors in children: the Bogalusa Heart Study. *J Pediatr.* 1995;127:868–874
15. Freedman DS, Dietz WH, Srinivasan SR, Berenson GS. The relation of overweight to cardiovascular risk factors among children and adolescents: the Bogalusa heart study. *Pediatrics.* 1999;103:1175–1182
16. Must A, Jacques PF, Dallal GE, Bajema CJ, Dietz WH. Long-term morbidity and mortality of overweight adolescents. A follow-up of the Harvard Growth Study of 1922 to 1935. *N Engl J Med.* 1992;327: 1350–1355
17. Clarke WR, Woolson RF, Lauer RM. Changes in ponderosity and blood pressure in childhood: the Muscatine Study. *Am J Epidemiol.* 1986;124: 195–206
18. Johnson AL, Cornoni JC, Cassel JC, Tyroler HA, Heyden S, Hames CG. Influence of race, sex and weight on blood pressure behavior in young adults. *Am J Cardiol.* 1975;35:523–530
19. Morrison JA, Laskerzewski PM, Rauh JL, et al. Lipids, lipoproteins, and sexual maturation during adolescence: the Princeton Maturation Study. *Metabolism.* 1979;28:641–649
20. Shinha R, Fisch G, Teague B, et al. Prevalence of impaired glucose tolerance among children and adolescents with marked obesity. *N Engl J Med.* 2002;346:802–810
21. Pinhas-Hamiel O, Dolan LM, Daniels SR, Standiford D, Khoury PR, Zeitler P. Increased incidence of non-insulin-dependent diabetes mellitus among adolescents. *J Pediatr.* 1996;128:608–615
22. Richards GE, Cavallo A, Meyer WJ III, et al. Obesity, acanthosis nigricans, insulin resistance, and hyperandrogenemia: pediatric perspective and natural history. *J Pediatr.* 1985;107:893–897
23. Strauss RS. Childhood obesity and self-esteem. *Pediatrics.* 2000;105(1). Available at: http://www.pediatrics.org/cgi/content/full/105/1/e15
24. Davison KK, Birch LL. Weight status, parent reaction, and self-concept in five-year-old girls. *Pediatrics.* 2001;107:46–53
25. Mitchell BD, Kammerer CM, Reinhart LJ, Stern MP. NIDDM in Mexican-American families. Heterogeneity by age of onset. *Diabetes Care.* 1994;17:567–573
26. Pugliese MT, Lifshitz F, Grad G, Fort P, Marks-Katz M. Fear of obesity. A cause of short stature and delayed puberty. *N Engl J Med.* 1983;309: 513–518
27. American Academy of Pediatrics, Section on Pediatric Pulmonology, Subcommittee on Obstructive Sleep Apnea Syndrome. Clinical practice guideline: diagnosis and management of childhood obstructive sleep apnea syndrome. *Pediatrics.* 2002;109:704–712
28. Rodriguez MA, Winkleby MA, Ahn D, Sundquist J, Kraemer HC. Identification of population subgroups of children and adolescents with high asthma prevalence: findings from the Third National Health and Nutrition Examination Survey. *Arch Pediatr Adolesc Med.* 2002;156: 269–275
29. Riley DJ, Santiago TV, Edelman NH. Complications of obesity-hypoventilation syndrome in childhood. *Am J Dis Child.* 1976;130: 671–674
30. Boxer GH, Bauer AM, Miller BD. Obesity-hypoventilation in childhood. *J Am Acad Child Adolesc Psychiatry.* 1988;27:552–558
31. Mallory GB Jr, Fiser DH, Jackson R. Sleep-associated breathing disorders in obese children and adolescents. *J Pediatr.* 1989;115:892–897
32. Silvestri JM, Weese-Mayer DE, Bass MT, Kenny AS, Hauptman SA, Pearsall SM. Polysomnography in obese children with a history of sleep-associated breathing disorders. *Pediatr Pulmonol.* 1993;16:124–129
33. Dietz WH, Gross WL, Kirkpatrick JA Jr. Blount disease (tibia vara): another skeletal disorder associated with childhood obesity. *J Pediatr.* 1982;101:735–737
34. Loder RT, Aronson DD, Greenfield ML. The epidemiology of bilateral slipped capital femoral epiphysis. A study of children in Michigan. *J Bone Joint Surg.* 1993;75:1141–1147
35. Rashid M, Roberts EA. Nonalcoholic steatohepatitis in children. *J Pediatr Gastroenterol Nutr.* 2000;30:48–53
36. Guo SS, Chumlea WC. Tracking of body mass index in children in relation to overweight in adulthood. *Am J Clin Nutr.* 1999;70(suppl): 145S–148S
37. Wisemandle W, Maynard LM, Guo SS, Siervogel RM. Childhood

weight, stature, and body mass index among never overweight, early-onset overweight and late-onset overweight groups. *Pediatrics*. 2000; 106(1). Available at: http://www.pediatrics.org/cgi/content/full/106/1/e14

38. Wolf AM, Colditz GA. Current estimates of the economic cost of obesity in the United States. *Obes Res*. 1998;6:97–106

39. Becque MD, Katch VL, Rocchini AP, Marks CR, Moorehead C. Coronary risk incidence of obese adolescents: reduction by exercise plus diet intervention. *Pediatrics*. 1988;81:605–612

40. Sothern MS, von Almen TK, Schumacher H, et al. An effective multi-disciplinary approach to weight reduction in youth. *Ann N Y Acad Sci*. 1993;699:292–294

41. Jacobson MS, Copperman N, Haas T, Shenker IR. Adolescent obesity and cardiovascular risk: a rational approach to management. *Ann N Y Acad Sci*. 1993;699:220–229

42. Epstein LH, Myers MD, Raynor HA, Saelens BE. Treatment of pediatric obesity. *Pediatrics*. 1998;101(suppl):554–570

43. Harrell JS, Gansky SA, McMurray RG, Bangdiwala SI, Frauman AC, Bradley CB. School-based interventions improve heart health in children with multiple cardiovascular disease risk factors. *Pediatrics*. 1998; 102:371–380

44. Willi SM, Oexamnn MJ, Wright NM, Collup NA, Key LL Jr. The effects of a high protein, low-fat, ketogenic diet on adolescents with morbid obesity: body composition, blood chemistries, and sleep abnormalities. *Pediatrics*. 1998;101:61–67

45. Epstein LH, Valoski A, Wing RR, McCurley J. Ten-year follow-up of behavioral family-based treatment for obese children. *JAMA*. 1990;264: 2519–2523

46. Wadden TA, Foster GD, Letizia KA. One-year behavioral treatment of obesity: comparison of moderate and severe caloric restriction and the effects of weight maintenance therapy. *J Consult Clin Psychol*. 1994;62: 165–171

47. Rosenbaum M, Leibel RL, Hirsch J. Obesity. *N Engl J Med*. 1997;337: 396–407

48. Rosenbaum M, Leibel RL. The physiology of body weight regulation: relevance to the etiology of obesity in children. *Pediatrics*. 1998; 101(suppl):525–539

49. Ritzen EM, Lindgren AC, Hagenas L, Marcus C, Muller J, Blichfeldt S. Growth hormone treatment of patients with Prader-Willi syndrome. Swedish Growth Hormone Advisory Group. *J Pediatr Endocrinol Metab*. 1999 Apr;12(suppl):345–349

50. Whitman BY, Myers S, Carrel A, Allen D. The behavioral impact of growth hormone treatment for children and adolescents with Prader-Willi syndrome: a 2-year, controlled study. *Pediatrics*. 2002;109(2). Available at: http://www.pediatrics.org/cgi/content/full/109/2/e35

51. Carrel AL, Myers SE, Whitman BY, Allen DB. Sustained benefits of growth hormone on body composition, fat utilization, physical strength and agility, and growth in Prader-Willi syndrome are dose-dependent. *J Pediatr Endocrinol Metab*. 2001;14:1097–1105

52. Stunkard AJ, Harris JR, Pedersen NL, McClearn GE. The body mass index of twins who have been reared apart. *N Engl J Med*. 1990;322: 1483–1487

53. Bouchard C, Tremblay A, Despres JP, et al. The response to long-term overfeeding in identical twins. *N Engl J Med*. 1990;322:1477–1482

54. Whitaker RC, Wright JA, Pepe MS, Seidel KD, Dietz WH. Predicting obesity in young adulthood from childhood and parental obesity. *N Engl J Med*. 1997;337:869–873

55. Agras SW, Kraemer HC, Berkowitz RI, Hammer LD. Influence of early feeding style on adiposity at 6 years of age. *J Pediatr*. 1990;116:805–809

56. von Kries R, Koletzko B, Sauerwald T, et al. Breast feeding and obesity: cross sectional study. *BMJ*. 1999;319:147–150

57. Gilman MW, Rifas-Shiman SL, Camargo CA Jr, et al. Risk of overweight among adolescents who were breastfed as infants. *JAMA*. 2001;285: 2461–2467

58. Hediger ML, Overpeck MD, Kuczmarski RJ, Ruan WJ. Association between infant breastfeeding and overweight in young children. *JAMA*. 2001;285:2453–2460

59. Heald FP. Natural history and physiological basis of adolescent obesity. *Fed Proc*. 1966;25:1–3

60. Travers SH, Jeffers BW, Bloch CA, Hill JO, Eckel RH. Gender and Tanner stage differences in body composition and insulin sensitivity in early pubertal children. *J Clin Endocrinol Metab*. 1995;80:172–178

61. Adair LS, Gordon-Larsen P. Maturational timing and overweight prevalence in US adolescent girls. *Am J Public Health*. 2001;91:642–644

62. Irwin CE Jr, Igra V, Eyre S, Millstein S. Risk-taking behavior in adolescents: the paradigm. *Ann N Y Acad Sci*. 1997;817:1–35

63. Alaimo K, Olson CM, Frongillo EA Jr. Low family income and food insufficiency in relation to overweight in US children: is there a paradox? *Arch Pediatr Adolesc Med*. 2001;155:1161–1167

64. Strauss RS, Knight J Influence of the home environment on the development of obesity in children. *Pediatrics*. 1999;103(6). Available at: http://www.pediatrics.org/cgi/content/full/103/6/e85

65. Birch LL, Fisher JO. Mothers' child-feeding practices influence daughters' eating and weight. *Am J Clin Nutr*. 2000;71:1054–1061

66. Klesges RC, Stein RJ, Eck LH, Isbell TR, Klesges LM. Parental influence on food selection in young children and its relationships to childhood obesity. *Am J Clin Nutr*. 1991;53:859–864

67. Ray JW, Klesges RC. Influences on the eating behavior of children. *Ann N Y Acad Sci*. 1993;699:57–69

68. Fisher JO, Birch LL. Fat preferences and fat consumption of 3- to 5-year-old children are related to parental adiposity. *J Am Diet Assoc*. 1995;95:759–764

69. Neumark-Sztainer D, Story M, Resnick MD, Blum RW. Correlates of inadequate fruit and vegetable consumption among adolescents. *Prev Med*. 1996;25:497–505

70. Krebs-Smith SM, Cook A, Subar AF, Cleveland L, Friday J, Kahle LL. Fruit and vegetable intakes of children and adolescents in the United States. *Arch Pediatr Adolesc Med*. 1996;150:81–86

71. Kennedy E, Powell R. Changing eating patterns of American children: a view from 1996. *J Am Coll Nutr*. 1997;16:524–529

72. Berkey CS, Rockett HR, Field AE, et al. Activity dietary intake, and weight changes in a longitudinal study of preadolescent and adolescent boys and girls *Pediatrics*. 2000;105(4). Available at: http://www.pediatrics.org/cgi/content/full/105/4/e56

73. Anderson RE, Crespo CJ, Bartlett SJ, Cheskin LJ, Pratt M. Relationship of physical activity and television watching with body weight and level of fatness among children: results from the Third National Health and Nutrition Examination Survey. *JAMA*. 1998;279:938–942

74. Dennison BA, Erb TA, Jenkins PL. Television viewing and television in bedroom associated with overweight risk among low-income preschool children. *Pediatrics*. 2002;109:1028–1035

75. Pate RR, Ross JG. The National Children and Youth Fitness Study II: factors associated with health-related fitness. *J Physical Educ Recreation Dance*. 1987;58:93–96

76. Dietz WH Jr, Gortmaker SL. Do we fatten our children at the TV set? Obesity and television viewing in children and adolescents. *Pediatrics*. 1985;75:807–812

77. Gortmaker SL, Must A, Sobol AM, Peterson K, Colditz GA, Dietz WH. Television viewing as a cause of increasing obesity among children in the United States, 1986–1990. *Arch Pediatr Adolesc Med*. 1996;150:356–362

78. Tucker LA. The relationship of television viewing to physical fitness and obesity. *Adolescence*. 1986;21:797–806

79. Robinson TN, Hammer LD, Killen JD, et al. Does television viewing increase obesity and reduce physical activity? Cross-sectional and longitudinal analyses among adolescent girls. *Pediatrics*. 1993;91:273–280

80. Robinson T. Reducing children's television viewing to prevent obesity: a randomized controlled trial. *JAMA*. 1999;282:1561–1567

81. Miller LA, Grunwald G, Johnson SL, Krebs NF. Disease severity at time of referral for pediatric failure to thrive and obesity: time for a paradigm shift? *J Pediatr*. 2002;141:121–124

82. Jain A, Sherman SN, Chamberlin DL, Carter Y, Powers SW, Whitaker RC. Why don't low-income mothers worry about their preschoolers being overweight? *Pediatrics*. 2001;107:1138–1146

83. Nawaz H, Adams ML, Katz DL. Physician-patient interactions regarding diet, exercise, and smoking. *Prev Med*. 2000;31:652–657

84. Calfas KJ, Long BJ, Sallis JF, Wooten WJ, Pratt M, Patrick K. A controlled trial of physician counseling to promote the adoption of physical activity. *Prev Med*. 1996;25:225–233

85. Lu MC, Lange L, Slusser W, Hamilton J, Halfon N. Provider encouragement of breast-feeding: evidence from a national survey. *Obstet Gynecol*. 2001;97:290–295

86. Epps RP, Manley MW. The clinician's role in preventing smoking initiation. *Med Clin North Am*. 1992;76:439–449

87. Ludwig DS, Peterson KE, Gortmaker SL. Relation between consumption of sugar-sweetened drinks and childhood obesity: a prospective, observational analysis. *Lancet*. 2001;357:505–508

88. Tershakovec AM, Watson MH, Wenner WJ Jr, Marx AL. Insurance reimbursement for the treatment of obesity in children. *J Pediatr*. 1999; 134:573–578

ADDITIONAL RESOURCES

American Academy of Pediatrics, Committee on Nutrition. Cholesterol in childhood. *Pediatrics*. 1998;101:141–147

American Academy of Pediatrics, Committee on Sports Medicine and Fitness and Committee on School Health. Physical fitness and activity in schools. *Pediatrics.* 2000;105:1156–1157

Centers for Disease Control and Prevention. *2000 CDC Growth Charts: United States.* Atlanta, GA: Centers for Disease Control and Prevention; 2000. Available at: http://www.cdc.gov/growthcharts

Jacobson MS, Rees J, Golden NH, Irwin C. Adolescent nutritional disorders. *Ann N Y Acad Sci.* 1997;817

National Association for Sports and Physical Activity Web site. Available at: http://www.aahperd.org

National Institutes of Health, National Heart, Lung, and Blood Institute. *The Practical Guide: Identification, Evaluation, and Treatment of Overweight and Obesity in Adults.* Rockville, MD: National Heart, Lung, and Blood Institute; 2000. NIH Publ. No. 00-4084

Story M, Holt K, Sofka D, eds. *Bright Futures in Practice: Nutrition.* Arlington, VA: National Center for Education in Maternal and Child Health; 2000

US Department of Health and Human Services, Office of Public Health and Science, Office of Disease Prevention and Health Promotion, Public Health Foundation. *Healthy People 2010 Toolkit: A Field Guide to Health Planning.* Washington, DC: Public Health Foundation; 2002. Available at: http://www.health.gov/healthypeople/state/toolkit or by calling toll-free 877/252–1200 (Item RM-005)

Weight-control Information Network Web site. Available at: http://www.niddk.nih.gov/health/nutrit/win.htm

All policy statements from the American Academy of Pediatrics automatically expire 5 years after publication unless reaffirmed, revised, or retired at or before that time.

AMERICAN ACADEMY OF PEDIATRICS

POLICY STATEMENT
Organizational Principles to Guide and Define the Child Health Care System and/or Improve the Health of All Children

Committee on School Health

Soft Drinks in Schools

ABSTRACT. This statement is intended to inform pediatricians and other health care professionals, parents, superintendents, and school board members about nutritional concerns regarding soft drink consumption in schools. Potential health problems associated with high intake of sweetened drinks are 1) overweight or obesity attributable to additional calories in the diet; 2) displacement of milk consumption, resulting in calcium deficiency with an attendant risk of osteoporosis and fractures; and 3) dental caries and potential enamel erosion. Contracts with school districts for exclusive soft drink rights encourage consumption directly and indirectly. School officials and parents need to become well informed about the health implications of vended drinks in school before making a decision about student access to them. A clearly defined, district-wide policy that restricts the sale of soft drinks will safeguard against health problems as a result of overconsumption.

BACKGROUND AND INFORMATION

Overweight

Overweight is now the most common medical condition of childhood, with the prevalence having doubled over the past 20 years. Nearly 1 of every 3 children is at risk of overweight (defined as body mass index [BMI] between the 85th and 95th percentiles for age and sex), and 1 of every 6 is overweight (defined as BMI at or above the 95th percentile).[1] Complications of the obesity epidemic include high cholesterol, high blood pressure, type 2 diabetes mellitus, coronary plaque formation, and serious psychosocial implications.[2-6] Annually, obesity-related diseases in adults and children account for more than 300 000 deaths and more than $100 billion per year in treatment costs.[7-9]

Soft Drinks and Fruit Drinks

In the United States, children's daily food selections are excessively high in discretionary, or added, fat and sugar.[10-15] This category of fats and sugars accounts for 40% of children's daily energy intake.[10] Soft drink consumers have a higher daily energy intake than nonconsumers at all ages.[16] Sweetened drinks (fruitades, fruit drinks, soft drinks, etc) constitute the primary source of added sugar in the daily diet of children.[17] High-fructose corn syrup, the principle nutrient in sweetened drinks, is not a problem food when consumed in smaller amounts, but each 12-oz serving of a carbonated, sweetened soft drink contains the equivalent of 10 teaspoons of sugar and 150 kcal. Soft drink consumption increased by 300% in 20 years,[12] and serving sizes have increased from 6.5 oz in the 1950s to 12 oz in the 1960s and 20 oz by the late 1990s. Between 56% and 85% of children in school consume at least 1 soft drink daily, with the highest amounts ingested by adolescent males. Of this group, 20% consume 4 or more servings daily.[16]

Each 12-oz sugared soft drink consumed daily has been associated with a 0.18-point increase in a child's BMI and a 60% increase in risk of obesity, associations not found with "diet" (sugar-free) soft drinks.[18] Sugar-free soft drinks constitute only 14% of the adolescent soft drink market.[19] Sweetened drinks are associated with obesity, probably because overconsumption is a particular problem when energy is ingested in liquid form[20] and because these drinks represent energy added to, not displacing, other dietary intake.[21-23] In addition to the caloric load, soft drinks pose a risk of dental caries because of their high sugar content and enamel erosion because of their acidity.[24]

Calcium

Milk consumption decreases as soft drinks become a favorite choice for children, a transition that occurs between the third and eighth grades.[12,15] Milk is the principle source of calcium in the typical American diet.[11] Dairy products contain substantial amounts of several nutrients, including 72% of calcium, 32% of phosphorus, 26% of riboflavin, 22% of vitamin B_{12}, 19% of protein, and 15% of vitamin A in the US food supply.[25] The percent daily value for milk is considered either "good" or "excellent" for 9 essential nutrients depending on age and gender. Intake of protein and micronutrients is decreased in diets low in dairy products.[19,26] The resulting diminished calcium intake jeopardizes the accrual of maximal peak bone mass at a critical time in life, adolescence.[27] Nearly 100% of the calcium in the body resides in bone.[27] Nearly 40% of peak bone mass is accumulated during adolescence. Studies suggest that a 5% to 10% deficit in peak bone mass may result in a 50% greater lifetime prevalence of hip fracture,[28] a problem certain to worsen if steps are not taken to improve calcium intake among adolescents.[29]

STATEMENT OF PROBLEM

Soft drinks and fruit drinks are sold in vending machines, in school stores, at school sporting events, and at school fund drives. "Exclusive pouring rights" contracts, in which the school agrees to promote one brand exclusively in exchange for money, are being signed in an increasing number of school districts across the country,[30] often with bonus incentives tied to sales.[31] Although they are a new phenomenon, such contracts already have provided schools with more than $200 million in unrestricted revenue.

Some superintendents, school board members, and principals claim that the financial gain from soft drink contracts is an unquestioned "win" for students, schools, communities, and taxpayers.[31,32] Parents and school authorities generally are uninformed about the potential risk to the health of their children that may be associated with the unrestricted consumption of soft drinks. The decision regarding which foods will be sold in schools more often is made by school district business officers alone rather than with input from local health care professionals.

Subsidized school lunch programs are associated with a high intake of dietary protein, complex carbohydrates, dairy products, fruits, and vegetables.[16] The US Department of Agriculture, which oversees the National School Lunch Program, is concerned that foods with high sugar content (especially foods of minimal nutritional value, such as soft drinks) are displacing nutrients within the school lunch program, and there is evidence to support this.[26]

There are precedents for using optimal nutrition standards to create a model district-wide school nutrition policy,[33] but this is not yet a routine practice in most states. The discussion engendered by the creation of such a policy would be an important first step in establishing an ideal nutritional environment for students.

RECOMMENDATIONS

1. Pediatricians should work to eliminate sweetened drinks in schools. This entails educating school authorities, patients, and patients' parents about the health ramifications of soft drink consumption. Offerings such as real fruit and vegetable juices, water, and low-fat white or flavored milk provide students at all grade levels with healthful alternatives. Pediatricians should emphasize the notion that every school in every district shares a responsibility for the nutritional health of its student body.

2. Pediatricians should advocate for the creation of a school nutrition advisory council comprising parents, community and school officials, food service representatives, physicians, school nurses, dietitians, dentists, and other health care professionals. This group could be one component of a school district's health advisory council. Pediatricians should ensure that the health and nutritional interests of students form the foundation of nutritional policies in schools.

3. School districts should invite public discussion before making any decision to create a vended food or drink contract.

4. If a school district already has a soft drink contract in place, it should be tempered such that it does not promote overconsumption by students.
   - Soft drinks should not be sold as part of or in competition with the school lunch program, as stated in regulations of the US Department of Agriculture.[34]
   - Vending machines should not be placed within the cafeteria space where lunch is sold. Their location in the school should be chosen by the school district, not the vending company.
   - Vending machines with foods of minimal nutritional value, including soft drinks, should be turned off during lunch hours and ideally during school hours.
   - Vended soft drinks and fruit-flavored drinks should be eliminated in all elementary schools.
   - Incentives based on the amount of soft drinks sold per student should not be included as part of exclusive contracts.
   - Within the contract, the number of machines vending sweetened drinks should be limited. Schools should insist that the alternative beverages listed in recommendation 1 be provided in preference over sweetened drinks in school vending machines.
   - Schools should preferentially vend drinks that are sugar-free or low in sugar to lessen the risk of overweight.

5. Consumption or advertising of sweetened soft drinks within the classroom should be eliminated.

Committee on School Health, 2002–2003
Howard L. Taras, MD, Chairperson
Barbara L. Frankowski, MD, MPH
Jane W. McGrath, MD
Cynthia J. Mears, DO
*Robert D. Murray, MD
Thomas L. Young, MD

Liaisons
Janis Hootman, RN, PhD
   National Association of School Nurses
Janet Long, MEd
   American School Health Association
Jerald L. Newberry, MEd
   National Education Association, Health Information
Mary Vernon-Smiley, MD, MPH
   Centers for Disease Control and Prevention

Staff
Su Li, MPA

*Lead author

REFERENCES

1. American Academy of Pediatrics, Committee on Nutrition. Prevention of pediatric overweight and obesity. *Pediatrics*. 2003;112:424–430
2. Freedman DS, Dietz WH, Srinivasan SR, Berenson GS. The relation of overweight to cardiovascular risk factors among children and adolescents: the Bogalusa Heart Study. *Pediatrics*. 1999;103:1175–1182
3. Pinhas-Hamiel O, Dolan LM, Daniels SR, Standiford D, Khoury PR, Zeitler P. Increased incidence of non-insulin-dependent diabetes mellitus among adolescents. *J Pediatr*. 1996;128:608–615
4. Ludwig DS, Ebbeling CB. Type 2 diabetes mellitus in children: primary care and public health considerations. *JAMA*. 2001;286:1427–1430

AMERICAN ACADEMY OF PEDIATRICS   153

5. Dietz W. Health consequences of obesity in youth: childhood predictors of adult disease. *Pediatrics*. 1998;101:518–525

6. Davison KK, Birch LL. Weight status, parent reaction, and self-concept in five-year-old girls. *Pediatrics*. 2001;107:46–53

7. Allison DB, Fontaine KR, Manson JE, Stevens J, VanItallie TB. Annual deaths attributable to obesity in the United States. *JAMA*. 1999;282: 1530–1538

8. Must A, Spadano J, Coakley EH, Field AE, Colditz G, Dietz WH. The disease burden associated with overweight and obesity. *JAMA*. 1999; 282:1523–1529

9. Blumenthal D. Controlling health care expenditures. *N Engl J Med*. 2001;344:766–769

10. Muñoz KA, Krebs-Smith SM, Ballard-Barbash R, Cleveland LE. Food intakes of US children and adolescents compared with recommendations. *Pediatrics*. 1997;100:323–329

11. Subar AF, Krebs-Smith SM, Cook A, Kahle LL. Dietary sources of nutrients among US children, 1989–1991. *Pediatrics*. 1998;102:913–923

12. Calvadini C, Siega-Riz AM, Popkin BM. US adolescent food intake trends from 1965 to 1996. *Arch Dis Child*. 2000;83:18–24

13. Borrud LG, Enns CW, Mickle S. What we eat in America: USDA surveys food consumption changes. *Food Rev*. 1996;19:14–19. Available at: http://www.ers.usda.gov/publications/foodreview/sep1996/ sept96d.pdf. Accessed February 12, 2003

14. Borrud LG, Mickle S, Nowverl A, Tippett K. *Eating Out in America: Impact on Food Choices and Nutrient Profiles*. Beltsville, MD: Food Surveys Research Group, US Department of Agriculture; 1998. Available at: http://www.barc.usda.gov/bhnrc/foodsurvey/Eatout95.html. Accessed February 12, 2003

15. Lytle LA, Seifert S, Greenstein J, McGovern P. How do children's eating patterns and food choices change over time? Results from a cohort study. *Am J Health Promot*. 2000;14:222–228

16. Gleason P, Suitor C. *Children's Diets in the Mid-1990s: Dietary Intake and Its Relationship with School Meal Participation*. Alexandria, VA: US Department of Agriculture, Food and Nutrition Service, Office of Analysis, Nutrition and Evaluation; 2001. Available at: http://www.fns.usda. gov/oane/menu/published/cnp/files/childiet.pdf. Accessed February 12, 2003

17. Guthrie JF, Morton JF. Food sources of added sweeteners in the diets of Americans. *J Am Diet Assoc*. 2000;100:43–51

18. Ludwig DS, Peterson KE, Gortmaker SL. Relation between consumption of sugar-sweetened drinks and childhood obesity: a prospective observational analysis. *Lancet*. 2001;357:505–508

19. Harnack L, Stang J, Story M. Soft drink consumption among US children and adolescents: nutritional consequences. *J Am Diet Assoc*. 1999; 99:436–441

20. Mattes RD. Dietary compensation by humans for supplemental energy provided as ethanol or carbohydrates in fluids. *Physiol Behav*. 1996;59: 179–187

21. Bellisle F, Rolland-Cachera M-F. How sugar-containing drinks might increase adiposity in children. *Lancet*. 2001;357:490–491

22. Tordoff MG, Alleva AM. Effect of drinking soda sweetened with aspartame or high-fructose corn syrup on food intake and body weight. *Am J Clin Nutr*. 1990;51:963–969

23. De Castro JM, Orozco S. Moderate alcohol intake and spontaneous eating patterns of humans: evidence of unregulated supplementation. *Am J Clin Nutr*. 1990;52:246–253

24. Heller K, Burt BA, Eklund SA. Sugared soda consumption and dental caries in the United States. *J Dent Res*. 2001;80:1949–1953

25. Gerrior S, Bente L. *Nutrient Content of the US Food Supply, 1909–97*. Home Economics Research Report No. 54. Washington, DC: Center for Nutrition Policy and Promotion, US Department of Agriculture; 2001. Available at: http://www.usda.gov/cnpp/Pubs/Food%20Supply/ foodsupplyrpt.pdf. Accessed February 12, 2003

26. Johnson RK, Panely C, Wang MQ. The association between noon beverage consumption and the diet quality of school-age children. *J Child Nutr Manage*. 1998;22:95–100

27. American Academy of Pediatrics, Committee on Nutrition. Calcium requirements of infants, children, and adolescents. *Pediatrics*. 1999;104: 1152–1157

28. Wyshak G. Teenaged girls, carbonated beverage consumption, and bone fractures. *Arch Pediatr Adolesc Med*. 2000;154:610–613

29. NIH Consensus Development Panel on Osteoporosis Prevention, Diagnosis, and Therapy. Osteoporosis: prevention, diagnosis, and therapy. *JAMA*. 2001;285:785–795

30. Henry T. Coca-cola rethinks school contracts. Bottlers asked to fall in line. *USA Today*. March 14, 2001:A01

31. Nestle M. Soft drink "pouring rights": marketing empty calories to children. *Public Health Rep*. 2000;115:308–319

32. Zorn RL. The great cola wars: how one district profits from the competition for vending machines. *Am Sch Board J*. 1999;186:31–33

33. Stuhldreher WL, Koehler AN, Harrison MK, Deel H. The West Virginia Standards for School Nutrition. *J Child Nutr Manage*. 1998;22:79–86

34. National School Lunch Program Regulations. 7 CFR §210.11 (2002). Competitive food services

---

All policy statements from the American Academy of Pediatrics automatically expire 5 years after publication unless reaffirmed, revised, or retired at or before that time.

AMERICAN ACADEMY OF PEDIATRICS

Committee on Nutrition

The Use and Misuse of Fruit Juice in Pediatrics

ABSTRACT. Historically, fruit juice was recommended by pediatricians as a source of vitamin C and an extra source of water for healthy infants and young children as their diets expanded to include solid foods with higher renal solute. Fruit juice is marketed as a healthy, natural source of vitamins and, in some instances, calcium. Because juice tastes good, children readily accept it. Although juice consumption has some benefits, it also has potential detrimental effects. Pediatricians need to be knowledgeable about juice to inform parents and patients on its appropriate uses.

ABBREVIATIONS. FDA, Food and Drug Administration; AAP, American Academy of Pediatrics.

INTRODUCTION

In 1997, US consumers spent almost $5 billion on refrigerated and bottled juice.[1] Mean juice consumption in America is more than 2 billion gal/y or 9.2 gal/y per person.[2] Children are the single largest group of juice consumers. Children younger than 12 years account for only about 18% of the total population but consume 28% of all juice and juice drinks.[3] By 1 year of age, almost 90% of infants consume juice. The mean daily juice consumption by infants is approximately 2 oz/d, but 2% consume more than 16 oz/d, and 1% of infants consume more than 21 oz/d.[2,4,5] Toddlers consume a mean of approximately 6 oz/d.[2] Ten percent of children 2 to 3 years old and 8% of children 4 to 5 years old drink on average more than 12 oz/d.[2] Adolescents consume the least, accounting for only 10% of juice consumption.

DEFINITIONS

To be labeled as a fruit juice, the Food and Drug Administration (FDA) mandates that a product be 100% fruit juice. For juices reconstituted from concentrate, the label must state that the product is reconstituted from concentrate. Any beverage that is less than 100% fruit juice must list the percentage of the product that is fruit juice, and the beverage must include a descriptive term, such as "drink," "beverage," or "cocktail." In general, juice drinks contain between 10% and 99% juice and added sweeteners, flavors, and sometimes fortifiers, such as vitamin C or calcium. These ingredients must be listed on the label, according to FDA regulations.

COMPOSITION OF FRUIT JUICE

Water is the predominant component of fruit juice. Carbohydrates, including sucrose, fructose, glucose, and sorbitol, are the next most prevalent nutrient in juice. The carbohydrate concentration varies from 11 g/100 mL (0.44 kcal/mL) to more than 16 g/100 mL (0.64 kcal/mL). Human milk and standard infant formulas have a carbohydrate concentration of 7 g/100 mL.

Juice contains a small amount of protein and minerals. Juices fortified with calcium have approximately the same calcium content as milk but lack other nutrients present in milk. Some juices have high contents of potassium, vitamin A, and vitamin C. In addition, some juices and juice drinks are fortified with vitamin C. The vitamin C and flavonoids in juice may have beneficial long-term health effects, such as decreasing the risk of cancer and heart disease.[6,7] Drinks that contain ascorbic acid consumed simultaneously with food can increase iron absorption by twofold.[8,9] This may be important for children who consume diets with low iron bioavailability.

Juice contains no fat or cholesterol, and unless the pulp is included, it contains no fiber. The fluoride concentration of juice and juice drinks varies. One study found fluoride ion concentrations ranged from 0.02 to 2.8 parts per million.[10] The fluoride content of concentrated juice varies with the fluoride content of the water used to reconstitute the juice.

Grapefruit juice contains substances that suppress a cytochrome P-450 enzyme in the small bowel wall. This results in altered absorption of some drugs, such as cisapride, calcium antagonists, and cyclosporin.[11–13] Grapefruit juice should not be consumed when these drugs are used.

Some manufacturers specifically produce juice for infants. These juices do not contain sulfites or added sugars and are more expensive than regular fruit juice.

ABSORPTION OF CARBOHYDRATE FROM JUICE

The 4 major sugars in juice are sucrose, glucose, fructose, and sorbitol. Sucrose is a disaccharide that is hydrolyzed into 2 component monosaccharides, glucose and fructose, by sucrase present in the small bowel epithelium. Glucose is then absorbed rapidly via an active-carrier–mediated process in the brush border of the small bowel. Fructose is absorbed by a facilitated transport mechanism via a carrier but not against a concentration gradient. In addition, fructose may be absorbed by a disaccharidase-related transport system, because the absorption of fructose is more efficient in the presence of glucose, with maximal absorption occurring when fructose and glucose are present in equimolar concentrations.[14] Clinical studies have demonstrated this, with more apparent malabsorption when fructose concentration exceeds that of glucose (eg, apple and pear juice) than when the 2 sugars are present in equal concentrations (eg, white grape juice).[15,16] However, when provided in appropriate amounts (10 mL/kg of body weight), these different juices are absorbed equally as well.[17] Sorbitol is absorbed via passive diffusion at slow rates, resulting in much of the ingested sorbitol being unabsorbed.[18]

Carbohydrate that is not absorbed in the small intestine is fermented by bacteria in the colon. This bacterial fermentation results in the production of hydrogen, carbon dioxide, methane, and the short-chain fatty acids—acetic, propionic, and butyric. Some of these gases and fatty acids are reabsorbed through the colonic epithelium, and in this way, a portion of the malabsorbed carbohydrate can be scavenged.[19] Nonabsorbed carbohydrate presents an osmotic load to the gastrointestinal tract, which causes diarrhea.[20]

Malabsorption of carbohydrate in juice, especially when consumed in excessive amounts, can result in chronic diarrhea, flatulence, bloating, and abdominal pain.[21–27] Fructose and sorbitol have been implicated most commonly,[15,16,28–30] but the ratios of specific carbohydrates may also be important.[31] The malabsorption of carbohydrate that can result from large intakes of juice is the basis for some health care providers to recommend juice for the treatment of constipation.[32]

JUICE IN THE FOOD GUIDE PYRAMID

Fruit is 1 of the 5 major food groups in the Food Guide Pyramid.[33] It is recommended that children consuming approximately 1600 kcal/d (depending on size, 1–4 years old) should have 2 fruit servings and those consuming 2800 kcal/d (depending on size, 10–18 years old) should consume 4 fruit servings. Half of these servings can be provided in the form of fruit juice (not fruit drinks). A 6-oz glass of fruit juice equals 1 fruit serving. Fruit juice offers no nutritional advantage over whole fruit. In fact, fruit juice lacks the fiber of whole fruit. Kilocalorie for kilocalorie, fruit juice can be consumed more quickly than whole fruit. Reliance on fruit juice instead of whole fruit to provide the recommended daily intake of fruits does not promote eating behaviors associated with consumption of whole fruits.

MICROBIAL SAFETY OF JUICE

Only pasteurized juice is safe for infants, children, and adolescents. Pasteurized fruit juices are free of microorganisms. Unpasteurized juice may contain pathogens, such as *Escherichia coli* and *Salmonella* and *Cryptosporidium* organisms.[34] These organisms can cause serious disease, such as hemolytic-uremic syndrome, and should never be given to infants and children. Unpasteurized juice must contain a warning on the label that the product may contain harmful bacteria.[35]

INFANTS

The American Academy of Pediatrics (AAP) recommends that breast milk be the only nutrient fed to infants until 4 to 6 months of age.[36] For mothers who cannot breastfeed or choose not to breastfeed, a prepared infant formula can be used and is a complete source of nutrition. No additional nutrients are needed. There is no nutritional indication to feed juice to infants younger than 6 months. Offering juice before solid foods are introduced into the diet could risk having juice replace breast milk or infant formula in the diet. This can result in reduced intake of protein, fat, vitamins, and minerals such as iron, calcium, and zinc.[37] Malnutrition and short stature in children have been associated with excessive consumption of juice.[4,38]

After approximately 4 to 6 months of age, solid foods can be introduced into the diets of infants. The AAP recommends that single-ingredient foods be chosen and introduced 1 at a time at weekly intervals. Iron-fortified infant cereals or pureed meats are good choices for first weaning foods. Because foods high in iron are recommended as weaning foods, beverages that contain vitamin C do not offer a nutritional advantage for iron-sufficient individuals.

It is prudent to give juice only to infants who can drink from a cup (approximately 6 months or older). Teeth begin to erupt at approximately 6 months of age. Dental caries have also been associated with juice consumption.[39] Prolonged exposure of the teeth to the sugars in juice is a major contributing factor to dental caries. The AAP and the American Academy of Pedodontics recommendations state that juice should be offered to infants in a cup, not a bottle, and that infants not be put to bed with a bottle in their mouth.[40] The practice of allowing children to carry a bottle, cup, or box of juice around throughout the day leads to excessive exposure of the teeth to carbohydrate, which promotes development of dental caries.

Fruit juice should be used as part of a meal or snack. It should not be sipped throughout the day or used as a means to pacify an unhappy infant or child. Because infants consume fewer than 1600 kcal/d, 4 to 6 oz of juice per day, representing 1 food serving of fruit, is more than adequate. Infants can be encouraged to consume whole fruits that are mashed or pureed.

The AAP practice guideline on the management of acute gastroenteritis in young children recommends that only oral electrolyte solutions be used to rehydrate infants and young children and that a normal diet be continued throughout an episode of gastroenteritis.[41] Surveys show that many health care providers do not follow the recommended procedures for management of diarrhea.[42] The high carbohydrate content of juice (11–16 g %), compared with oral electrolyte solutions (2.5–3 g %), may exceed the intestine's ability to absorb carbohydrate, resulting in carbohydrate malabsorption. Carbohydrate malabsorption causes osmotic diarrhea, increasing the severity of the diarrhea already present.[43] Fruit juice is low in electrolytes. The sodium concentration is 1 to 3 mEq/L. Stool sodium concentration in children with acute diarrhea is 20 to 40 mEq/L. Oral electrolyte solutions contain 40 to 45 mEq/L of sodium. As a replacement for fluid losses, juice may predispose infants to development of hyponatremia.

In the past, there was concern that infants who were fed orange juice were likely to develop an allergy to it. The development of a perioral rash in some infants after being fed freshly squeezed citrus juice is most likely a contact dermatitis attributable to peel oils.[44] Diarrhea and other gastrointestinal symptoms observed in some infants were most likely attributable to carbohydrate malabsorption. Although allergies to fruit may develop early in life, they are uncommon.[45]

TODDLERS AND YOUNG CHILDREN

Most issues relevant to juice intake for infants are also are relevant for toddlers and young children. Fruit juice and fruit drinks are easily overconsumed by toddlers and young children because they taste good. In addition, they are conveniently packaged or can be placed in a bottle and carried around during the day. Because juice is viewed as nutritious, limits on consumption are not usually set by parents. Like soda, it can contribute to energy imbalance. High intakes of juice can contribute to diarrhea, overnutrition or undernutrition, and development of dental caries.

OLDER CHILDREN AND ADOLESCENTS

Juice consumption presents fewer nutritional issues for older children and adolescents, because they consume less of these beverages. Nevertheless, it seems prudent to limit juice intake to two 6-oz servings, or half of the recommended fruit servings each day. It is important to encourage consumption of the whole fruit for the benefit of fiber intake and a longer time to consume the same kilocalories.

Excessive juice consumption and the resultant increase in energy intake may contribute to the development of obesity. One study found a link between juice intake in excess of 12 oz/d and obesity.[4] Other studies, however, found that children who consumed greater amounts of juice were taller and had lower body mass index than those who consumed less juice[46] or found no relationship between juice intake and growth parameters.[47] More research is needed to better define this relationship.

CONCLUSIONS

1. Fruit juice offers no nutritional benefit for infants younger than 6 months.
2. Fruit juice offers no nutritional benefits over whole fruit for infants older than 6 months and children.
3. One hundred percent fruit juice or reconstituted juice can be a healthy part of the diet when consumed as part of a well-balanced diet. Fruit drinks, however, are not nutritionally equivalent to fruit juice.
4. Juice is not appropriate in the treatment of dehydration or management of diarrhea.

5. Excessive juice consumption may be associated with malnutrition (overnutrition and undernutrition).
6. Excessive juice consumption may be associated with diarrhea, flatulence, abdominal distention, and tooth decay.
7. Unpasteurized juice may contain pathogens that can cause serious illnesses.
8. A variety of fruit juices, provided in appropriate amounts for a child's age, are not likely to cause any significant clinical symptoms.
9. Calcium-fortified juices provide a bioavailable source of calcium but lack other nutrients present in breast milk, formula, or cow's milk.

RECOMMENDATIONS

1. Juice should not be introduced into the diet of infants before 6 months of age.
2. Infants should not be given juice from bottles or easily transportable covered cups that allow them to consume juice easily throughout the day. Infants should not be given juice at bedtime.
3. Intake of fruit juice should be limited to 4 to 6 oz/d for children 1 to 6 years old. For children 7 to 18 years old, juice intake should be limited to 8 to 12 oz or 2 servings per day.
4. Children should be encouraged to eat whole fruits to meet their recommended daily fruit intake.
5. Infants, children, and adolescents should not consume unpasteurized juice.
6. In the evaluation of children with malnutrition (overnutrition and undernutrition), the health care provider should determine the amount of juice being consumed.
7. In the evaluation of children with chronic diarrhea, excessive flatulence, abdominal pain, and bloating, the health care provider should determine the amount of juice being consumed.
8. In the evaluation of dental caries, the amount and means of juice consumption should be determined.
9. Pediatricians should routinely discuss the use of fruit juice and fruit drinks and should educate parents about differences between the two.

COMMITTEE ON NUTRITION, 1999–2000
Susan S. Baker, MD, PhD, Chairperson
William J. Cochran, MD
Frank R. Greer, MD
Melvin B. Heyman, MD
Marc S. Jacobson, MD
Tom Jaksic, MD, PhD
Nancy F. Krebs, MD

LIAISONS
Donna Blum-Kemelor, MS, RD
   US Department of Agriculture
William Dietz, MD, PhD
   Centers for Disease Control and Prevention
Gilman Grave, MD
   National Institute of Child Health and Human Development
Suzanne S. Harris, PhD
   International Life Sciences Institute

Van S. Hubbard, MD, PhD
  National Institute of Diabetes and Digestive
  and Kidney Diseases
Ann Prendergast, RD, MPH
  Maternal and Child Health Bureau
Alice E. Smith, MS, RD
  American Dietetic Association
Elizabeth Yetley, PhD
  Food and Drug Administration
Doris E. Yuen, MD, PhD
  Canadian Paediatric Society

SECTION LIAISONS
Scott C. Denne, MD
  Section on Perinatal Pediatrics
Ronald M. Lauer, MD
  Section on Cardiology

STAFF
Pamela Kanda, MPH

REFERENCES

1. Food Marketing Institute Information Service. *Food Institute Report.* Washington, DC: Food Marketing Institute Information Service; 1998

2. Agriculture Research Service. *Food and Nutrient Intakes by Individuals in the United States by Sex and Age, 1994–96.* Washington, DC: US Department of Agriculture; 1998. NFS Report No. 96-2

3. National Family Opinion Research. *Share of Intake Panel* [database]. Greenwich, CT: National Family Opinion Research. Cited by: Clydesdale FM, Kolasa KM, Ikeda JP. All you want to know about fruit juice. *Nutrition Today.* 1994;March/April:14–28

4. Dennison BA, Rockwell HL, Baker SL. Excess fruit juice consumption by preschool-aged children is associated with short stature and obesity. *Pediatrics.* 1997;99:15–22

5. Dennison BA. Fruit juice consumption by infants and children: a review. *J Am Coll Nutr.* 1996;15(suppl 5):4S–11S

6. Ames BN. Micronutrients prevent cancer and delay aging. *Toxicol Lett.* 1998;102–103:5–18

7. Hollman PC, Hertog MG, Katan MB. Role of dietary flavonoids in protection against cancer and coronary heart disease. *Biochem Soc Trans.* 1996;24:785–789

8. Fairweather-Tait S, Fox T, Wharf SG, Eagles J. The bioavailability of iron in different weaning foods and the enhancing effect of a fruit drink containing ascorbic acid. *Pediatr Res.* 1995;37:389–394

9. Abrams SA, O'Brien KO, Wen J, Liang LK, Stuff JE. Absorption by 1-year old children of an iron supplement given with cow's milk or juice. *Pediatr Res.* 1996;39:171–175

10. Kiritsy MC, Levy SM, Warren JJ, Guha-Chowdhury N, Heilman JR, Marshall T. Assessing fluoride concentrations of juices and juice-flavored drinks. *J Am Dent Assoc.* 1996;127:895–902

11. Bailey DG, Malcolm J, Arnold O, Spence JD. Grapefruit juice-drug interactions. *Br J Clin Pharmacol.* 1998;46:101–110

12. Gross AS, Goh YD, Addison RS, Shenfield GM. Influence of grapefruit juice on cisapride pharmacokinetics. *Clin Pharmacol Ther.* 1999;65:395–401

13. Fuhr U. Drug interactions with grapefruit juice. Extent, probable mechanism and clinical relevance. *Drug Saf.* 1998;18:251–272

14. Riby JE, Fujisawa T, Kretchmer N. Fructose absorption. *Am J Clin Nutr.* 1993;58(suppl 5):748S–753S

15. Smith MM, Davis M, Chasalow FI, Lifshitz F. Carbohydrate absorption from fruit juice in young children. *Pediatrics.* 1995;95:340–344

16. Nobigrot T, Chasalow FI, Lifshitz F. Carbohydrate absorption from one serving of fruit juice in young children: age and carbohydrate composition effects. *J Am Coll Nutr.* 1997;16:152–158

17. Lifshitz CH. Carbohydrate absorption from fruit juices in infants. *Pediatrics.* 2000;105(1). URL: http://www.pediatrics.org/cgi/content/full/105/1/e4

18. Southgate DA. Digestion and metabolism of sugar. *Am J Clin Nutr.* 1995;62(suppl 1):203S–211S

19. Lifshitz CH. Role of colonic scavengers of unabsorbed carbohydrate in infants and children. *J Am Coll Nutr.* 1996;15(suppl 5):30S–34S

20. Gryboski JD. Diarrhea from dietetic candies. *N Engl J Med.* 1966;275:718

21. Hyams JS, Leichtner AM. Apple juice: an unappreciated cause of chronic diarrhea. *Am J Dis Child.* 1985;139:503–505

22. Hyams JS, Etienne NL, Leichtner AM, Theuer RC. Carbohydrate malabsorption following fruit juice ingestion in young children. *Pediatrics.* 1988;82:64–68

23. Rumessen JJ, Gudmand-Hoyer E. Functional bowel disease: malabsorption and abdominal distress after ingestion of fructose, sorbitol, and fructose-sorbitol mixtures. *Gastroenterology.* 1988;95:694–700

24. Hoekstra JH, van den Aker JHL, Ghoos YF, Hartemink R, Kneepkens CM. Fluid intake and industrial processing in apple juice induced chronic non-specific diarrhea. *Arch Dis Child.* 1995;73:126–130

25. Ament ME. Malabsorption of apple juice and pear nectar in infants and children: clinical implications. *J Am Coll Nutr.* 1996;15(suppl 5):26S–29S

26. Davidson M, Wasserman R. The irritable colon of childhood (chronic non-specific diarrhea syndrome). *J Pediatr.* 1996;69:1027–1038

27. Lifshitz F, Ament ME, Kleinman RE, et al. Role of juice carbohydrate malabsorption in chronic nonspecific diarrhea in children. *J Pediatr.* 1992;120:825–829

28. Hoekstra JH, van Kempen AA, Kneepkens C. Apple juice malabsorption: fructose or sorbitol? *J Pediatr Gastroenterol Nutr.* 1993;16:39–42

29. Kneepkens CM, Jakobs C, Douwes AC. Apple juice, fructose and chronic nonspecific diarrhoea. *Eur J Pediatr.* 1989;148:571–573

30. Hoekstra JH, van den Aker JH, Hartemink R, Kneepkens CM. Fruit juice malabsorption: not only fructose. *Acta Paediatr.* 1995;84:1241–1244

31. Fujisawa T, Riby J, Kretchmer N. Intestinal absorption of fructose in the rat. *Gastroenterology.* 1991;101:360–367

32. Baker SS, Liptak GS, Colletti RB, et al. Constipation in infants and children: evaluation and treatment. *J Pediatr Gastroenterol Nutr.* 1999;29:612–626

33. US Department of Agriculture, Human Nutrition Information Service. *The Food Guide Pyramid.* Washington, DC: US Government Printing Office; 1992. Home and Garden Bull No. 252

34. Parish ME. Public health and nonpasteurized fruit juices. *Crit Rev Microbiol.* 1997;23:109–119

35. Food Labeling. Warning and Notice Statement: Labeling of Juice Products; Final Rule. 63 *Federal Register* 37029–37056 (1998) (codified at 21 CFR §101, 120)

36. American Academy of Pediatrics, Committee on Nutrition. Supplemental foods for infants. In: Kleinman RE, ed. *Pediatric Nutrition Handbook.* 4th ed. Elk Grove Village, IL: American Academy of Pediatrics; 1998:43–53

37. Gibson SA. Non-milk extrinsic sugars in the diets of pre-school children: association with intakes of micronutrients, energy, fat and NSP. *Br J Nutr.* 1997;78:367–378

38. Smith MM, Lifshitz F. Excess fruit juice consumption as a contributing factor in nonorganic failure to thrive. *Pediatrics.* 1994;93:438–443

39. Konig KG, Navia JM. Nutritional role of sugars in oral health. *Am J Clin Nutr.* 1995;62(suppl 1):275S–283S

40. American Academy of Pediatrics and American Academy of Pedodontics. Juice in ready-to-use bottles and nursing bottle carries. *AAP News and Comment.* 1978;29(1):11

41. American Academy of Pediatrics, Provisional Committee on Quality Improvement, Subcommittee on Acute Gastroenteritis. Practice parameter: the management of acute gastroenteritis in young children. *Pediatrics.* 1996;97:424–433

42. Bezerra JA, Stathos TH, Duncan B, Gaines JA, Udall JN Jr. Treatment of infants with acute diarrhea: what's recommended and what's practiced. *Pediatrics.* 1992;90:1–4

43. Cochran WJ, Klish WJ. Treating acute gastroenteritis in infants. *Drug Prot.* 1987;2:88–93

44. Ratner B, Untracht S, Malone J, Retsina M. Allergenicity of modified and processed food stuffs: IV. Orange: allergenicity of orange studied in man. *J Pediatr.* 1953;43:421–428

45. Blanco Quiros A, Sanchez Villares E. Pathogenic basis of food allergy treatment. In: Reinhardt D, Schmidt E, eds. *Food Allergy.* New York, NY: Raven Press; 1988:265–270

46. Alexy U, Sichert Hellert W, Kersting M, Manz F, Schoch G. Fruit juice consumption and the prevalence of obesity and short stature in German preschool children: results of the DONALD study. *J Pediatr Gastroenterol Nutr.* 1999;29:343–349

47. Skinner JD, Carruth BR, Moran J III, Houck K, Coletta F. Fruit juice intake is not related to children's growth. *Pediatrics.* 1999;103:58–64

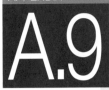

A.9 American Academy of Pediatrics Obesity Resources

American Academy of Pediatrics Institute for Healthy Childhood Weight

The American Academy of Pediatrics (AAP) Institute for Healthy Childhood Weight is an arm of the AAP solely dedicated to addressing obesity prevention, assessment, and treatment at the point of care, in communities, and with families. The Institute leverages AAP expertise to focus on translating policy, research, and best practices into action within health care, communities, and families.

URL: www.aap.org/healthyweight

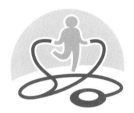

American Academy of Pediatrics
Institute for Healthy
Childhood Weight
WHERE LIFELONG RESULTS BEGIN

Pediatric ePractice: Optimizing Your Obesity Care (PeP)

Pediatric ePractice: Optimizing your Obesity Care is an innovative new Internet tool developed to help pediatricians prevent, assess, and treat obesity by facilitating access to resources and tools to support improved obesity care. It's a highly visual and interactive Web site designed to align with the pediatric workflow.

URL: www.pep.aap.org

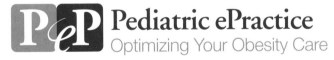

PeP Pediatric ePractice
Optimizing Your Obesity Care
From the American Academy of Pediatrics

American Academy of Pediatrics Section on Obesity

The mission of the Section is to improve the health and well-being of children and families by reducing the prevalence of childhood obesity and promoting healthy active living.

URL: http://aap.org/sections/obesity

Healthy Active Living for Families (HALF)— Growing Healthy

The Healthy Active Living for Families project incorporates parent feedback and expert recommendations into extensive Web-based healthy active living resources and widgets for families of infants, toddlers, and preschoolers. Content is age appropriate, plain language, strength based, and evidence informed.

URL: www.healthychildren.org/growinghealthy

Healthy Active Living for Families (HALF)— Implementation Guide

A Web-based Implementation Guide supports pediatricians and other health care professionals in using these materials and enhances their obesity prevention anticipatory guidance. The guide highlights opportunities for care in the context of parent concerns, the onset of risk behaviors, and evidence-based desired behaviors that foster healthy active living.

URL: www.aap.org/HALFIG

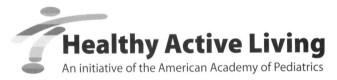

Healthy Active Living
An initiative of the American Academy of Pediatrics

AAP Patient Education: HealthyGrowth (Mobile App)

As a health care provider, you can use this app to create tailored patient information on healthy eating and active living for young children and their families. This app for iOS devices (iPad/iPhone) allows you and the parent to identify healthy active living topic areas that are important to the family during a patient encounter. The resulting personalized action strategies can be printed or e-mailed directly to the parent. The realistic action strategies were drawn from research with families.

URLs: iOS App Store: https://itunes.apple.com/us/app/aap-patient-education-healthygrowth/id648888362?mt=8

Google Play: https://play.google.com/store/apps/details?id=com.phonegap.aaphalf

Index